BIOLOGICAL APPROACHES TO THE CONTROLLED DELIVERY OF DRUGS

ANNALS OF THE NEW YORK ACADEMY OF SCIENCES
Volume 507

BIOLOGICAL APPROACHES TO THE CONTROLLED DELIVERY OF DRUGS

Edited by R. L. Juliano

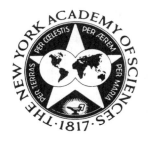

The New York Academy of Sciences
New York, New York
1987

Library of Congress Cataloging-in-Publication Data

Biological approaches to the controlled delivery of drugs.

(Annals of the New York Academy of Sciences; v. 507)

"Papers . . . presented at a conference entitled
Biological approaches to controlled drug delivery,
which was held by the New York Academy of Sciences
in New York City on January 13–15, 1987"—Contents p.
   Includes bibliographies and index.
   1. Drugs—Dosage forms—Congresses.   2. Drugs—
Metabolism—Congresses.   3. Prodrugs—Congresses.
I. Juliano, R. L.   II. New York Academy of Sciences.
III. Series.   [DNLM: 1. Delayed-Action Preparations—
congresses.   2. Dosage Forms—congresses.
W1 AN626YL v.507 / QV 785 B6148 1987]
Q11.N5 vol.507   [RS200]   500 s   87-34779
ISBN 0-89766-410-8   [615'.1]
ISBN 0-89766-409-4

SP
Printed in the United States of America
ISBN 0-89766-410-8 (cloth)
ISBN 0-89766-409-4 (paper)

ANNALS OF THE NEW YORK ACADEMY OF SCIENCES

Volume 507
December 22, 1987

BIOLOGICAL APPROACHES TO THE CONTROLLED DELIVERY OF DRUGS[a]

Editor and Conference Organizer
R. L. JULIANO

CONTENTS

[a]The papers in this volume were presented at a conference entitled Biological Approaches to Controlled Drug Delivery, which was held by the New York Academy of Sciences in New York City on January 13–15, 1987.

Financial assistance was received from:

- ALCON LABORATORIES, INC.
- AMERICAN CYANAMID/LEDERLE LABORATORIES
- BURROUGHS-WELLCOME COMPANY
- CIBA-GEIGY
- EASTMAN KODAK COMPANY
- GENENTECH INC.
- LILLY RESEARCH LABORATORIES
- MCNEIL PHARMACEUTICAL
- MERCK SHARP & DOHME RESEARCH LABORATORIES
- MERRELL DOW RESEARCH INSTITUTE
- NATIONAL CANCER INSTITUTE/NATIONAL INSTITUTES OF HEALTH
- OFFICE OF NAVAL RESEARCH (GRANT #N00014-87-C-0030)
- PFIZER ·CENTRAL RESEARCH
- PFIZER RESEARCH AND DEVELOPMENT
- SANDOZ CORPORATION
- SEARLE RESEARCH AND DEVELOPMENT
- SMITH KLINE AND FRENCH LABORATORIES
- U.S. ARMY MEDICAL RESEARCH AND DEVELOPMENT COMMAND
- THE UPJOHN COMPANY

Preface

R. L. JULIANO[a]

Department of Pharmacology
University of Texas Medical School
Houston, Texas 77096

Pharmacology is entering an exciting but challenging new era. Most of the drugs in our current therapeutic armamentarium are relatively simple molecules. Many of these drugs were discovered by broad-scale screening processes, and most have been produced by conventional organic synthetic routes. Generally these drugs display only a limited degree of precision or selectivity in their pharmacological effects; thus, therapeutic actions are attained, but these are most often accompanied by undesirable side effects.

I believe that we are now entering an era when it should be possible to create drugs that are far more selective, far more precise in their pharmacologic and therapeutic actions than any that have come before. In many cases these novel drug molecules will be larger, more complex, more information-rich structures than the drugs we customarily deal with. Often they will be similar to, or structurally analogous with, naturally occurring biological mediators such as hormones, growth factors, or autacoids. Often they will be produced by biotechnological approaches rather than by organic synthesis, although I am sure we will see a melding of these technologies in the future. It seems likely, at least in the early phases of developing these novel biopharmaceutical entities, that these molecules may be considerably less stable than "conventional" drugs and may be subject to degradation by proteases, nucleases, or other hydrolytic enzymes.

At present we know very little about the kinetic behavior, tissue distribution, and pharmacodynamic aspects of complex biomolecules be they peptides, oligonucleotides, or complex lipid autacoids. Cell biologists are beginning to unravel some of the intricacies of protein sorting at the subcellular level, but this information has not yet been applied to the design of peptide-based drugs. Further, there is a dearth of information on how (or indeed whether) complex biological molecules such as peptides, nucleic acids, or active lipophilic compounds can move from likely portals of drug administration to critical target sites within tissues and cells where the desired pharmacologic effects will take place.

This symposium is intended as a first step in addressing these concerns. I hope that it will serve to integrate emerging concepts in cell and molecular biology with practical pharmacologic and pharmaceutical concerns related to increasing the selectivity of new drugs and thus improving their therapeutic indices. The first part of the symposium deals with biological barriers to the transport of complex molecules. Thus, we explore various aspects of nonspecific and of receptor-mediated endocytosis. We examine the movement of molecules across epithelial and endothelial barriers, and learn of genetic mechanisms whereby cells can modulate their ability to transport drugs. Finally, we analyze approaches for enhancing polypeptide delivery using both gene-cloning techniques and pharmaceutical manipulations. The second part of the symposium examines two popular technologies for controlled or targeted delivery of drugs and macromolecules. The first approach involves microparticles such as protein

[a]Present address: Department of Pharmacology, University of North Carolina Medical School, Chapel Hill, North Carolina 27514.

microspheres, emulsions and liposomes, while the second involves monoclonal antibodies as therapeutic agents. Many of the opportunities, as well as many of the problems, associated with these two technologies will no doubt relate back to the analysis of biological barriers that was made earlier in this symposium. Finally, we consider two very promising general strategies for increasing drug selectivity: the first involves a number of distinct approaches, all of which use biochemical or molecular biological avenues for manipulating cells; the second involves prodrugs as an approach to drug targeting.

This symposium blends themes from cellular and molecular biology with those of drug design, pharmacology, and pharmaceutics. It is hoped that this volume will provide a fruitful venue of interaction for persons as diverse as basic biological scientists, clinicians, and pharmaceutical researchers. The efforts of these individuals will no doubt result in the emergence of novel, more sophisticated, and more selective therapeutic agents.

Viruses as Tools in Drug Delivery

ARI HELENIUS, STEPHEN DOXSEY,

AND IRA MELLMAN

Department of Cell Biology
Yale School of Medicine
New Haven, Connecticut 06510

The hydrophobic character of the lipid bilayer provides an effective barrier for polar macromolecules. Only in exceptional cases can proteins and nucleic acids pass across cellular membranes. Direct bilayer translocation of macromolecules is, in fact, not needed for most types of exchanges between membrane-bounded compartments. Incoming nutrients and signals are usually channeled into the cells as low molecular weight substances, through the mediation of ions, or by other mechanisms that do not involve translocation of macromolecules across the lipid bilayer. In cases where macromolecular translocation is unavoidable, such as during segregation of secretory proteins into the endoplasmic reticulum or transfer of cytoplasmically translated mitochondrial proteins into mitochondria, complex mechanisms appear to be involved.[1-3] The details of these mechanisms are not yet fully understood, but it seems that the proteins are transported across the bilayers in partially unfolded form at the expense of energy (FIGURE 1A).

Paradoxically, it appears easier for the cell to carry macromolecules and other membrane-impermeable substances over a barrier made up of two membranes than of one. If the donor and the acceptor compartments each have their own limiting membranes, the preferred mode of transport of macromolecules is either direct fusion of the two membranes with each other or vesicle transport from one to the other (FIGURE 1B).[4] Neither of these mechanisms requires translocation of the macromolecules across a lipid bilayer membrane. Whenever fusion and vesicle transport occurs in the cell, it can be assumed, however, that specific mechanisms regulate the movement of the vesicles, mediate the specific recognition between the membranes, and induce membrane perturbations that lead to fission and fusion reactions. Although thousands of fusion and fission reactions take place every minute in a normal eukaryotic cell, little is known about the specific mechanisms involved.

VIRUS ENTRY INTO CELLS

In transferring their genome and accessory proteins from the infected host cell to a uninfected cell, viruses face a difficult transport problem. Not only do they have to attach to specific target cells, but they must also transport their nucleocapsids (large, polar macromolecular assemblies) through at least one membrane. There are several ways in which the viruses have "solved" this problem. Research during the last few years has shed some light on the molecular mechanisms of some of them (see Refs. 5-8).

Nonenveloped viruses interact with the plasma membrane or the membranes of endocytic organelles and somehow induce direct transfer of the genome into the cytoplasm. *Bacteriophages* (such as T4), in particular, are known to possess intricate attachment and injection devices that allow them to deliver their DNA through both the inner and outer membranes of gram-negative bacteria.[9] For *nonenveloped animal*

1

viruses the entry mechanisms are less clear. Major advances in understanding their entry are, however, imminent since the crystal structure of some of these viruses is being elucidated and the cell biology of the early virus cell interactions is being studied in further detail.[10,11]

Enveloped animal viruses rely on membrane fission and membrane fusion to transfer their genomes into host cells. The virus membrane serves a "transport vesicle." It is very similar in its mission to transport vesicles observed intracellularly between compartments (cf. FIGURE 1B). In addition to this mode of transport some viruses actually use a variation on the theme: they employ the spike glycoproteins on the plasma membrane of the infected host cell to mediate fusion with the neighboring

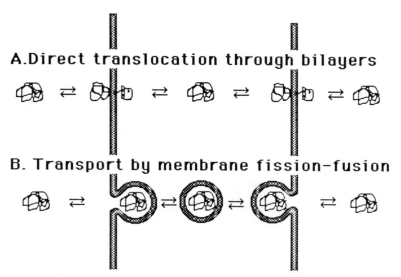

A. Direct translocation through bilayers

B. Transport by membrane fission-fusion

FIGURE 1. Transport of proteins between two membrane-bounded compartments. (**A**) Direct translocation of protein through a membrane is likely to involve unfolding and refolding. It therefore constitutes a less favorable mechanism for transport between two compartments. However, it is observed in many cases where transport must occur through a single membrane barrier. (**B**) When transport is mediated by a transport vesicle, no modifications in the transported proteins are needed. The formation of the transport vesicle and its fusion with the target membrane must be controlled events, but little is known about the mechanisms involved.

noninfected cells. In this case the fusion event transfers the genome from one cell to the next without involvement of any extracellular viruses.

VIRAL FUSION PROTEINS

The central factors in enveloped virus entry are the spike glycoproteins. They are crucial for viral morphogenesis in the infected cells; they mediate the interaction between the virus and cell surface receptors; and they are responsible for the fusion event. The location of the fusion event (the plasma membrane or endocytic vacuoles) is determined by the properties of the viral fusion factors. Fusion proteins that are active at neutral pH allow the viruses to fuse with the plasma membrane, whereas proteins that require acidic pH are activated only when the virus particles have been internalized into acidic endosomes or lysosomes.[7,12] The acid-requiring fusion factors appear to be more common than those functional at neutral pH. The mechanism whereby the virus is internalized into the acid compartments is usually a constitutive cellular function; receptor-mediated endocytosis via coated pits and coated vesicles.[13] The main advantage of entering via the endocytic pathway is that the nucleocapsids containing the viral genes are ushered from the cell surface through the membrane skeleton underlying the plasma membrane to a central location within the cytoplasm (M. Marsh, personal communication).

Some of the proteins responsible for the viral fusion activity have been studied in detail. Among the best characterized are the influenza virus hemagglutinin (HA), the Sendai virus F-protein and the Semliki Forest virus spike glycoprotein. The F-protein has pH-independent fusion activity, and the other two are activated at pH values between 6.1 and 5.0. Although quite different in structure and mode of action, the proteins possess certain similarities. They are integral membrane proteins anchored by single hydrophobic amino acid sequences close to the C-terminus; they are oligomeric; they all form projections in the viral membrane; and they occur in the viral membrane in 200 to 1000 copies. The properties that make them capable of fusing membranes are only partially understood. Each of them has in their projecting external domain a moiety that can interact with lipids in the target membrane. The HA and the F-proteins both have hydrophobic N-terminal peptides which are exposed during fusion.[13–15] The E1 subunit of the SFV spike has a site for interaction with cholesterol[16] and cholesterol is a requirement for fusion activity.[17]

Summarizing a large number of studies, one can presently conclude that the fusion proteins are at least transiently integrated or bound to both of the membranes during fusion and that they act as a bridge between them. One of their functions is to overcome the so-called *hydration force* that prevents the close approach of two hydrated polar membrane surfaces.[18] In addition they may destabilize the structure of the membranes at the local site of interaction. The nature of this destabilization event is presently unclear.

The molecular mechanism of fusion is obviously of great general and practical interest. There is virtually no molecular information about the numerous fusion events that operate continuously in the cell as part of normal cellular activities, during fertilization, cell division, myotube formation, and so on. The virus proteins provide, at present, the only well-characterized systems in which to study protein-mediated biological fusion events.

THE USE OF VIRAL FUSION PROTEINS FOR ARTIFICIAL DELIVERY

It is not surprising that numerous attempts have been made to harness the fusion activity of viral fusion proteins for artificial delivery of drugs and other substances into cells.[19,21,23] Three general approaches currently in use are shown in FIGURE 2. The fusion proteins can either be present in the membrane of the delivery vesicle (FIGURE 2A) or in the target cell membrane (FIGURE 2C). Alternatively, intact viruses can be used to bridge the target membrane and the delivery vesicle (FIGURE 2B). To achieve efficient binding and increase the probability of fusion, a high concentration of the appropriate receptor for the viral fusion protein should be present in the target membranes. In most cases the fusion proteins require acid pH for activation, and fusion can be induced by brief acid treatment. When pH-dependent viral proteins are used, fusion can be obtained simply by prolonged incubation at neutral pH. Each of the three approaches has limitations, and none has yet emerged as an accepted routine method for efficient bulk delivery. They all have, however, future potential for specific applications.

The *virosome approach* (FIGURE 2A) is most useful for the delivery of membrane lipids and other lipophilic compounds into the plasma membrane and perhaps the endosomal membrane of living cells.[19,20] Virosomes are reconstituted vesicles that contain viral spike glycoproteins. They may or may not contain entrapped molecules. Owing to the relatively small size of virosomes obtained by standard reconstitution methods, their volume is quite small.[15] They are consequently quite useful for implantation of lipids and lipid-soluble molecules into cellular membranes, but less than optimal for delivery of large amounts of soluble substances. The small size allows them to be internalized by coated vesicles and to be rapidly carried into the endosomes and lysosomes.[19,21] They are exposed to the acidic pH of these organelles and fuse. As a result, the contents of the virosomes will be delivered to the cytoplasm and the virosomal lipids implanted in the vacuolar membranes.

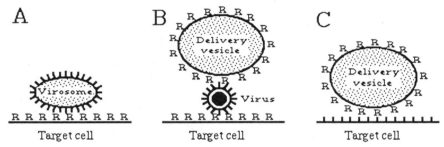

FIGURE 2. Three different ways to use spike glycoproteins in virus-mediated delivery. (A) The delivery vesicle contains the viral spike glycoproteins and the target cell the receptors. (B) The delivery vesicles and the target cells contain virus receptors. Viruses are used to fuse the two together. (C) The viral spike glycoproteins are expressed on the surface of the target cell plasma membrane. The receptors are present in the delivery vesicles.

A serious limiting factor has been the difficulty in obtaining virosomes with sufficiently high fusion activity. In most cases virosomes are inferior to intact viruses in their fusion activity. The proteins are either damaged during solubilization and isolation, or they do not insert correctly into the reconstituted membranes. This problem can be overcome by optimizing the solubilization and reconstitution procedure, as recently illustrated by studies on the vesicular stomatitis virus G-protein.[22]

The use of *viruses as a bridge* between delivery vesicle and target cell (FIGURE 2B) has certain advantages.[23] Since the only requirement imposed on the delivery vesicles is that they carry the viral receptors, one can use large, efficiently loaded vesicles. Most studies using this approach have employed loaded erythrocytes, Sendai virus, and tissue culture cells.[23] Our experience with Semliki Forest virus and influenza virus as fusion bridges has been discouraging, owing to the low efficiency of delivery. Although it is clear that a single virus particle can fuse with two membranes (i.e., a red cell and culture cell membrane), the conditions in which this becomes a frequent event are not yet easily obtained.

The third approach, which has recently been developed in our laboratory, depends on the expression of a *fusion protein on the target cell surface* and the use of a delivery vesicle that carries the appropriate receptor (FIGURE 2C). The location of fusion factor and receptor are thus reversed compared to the situation during normal virus entry. We are currently using loaded erythrocytes as carriers and HA-expressing cells as recipients.[24,26] The HA is synthesized by the target cells for delivery after infection or by the use of the appropriate expression vector systems that give high and efficient expression in tissue culture cells.[15,25] A similar method has been used by van Meer *et al.*[26] for the implantation of lipids into the plasma membrane of tissue culture cells.

The advantages of this system are several: (1) A variety of delivery vesicles can be used. They can either be small liposomes or large red cells; they can contain labeled lipid; or they may be loaded with soluble proteins. (2) Fusion is very efficient. Using red cells as delivery vesicles, we find that 80–95% of the cells in a monolayer receive test molecules. This permits the biochemical analysis of the fate and effect of a variety of delivered molecules. (3) Large numbers of proteins can be delivered. With a relatively small protein that is efficiently loaded into red cells, the delivery can be as high as 200 million copies per cell. (4) The fusion procedure is not deleterious to the target cells. (4) Delivery is easily controlled and highly reproducible.

The main disadvantage of the approach is that the HA must be present in large copy numbers on the cell surface. Sufficiently high expression can only be achieved by the use of certain expression vector systems available for HA such as SV40 late replacement vectors and papilloma virus vectors.[25,26] This restricts the potential target cell repertoire. Cells infected with influenza virus, which has a wide host range, can also be used as target cells, but the cells succumb to cytopathic effects after about 10 hours of infection.[24] At the present time, there is only one cell line (derived from 3T3 NIH mouse fibroblasts) that constitutively expresses sufficient amounts of HA to allow effective delivery.[24,25] A second obvious disadvantage of this delivery scheme is that it requires acidification of the extracellular medium, is thereby effectively limited to use in tissue culture.

In spite of these limitations, the procedure shown in FIGURE 2C seems the most promising. It is in routine use in our laboratory for the study of a variety of cellular biological and virological questions. We have just completed a study in which we could show that antibodies to the heavy chain of clathrin inhibited endocytic uptake of Semliki Forest virus.[27] This provided direct evidence for a role of clathrin in receptor-mediated endocytosis.

REFERENCES

1. WALTER, P., R. GILMORE & G. BLOBEL. 1984. Protein translocation across the endoplasmic reticulum. Cell **38:** 5–8.
2. HURT, E. C. 1986. How proteins find their way into mitochondria and intramitochondrial compartments. Trends Biochem. **11:** 204–207.
3. WICKNER, W. T. & H. F. LODISH. 1985. Multiple mechanisms of protein insertion into and across membranes. Science **230:** 400–207.
4. PALADE, G. 1975. Intracellular aspects of the process of protein secretion. Science **189:** 347–358.
5. HELENIUS, A., M. MARSH & J. WHITE. 1980. The entry of viruses into animal cells. Trends in Biochemical Sciences **5:** 104–106.
6. MARSH, M. 1984. The entry of enveloped viruses into cells by endocytosis. Biochem J. **218:** 1–10.
7. WHITE, J., M. KIELIAN & A. HELENIUS. 1983. Membrane fusion proteins of enveloped animal viruses. Q. Rev. Biophys. **16:** 151–195.
8. DIMMOCK, N. J. 1983. Initial stages in infection with animal viruses. J. Gen. Virol. **59:** 1–22.

9. CROWTER, R. A. Y. KIKUCHI, E. V. LENK & J. KING. 1977. Molecular reorganization in the hexagon to star transition of the baseplate of the bacteriophage T4. J. Mol. Biol. **116:** 489–523.
10. HARRISON, S. C. 1986. Alphavirus struture. *In* The Togaviridae and Flavivirida. S. Schlesinger & M. J. Schlesinger, Eds. Chapter **2:** 21–34. Plenum Publishing Corp. New York.
11. HOGLE, J. 1985. 3-dimensional structure of polio virus at 2.9 Å resolution. Science **229:** 1358–1365.
12. HELENIUS, A., J. KARTENBECK, K. SIMONS & E. FRIES. 1980. On the entry of Semliki Forest virus into BHK-21 cells. J. Cell Biol. **84:** 404–420.
13. SKEHEL, J. J., P. M. BAYLEY, E. B. BROWN, S. R. MARTIN, M. D. WATERFIELD, J. M. WHITE, I. A. WILSON & D. C. WILEY. 1982. Changes in the conformation of influenza virus hemagglutinin at the pH optimum of virus-mediated membrane fusion. Proc. Natl. Acad. Sci. USA **79:** 968–972.
14. DOMS, R. W., M.-J. GETHING, J. HENNEBERRY, J. WHITE & A. HELENIUS. 1986. Analysis of a variant influenza hemagglutinin that induces fusion at elevated pH. J. Virol. **57:** 603–613.
15. GETHING, M.-J. & J. SAMBROOK. 1981. Cell-surface expression of influenza haemagglutinin from a cloned DNA copy of the RNA gene. Nature **293:** 620–625.
16. KIELIAN, M. C. & A. HELENIUS. 1985. pH-induced alterations in the fusogenic spike protein of Semliki Forest virus. J. Cell Biol. **101:** 2284–2291.
17. WHITE, J. & A. HELENIUS. 1980. pH-dependent fusion between the Semliki Forest virus membrane and liposomes. Proc. Natl. Acad. Sci. USA **77:** 3273–3277.
18. RAND, R. P. 1981. Interacting phospholipid bilayers: Measured forces and induced structural changes. Annu. Rev. Biophys. Bioeng. **10:** 277–314.
19. FURUSAWA, M. 1980. Cellular microinjection by cell fusion: Technique and applications in biology and medicine. Int. Rev. Cytol. **62:** 29–67.
20. MARSH, M., E. BOLZAU, J. WHITE & A. HELENIUS. 1983. Interactions of Semliki Forest virus spike glycoprotein rosettes and vesicles with cultured cells. J. Cell Biol. **96:** 455–461.
21. KULKA, R. G. & A. LOYTER. 1979. The use of fusion methods for the microinjection of animal cells. Curr. Topics Membr. Transport **12:** 365–430.
22. METSIKKÖ, K., G. VAN MEER & K. SIMONS. 1986. Reconstitution of the fusogenic activity of vesicular stomatitis virus. **5:** 3429–3435.
23. SCHLEGEL, R. A. & M. C. RECHSTEINER. 1986. Erythrocyte-mediated transfer methods. *In* Microinjection and Organelle Transplantation Techniques: Methods and Applications. J. E. Celis, A. Graessmann & A. Loyter, Eds. Academic Press. New York.
24. DOXSEY, S., A. HELENIUS & J. WHITE. 1985. An efficient method for introducing macromolecules into living cells. J. Cell Biol. **101:** 19–27.
25. SAMBROOK, J. L. RODGERS, J. WHITE, & M.-J. GETHING. 1985. Lines of BPV-transformed murine cells that constitutively express influenza virus hemagglutinin. EMBO J. **4:** 91–103.
26. VAN MEER, G. & K. SIMONS. 1983. An efficient method for introducing defined lipids into the plasma membrane of mammalian cells. J. Cell Biol. **83:** 1–10.
27. DOXSEY, S. J., F. M. BRODSKY, G. S. BLANK & A. HELENIUS. 1987. J. Cell Biol. **50:** 453–463.

Multidrug Resistance and P-Glycoprotein Expression

VICTOR LING

The Ontario Cancer Institute
Toronto, Ontario, Canada M4X 1K9

Multidrug resistance (MDR) describes a complex phenotype whose predominant feature is resistance to a wide range of structurally unrelated cytotoxic agents, many of which are anticancer drugs.[1,2] The phenotype is frequently found in mammalian cell lines and transplantable tumors selected for resistance to a single drug. Although the drugs to which a particular MDR line may be resistant cannot be readily predicted, cross resistance to the anthracyclines and the vinca alkaloids is often observed. Cross resistance to the alkylating agents and the antimetabolites occurs less frequently, and then usually at a lower level. Reduced drug accumulation appears to correlate with the resistance expressed. Thus, understanding the basis of the MDR phenotype may provide fundamental insights as to how mammalian cells regulate the intracellular levels of a wide diversity of compounds. In addition, and of particular clinical relevance, is the realization that tumor cells acquiring the MDR phenotype may be rendered nonresponsive, even to a combination of different drugs.

A wide variety of biochemical changes have been detected in MDR cell lines.[2] The consistent change is the increased expression of P-glycoprotein, a plasma membrane glycoprotein of approximately 170,000 daltons. Monoclonal antibodies developed against P-glycoprotein detect the presence of this membrane component in different MDR human and animal tumor cell lines.[3] The level of P-glycoprotein expression correlates with the degree of drug resistance. Significant levels of P-glycoprotein have also been detected in some biopsy specimens from patients with ovarian carcinomas,[4] sarcomas,[12] and leukemia.[13] These findings indicate that P-glycoprotein is a highly conserved molecule and that multidrug-resistant tumor cells can occur in a wide variety of human malignancies. Further studies will be required to determine what role these cells play in the overall response of the patient.

P-glycoprotein appears to be encoded by a small family of closely related genes.[5] In many MDR lines, increased P-glycoprotein expression is accompanied by gene amplification. The co-amplification and increased expression of other different flanking genes are frequently observed.[6] Thus it is likely that increased expression of the complement of co-amplified flanking genes contributes to the plethora of changes observed in different MDR lines. However, gene transfection studies indicate that transfer of the P-glycoprotein gene alone is sufficient to mediate multidrug resistance.[7,8]

Structural analysis of P-glycoprotein cDNAs from mouse, human, and hamster indicates that this protein is highly conserved.[9–11] A striking homology between P-glycoprotein and a bacterial hemolysin transport protein (HlyB protein) is observed.[11] P-glycoprotein can be viewed as a tandem duplication of the HlyB protein. The hydropathy profiles of the two proteins are similar and reveal an extensive transmembrane region, resembling those found in pore-forming plasma membrane proteins. A model is proposed for multidrug resistance in which P-glycoprotein functions as an energy-dependent export pump to reduce intracellular levels of anticancer drugs. It is envisioned that the cytoplasmic domain couples energy from

7

ATP to export drugs through a channel formed by the transmembrane segments of P-glycoprotein.

REFERENCES

1. LING V., J. GERLACH & N. KARTNER. 1984. Multidrug resistance. Breast Cancer Res. Treat. **4:** 89–94.
2. GERLACH, J. N. KARTNER, D. BELL & V. LING 1986. Multidrug resistance. Cancer Surv. **5:** 25–46.
3. KARTNER, N., D. EVERNDEN-PORELLE, G. BRADLEY & V. LING 1985. Monoclonal antibodies detecting P-glycoprotein in multidrug-resistant cell lines. Nature **316:** 820–823.
4. BELL, D., J. GERLACH, N. KARTNER, R. BUICK & V. LING. 1985. Detection of P-glycoprotein in ovarian cancer: A molecular marker associated with multidrug resistance. J. Clin. Oncol. **3:** 311–315.
5. RIORDAN, J., K. DEUCHARS, N. KARTNER, N. ALON, J. TRENT & V. LING. 1985. Amplification of P-glycoprotein gene in multidrug-resistant mammalian cell lines. Nature **316:** 817–819.
6. VAN DER BLIEK, A. M., T. VAN DER VELDE-KOERTS, V. LING & P. BORST. 1986. Overexpression and amplification of five genes in a multidrug-resistant Chinese hamster ovary cell line. Mol. Cell. Biol. **6:** 1671–1678.
7. GROS, P., Y. B. NERICEH, J. M. CROOP & D. E. HOUSEMAN. 1986. Isolation and expression of a complementary DNA that confers multidrug resistance. Nature **323:** 728–731.
8. DEUCHARS, K. L., R-P.DU, M. NAIK, D. EVERNDEN-PORELLE, N. KARTNER, A. M. VAN DER BLIEK & V. LING. 1987. Expression of hamster P-glycoprotein and multidrug resistance in DNA-mediated transformants of mouse LTA cells. Mol. Cell. Biol. **7:** 718–724.
9. GROS, P., J. CROOP & D. HOUSMAN. 1986. Mammalian multidrug resistance gene: Complete cDNA sequence indicates strong homology to bacterial transport proteins. Cell **47:** 371–380.
10. CHEN, C., J. E. CHIN, K. VEDA, D. P. CLARKE, I. PASTAN, M. M. GROHESMAN & I. B. RONINSON. 1986. Internal duplication and homology with bacterial transport proteins in the *mdr-1* (P-glycoprotein) gene grom multidrug-resistant human cells. Cells **47:** 381–389.
11. GERLACH, J. H., J. A. ENDICOTT, P. F. JURANKA, G. HENDERSON, F. SARANGI, K. L. DEUCHARS & V. LING. 1986. Homology between P-glycoprotein and a bacterial hemolysin transport protein suggests a model for multidrug resistance. Nature **324:** 485–489.
12. GERLACH, J. H., D. R. BELL, C. KARAKOUSIS, H. K. SLOCUM, N. KARTNER, Y. M. RUSTUM, V. LING & R. M. BAKER. 1987. P-glycoprotein in human sarcoma: Evidence for multidrug resistance. J Clin. Oncol. In press.
13. MA, D. D. F., R. A. DAVEY, D. H. HARMON, J. P. ISBISTER, R. D. SCURR, S. M. MACKERTICH, G. DOWDEN & D. R. BELL. 1987. Detection of a multidrug resistant phenotype in acute non-lymphoblastic leukemia. Lancet (Jan. 17): 135–137.

Bovine Brain Microvessel Endothelial Cell Monolayers as a Model System for the Blood-Brain Barrier[a]

KENNETH L. AUDUS AND RONALD T. BORCHARDT[b]

Department of Pharmaceutical Chemistry
The University of Kansas
Lawrence, Kansas 66045-2504

INTRODUCTION

The blood–brain barrier (BBB) is made up of brain microvessel endothelial cells (BMECs) characterized by tight intercellular junctions, minimal pinocytic activity, and the absence of fenestra.[1,2] These characteristics endow BMECs with the ability to restrict passage of most small polar blood-borne molecules (e.g., neurotransmitter catecholamines, small peptides) and macromolecules (e.g., proteins) from the cerebrovascular circulation to the brain.[3–5] There are, however, specific BBB mechanisms to facilitate the passage of certain small polar blood-borne molecules recognized as nutrients (such as glucose and amino acids) to the brain.[6] Moreover, recent evidence suggests that carrier mechanisms exist for transporting peptides and proteins (i.e., enkephalins and insulin) across the BBB.[7,8]

The BBB also constitutes a significant metabolic barrier to many blood-borne molecules. For example, leucine aminopeptidase, angiotensin-converting enzyme, acetylcholinesterase, butyrylcholinesterase, and alkaline phosphatase enzyme activities are associated with the BBB.[9] In addition, BMECs exhibit all of the enzymes for both synthesis and degradation of catecholamine neurotransmitters.[10]

Within the cerebrovasculature then, the BBB is a dynamic regulatory interface[11] that poses a formidable barrier to delivery of pharmacologic substances to the central nervous system. The strategy in our laboratories has been to use an *in vitro* model to define more precisely BBB permeability and metabolic mechanisms and their regulation by endogenous and environmental factors at the cellular level. By more precisely defining the fundamental characteristics of the BBB's function and regulation at the cellular level, a more efficient and selective delivery of therapeutic agents to the CNS might be realized.

THE BLOOD–BRAIN BARRIER *IN VITRO*

The complexity of the intact animal as an experimental model in studying permeability and metabolism may preclude valid interpretation of cellular level

[a]This work was supported by grants from the Upjohn Company, Kalamazoo, Michigan; INTERx, a subsidiary of Merck & Company, Lawrence, Kansas; The American Heart Association—Kansas Affiliate, Inc.; and the Alzheimer's Disease and Related Disorders Association, Inc.
[b]To whom all correspondence should be addressed.

9

processes specifically associated with the BBB. Two types of *in vitro* models have been developed to conduct studies of BBB function at the cellular level.[12] The first model has generally consisted of suspensions of isolated microvessel endothelial cells from gray matter of the cerebral cortex. This model has been extremely important in the characterization of amino acid transport systems, endothelial cell polarity, and the biochemistry of the BBB.[12] However, the disadvantages of this model include the inability to adequately assess *transcellular* transport processes and the existence of a defect in energy metabolism.[13]

Since it was first demonstrated that BMECs could be maintained in tissue culture by Panula *et al.,*[14] both primary and passaged cultures of isolated BMECs have subsequently been used as a second type of *in vitro* BBB model system.[15-17] The principal advantage of the culture models over isolated microvessels is that under appropriate experimental conditions, it is possible to study *transcellular* transport processes.

With some modifications, the primary culture system first described by Bowman *et al.*[16] has been developed and extensively characterized in our laboratories.[17-21] BMECs are isolated from bovine cerebral gray matter by a two-step enzymatic dispersion treatment with dispase and a collagenase/dispase mixture. The enzymatic treatment is followed by centrifugation over a pre-established 50% Percoll gradient to provide a

TABLE 1. Protocol for Isolation of Bovine Brain Microvessel Endothelial Cells[17]

Remove surface vessels and meninges from two bovine brains (Brain material bathed in Minimum Essential Medium; MEM)

Cut away (aspirate) cerebral gray matter, mince into 1–2 mm cubes

Dilute minced material to 500 ml (w/MEM) containing dispase (final concentration 0.5%). Incubate 3 hr at 37°C in shaking bath (adjust pH after first 30 minutes)

Centrifuge 1000 × *g* for 10 min; discard supernatant; resuspend pellets in 500 ml of 13% dextran (avg. MW 70,000)

Centrifuge 5800 × *g* for 10 min; discard supernatant fat, cell debris, and myelin floating on dextran; resuspend crude microvessel pellet in 20 ml collagenase/dispase (final concentration 1 mg/ml). Incubate for 5 hr at 37°C in shaking bath

Centrifuge 1000 × *g* for 10 min; discard supernatant; resuspend microvessels in 8 ml MEM; layer suspension over a 50% Percoll gradient

Centrifuge 1000 × *g* for 10 min; remove band 2 from gradient; wash with culture medium, aliquot, and freeze (−70°C) in medium supplemented with 20% plasma-derived horse serum and 10% DMSO

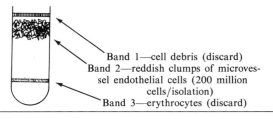

Band 1—cell debris (discard)
Band 2—reddish clumps of microvessel endothelial cells (200 million cells/isolation)
Band 3—erythrocytes (discard)

TABLE 2. Preparation of Growth Surfaces for Primary Cultures of Brain Microvessel Endothelial Cells[17] [a]

Growth surfaces are coated with rat-tail collagen (3 mg/ml aqueous acetic acid)
↓
Collagen-coated surfaces are exposed to ammonia fumes for 3–5 minutes
↓
Collagen-coated surfaces placed under UV light for 60–90 minutes to sterilize
↓
Collagen-coated surface is wetted with human fibronectin (0.04 mg/ml) for 30 minutes
↓
Growth surface ready for seeding cells at a density of 50,000 cells/cm²

Culture Medium:
45% Minimum Essential Medium (Eagle's)
45% F-12 Ham Nutrient Mix
10% Plasma-Derived Horse Serum
100 μg/ml Penicillin G
100 μg/ml Streptomycin
2.5 μg/ml Amphotericin B
100 μg/ml Heparin
10 mM HEPES, pH 7.4
13 mM Sodium Bicarbonate
50 μg/ml Polymyxin B[b]

[a]Method is applicable to all potential growth surfaces including plastic dishes, regenerated cellulose, and polycarbonate membranes.
[b]First three days of culture only.

homogenous isolate of BMECs.[17] Isolated BMECs are generally frozen at $-70°C$ for use as needed. TABLE 1 provides a more detailed outline of the protocol for isolation of BMECs. Thawed cells can be washed and seeded onto a fibronectin-treated growth surface that has previously been coated with rat-tail collagen. TABLE 2 describes the procedures for seeding BMECs onto appropriate growth surfaces and lists the components of the appropriate growth medium. Endothelial cells held together by tight intercellular junctions in short segments of microvessels, as shown in FIGURE 1, atttach, spread, and grow to form a complete monolayer approximately 10 days after seeding.[17] The cells have been conveniently grown up in plastic culture dishes for biochemical and histologic studies, on permeable, optically clear, 15-mm diameter regenerated cellulose membranes (MW cutoff 160,000), or on permeable, translucent polycarbonate filters (0.45–5-μm pore), for transendothelial permeability studies.

The BMEC monolayers are morphologically similar to BBB endothelial cells *in vivo,* exhibiting a continuous layer of closely apposed cells with few pinocytic vesicles and lacking fenestra.[17] FIGURE 2 presents a cross section of a monolayer showing typical morphologic arrangement of two endothelial cells. Enzymes considered specific for the BBB endothelium—gamma-glutamyl transpeptidase and alkaline phosphatase—have been demonstrated in these BMEC monlayers by both histochemical and biochemical methods.[17,19] Markers for cells of endothelial origin, angiotensin-converting enzyme, and factor VIII antigen, have also been demonstrated in this model.[17,19] TABLE 3 summarizes the enzymes identified to date to be associated with the *in vitro* model.

The transendothelial passage of selected substances has been investigated using a

Side-Bi-Side diffusion cell apparatus. As diagrammed in FIGURE 3, experiments were conducted with monolayers grown on either regenerated cellulose or polycarbonate membranes that were inserted into a Side-Bi-Side diffusion cell. The apparatus provides for a water-jacketed 3.4-ml chamber on both sides of the monolayer. The system can be thermostatically regulated with an external water bath and each chamber is stirred with a magnetic stir bar at a constant speed with synchronized stir motors. At various times after one chamber, the donor chamber, is pulsed with a test substance, an aliquot is removed from the other chamber for analysis. The apparatus thus provides for the study of the transendothelial passage of molecules.[18]

The bidirectional, large-neutral amino acid transport system characteristic of the BBB *in vivo* has been characterized in this *in vitro* model system.[18] Transendothelial

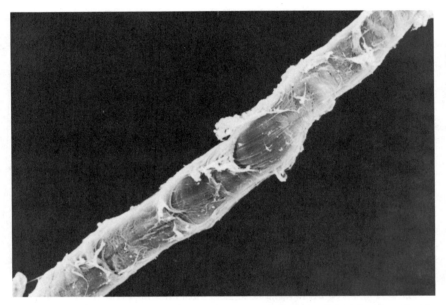

FIGURE 1. Bovine brain microvessel isolated by enzymatic dispersion.[17] (Original magnification ×640; reduced by 33%.)

flux of radiolabeled leucine across the monolayers was found to be a saturable process with an apparent K_m of 0.18 mM, inhibited by other large-neutral amino acids, bidirectional, and stereospecific.[18] The BBB choline carrier system is also present in this *in vitro* model. The choline carrier *in vitro* has been observed to be a bidirectional, competitive, and saturable carrier with kinetic parameters similar to those described for the *in vivo* BBB carrier (A. Trammel and R. T. Borchardt, unpublished results).

Molecules known to passively cross the BBB cross the monolayers in a manner that is nonsaturable, noncompetitive, and is related directly to the octanol/buffer partition coefficient and indirectly to the molecular weight of the substance.[20] Both carrier and passive permeability processes present in the model system are similar to those found in the BBB *in vivo*.[3,4,6]

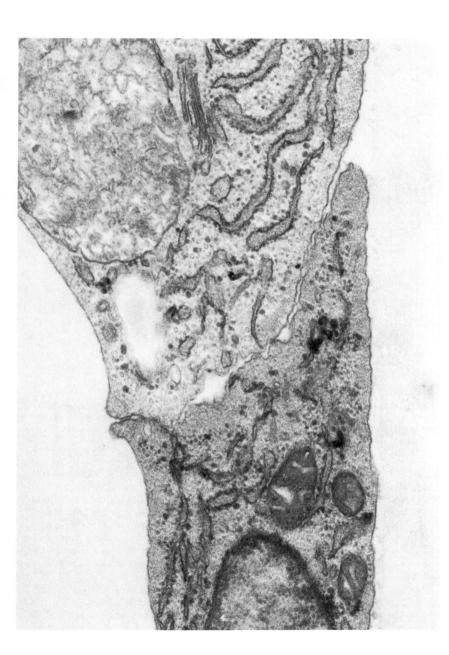

FIGURE 2. Cross section of a monolayer of brain microvessel endothelial cells (T. Raub and K.L. Audus, unpublished results). Endothelial cells are closely apposed, with no fenestra and few pinocytic vesicles. An abundance of mitochondria characteristic of the BBB is also observed in these cells.

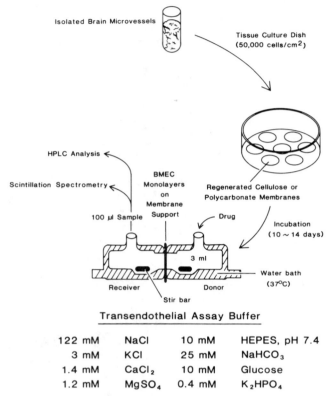

FIGURE 3. Outline of transendothelial transport study design.[18] Brain microvessels are seeded and grown to monolayers on either regenerated cellulose or polycarbonate membranes and mounted in a Side-Bi-Side diffusion cell. Typical components of the assay buffer are listed.

One apparent difference between the permeability properties of the *in vitro* system and the BBB *in vivo* is the *in vitro* system's leakiness to small membrane-impermeant molecules such as sucrose.[20] This difference could be due to the less complex tight junctions observed in primary cultures[22] and/or may be related to the absence of required factors in the artificial culture environment. Alternatively, the leakiness may result from the clamping of the monolayers in the diffusion cell's causing damage to peripheral cells of the monolayers. Therefore, for permeability studies, a membrane-impermeant molecule is always used to assess and correct for background leakiness in the system.[18]

The primary mechanism for facilitation of the transcellular movement of macro-molecules is transcytosis.[23] However, pinocytic activity, and therefore, transcytosis, has been shown to be minimal at the BBB.[1,2] Previous work has also suggested that BBB permeability and perhaps pinocytic activity may be under the control of circulating endogenous and environmental factors.[24–28] In our laboratories, the extent of pinocytic activity at the BBB is currently being reexamined both qualitatively and quantitatively with markers for fluid-phase (e.g., Lucifer yellow) and adsorptive-phase (e.g., lectins) endocytosis. Although overall endocytic activity is low but significant, adsorptive phase endocytosis has been found to be much greater than fluid-phase endocytosis in the model (T. Raub and K.L. Audus, unpublished results). The low overall endocytic activity of BMECs was consistent with present knowledge of endocytosis at the BBB *in vivo.*

The transcellular passage of insulin, a protein that presumably crosses the BBB by a receptor-mediated mechanism,[7] and albumin, a protein that leaks across the BBB in certain pathologic conditions,[25,26] is also being studied with the *in vitro* model. Both insulin and insulin-like growth factor-1 binding sites have been identified on the cultured BMECs (B.T. Keller and R.T. Borchardt, unpublished results). The binding sites of the BMECs have binding characteristics similar to those of insulin binding sites associated with isolated human brain microvessels.[7] Preliminary work also confirms that characteristics of reduced BBB permeability to macromolecules such as albumin are retained in the model system (K. Smith and R.T. Borchardt, unpublished results).

Additional studies will address the regulation of the permeability of the *in vitro* BBB to macromolecules by endogenous factors, such as glucocorticoids, vasoactive peptides, and a ubiquitous environmental factor, aluminum. Glucocorticoid-induced reclosing of the BBB after opening by hyperosmotic treatment or pathologic factors suggests that glucocorticoids may represent endogenous factors for regulating BBB permeability.[27] Similarly, vasoactive peptides may represent potential endogenous regulators of BBB permeability. For instance, the vasoactive peptide, angiotensin, has been shown to increase or decrease BBB permeability depending upon the plasma

TABLE 3. Some Biochemical Characteristics of Brain Microvessel Endothelial Cells (BMECs)

	Isolated Microvessels[9]	Cultured BMECs[17-19,21]
Specific BMEC enzymes		
Alkaline phosphatase	+	+
Gamma-glutamyl transpeptidase	+	+
Endothelial cell markers		
Angiotensin-converting enzyme	+	+
Factor VIII antigen	+	+
Other BMEC-associated enzymes		
Monoamine oxidase	+	+
Monoamine oxidase-A	+	+
Monoamine oxidase-B	?	+
Catechol-*o*-methyltransferase	+	+
Catechol-*o*-methyltransferase membrane bound	?	+
Catechol-*o*-methyltransferase cytosolic	?	−
Phenol sulfotransferase (thermostable)	?	+
Phenol sulfotransferase (thermolabile)	?	−
Acetylcholine esterase	+	+[a]
Butyrylcholine esterase	+	+[a]
Leucine aminopeptidase	+	+
Leucine aminopeptidase (membrane-bound)	?	+
Leucine aminopeptidase (cytosolic)	?	+

NOTE: + = significant activity; − = no significant activity; ? unknown.
[a]Unpublished results of A. Trammel and R. T. Borchardt.

concentration of the peptide.[29] In experimental animal models, aluminum has been shown to transiently increase blood–brain barrier permeability to peptides and small molecules.[28,30] Metal effects on BBB permeability and cellular metabolism have been suggested to be relevant in pathologic processes leading to neurotoxicity and certain dementias.[28,31] Studies with the model system suggest that low concentrations of aluminum significantly alter BMEC metabolism.[32]

APPLICATIONS OF THE *IN VITRO* BLOOD–BRAIN BARRIER MODEL FOR STUDYING DRUG DELIVERY TO THE CNS

Drugs that are analogs of nutrients may enter the central nervous system by carriers at the BBB. For example, alpha-methyldopa, a commonly used centrally acting antihypertensive drug, is believed to cross the BBB by the neutral amino acid carrier. Supporting evidence comes from *in vivo* models, which demonstrate that by changing blood levels of amino acids by manipulation of diet, the antihypertensive effectiveness of alpha-methyldopa is altered.[33] Similarly, baclofen, an antispasmodic agent, probably crosses the BBB via the neutral amino acid carrier. Although direct evidence for this supposition is apparently not available, it is known that baclofen crosses intestinal mucosa by an amino acid carrier and does not have a measurable octanol partition coefficient.[34] Alpha-methyldopa and baclofen transport across the BBB by the amino acid carrier is supported by evidence obtained with the *in vitro* model. For example, a dose-dependent inhibition by both baclofen and alpha-methyldopa of the transendothelial transport of radiolabeled leucine has been observed across the monolayers of the model.[18] The characteristics of the neutral amino acid carrier as well as the amine or choline carrier of the BBB continue to be studied in our laboratories as potential mechanisms for enhancing drug delivery systems to the CNS.

Recent evidence suggests that peptides and proteins may cross the BBB to a limited degree.[7,24] Examples of proteins that may cross the BBB include insulin and transferrin. Specific insulin and insulin-like growth factor binding sites have been characterized on human brain microvessel endothelial cells.[7,35] Because binding-site-mediated endocytosis and exocytosis of insulin can be shown,[36] these studies suggest, but do not fully demonstrate, that insulin undergoes transendothelial transport. Similarly, specific transferrin binding sites have been found to be distributed throughout the cerebrovasculature.[37] A recent study indicates that, in fact, transferrin is trancytosed across the BBB by a receptor-mediated mechanism.[38] Although this is a more controversial area of research, significant amounts of smaller peptides are believed to cross the BBB by passive mechanisms.[39,40] However, small tyrosinated peptides were found to cross the BBB by a carrier-mediated mechanism (from brain to blood) in a recent study.[8] Further studies are needed to determine the precise nature of the passage of small peptides across the blood–brain barrier. Since these macromolecules represent potential drug carriers or therapeutic entities themselves, a significant amount of our research is devoted to understanding the interactions of peptides and proteins with the BBB. The overall goal of this research is to identify specific mechanisms which may provide for efficient and selective delivery of therapeutic macromolecules to the BBB endothelium and subsequently, to the central nervous system.

Previous work in our laboratories has established the existence of significant carboxy- and amino-peptidase activity in the model system.[19,21] Additional studies in this area are now concerned with how certain enkephalins and other neuropeptides are degraded and to what extent. This information is quite relevant to the ability of the cerebrovasculature to regulate levels of circulating peptides or proteins which might otherwise be available to penetrate the blood–brain barrier.

SUMMARY

Investigation of blood–brain barrier permeability and metabolic processes, and their regulation by endogenous or exogenous factors, will be important for development of efficient and selective delivery of therapeutic agents to the central nervous system. Primary cultures of brain microvessel endothelial cells offer a potentially powerful tool for studying at the cellular level the biochemical mechanisms regulating BBB function. Using this *in vitro* model, our studies are directed at characterization of the BBB processes that might be exploited as new schemes for drug delivery to the central nervous system.

REFERENCES

1. REESE, T. S. & M. J. KARNOVSKY. 1967. Fine structural localization of blood–brain barrier to exogenous peroxidase. J. Cell Biol. **34:** 207–217.
2. BRIGHTMAN, M. W. & T. S. REESE. 1969. Junctions between intimately apposed cell membranes in the vertebrate brain. J. Cell Biol. **40:** 648–677.
3. CRONE, C. 1965. The permeability of brain capillaries to nonelectrolytes. Acta Physiol. Scand. **64:** 407–417.
4. RAPOPORT, S. I., K. OHNO & K. D. PETTIGREW. 1979. Drug entry into the brain. Brain Res. **172:** 354–359.
5. CORNFORD, E. M., L. D. BRAUN, P. D. CRANE & W. OLDENDORF. 1978. Blood–brain barrier restriction of peptides and the low uptake of enkephalins. Endocrinology **103:** 1297–1303.
6. PARDRIDGE, W. M. & W. H. OLDENDORF. 1977. Transport of metabolic substrates through the blood–brain barrier. J. Neurochem. **28:** 5–12.
7. PARDRIDGE, W. M. 1986. Receptor-mediated peptide transport through the blood–brain barrier. Endocrine Rev. **7:** 314–330.
8. BANKS, W. A., A. J. KASTIN, A. J. FISCHMAN, D. H. COY & S. L. SRAUSS. 1986. Carrier-mediated transport of enkephalins and N-tyr-MIF-1 across the blood–brain barrier. Am. J. Physiol. **251:** E477–E482.
9. SPATZ, M. & B. B. MRSULJA. 1982. Progress in cerebral microvascular studies related to the function of the blood–brain barrier. Adv. Cell. Neurobiol. **3:** 311–337.
10. LAI, F. M., S. UDENFRIEND & S. SPECTOR. 1975. Presence of norepinephrine and related enzymes in isolated brain microvessels. Proc. Natl. Acad. Sci. USA **72:** 4622–4625.
11. CORNFORD, E. M. 1985. The blood–brain barrier, a dynamic regulatory interface. Mol. Physiol. **7:** 219–260.
12. JOO, F. 1985. The blood–brain barrier in vitro: Ten years of research on microvessels isolated from brain. Neurochem. Int. **7:** 1–25.
13. LASBENNES, F. & J. GAYET, 1984. Capacity for energy metabolism in microvessels isolated from rat brain. Neurochem. Res. **9:** 1–10.
14. PANULA, P., F. JOO & L. RECHARDT. 1978. Evidence for the presence of viable endothelial cells in cultures derived from dissociated rat brain. Experientia **34:** 95–96.
15. DEBAULT, L. E., E. HENRIQUEZ, M. N. HART & P. A. CANCILLA. 1981. Cerebral microvessels and derived cells in tissue culture: II. Establishment, identification, and preliminary characterization of an endothelial cell line. In Vitro **17:** 480–494.
16. BOWMAN, P. D., A. L. BETZ, J. S. WOLINSKY, J. B. PENNEY, R. R. SHIVERS & G. W. GOLDSTEIN. 1981. Primary culture of capillary endothelium from rat brain. In Vitro **17:** 353–362.
17. AUDUS, K. L. & R. T. BORCHARDT. 1986. Characterization of an in vitro blood–brain

barrier model system for studying drug transport and metabolism. Pharm. Res. **3:** 81–87.

18. AUDUS, K. L. & R. T. BORCHARDT. 1986. Characteristics of the large neutral amino acid transport system of bovine brain microvessel endothelial cell monolayers. J. Neurochem. **47:** 484–488.
19. BARANCZYK-KUZMA, A., K. L. AUDUS & R. T. BORCHARDT. 1986. Catecholamine-metabolizing enzymes of bovine brain microvessel endothelial cell monolayers. J. Neurochem. **46:** 1956–1960.
20. RIM, S., K. L. AUDUS & R. T. BORCHARDT. 1986. Relationship of octanol/buffer and octanol/water partition coefficients to transcellular diffusion across brain microvessel endothelial cell monolayers. Int. J. Pharm. **32:** 79–84.
21. BARANCZYK-KUZMA, A. & K. L. AUDUS. 1987. Characteristics of aminopeptidase activity from bovine brain microvessel endothelium. J. Cerebr. Blood Flow Metab. (In press).
22. GOLDSTEIN, G. W. 1986. In vitro studies of the blood–brain barrier. Polym. Prep. **27:** 425.
23. MOSTOV, K. E. & SIMISTER, N. E. 1985. Transcytosis. Cell **43:** 389–390.
24. BANKS, W. A. & A. J. KASTIN. 1985. Permeability of the blood–brain barrier to neuropeptides; The case for penetration. Psychoneuroendocrinology **10:** 385–399.
25. ZIYLAN, Z. Y., G. AGCIOGLU & N. GOKHAN. 1984. Effect of dexamethasone on the opening and reclosure time of the blood–brain barrier during acute drug-induced hypertension. IRCS Med. Sci. **12:** 1095–1096.
26. EISENBERG, H. M., C. F. BARLOW & A. V. LORENZO. 1970. Effect of dexamethasone on altered brain vascular permeability. Arch. Neurol. **23:** 18–22.
27. LONG, J. B. & J. W. HOLADAY. 1985. Blood–brain barrier: Endogenous modulation by adrenal-cortical function. Science **227:** 1580–1583.
28. KIM, Y. S., M. H. LEE & H. M. WISNIEWSKI. 1986. Aluminum induced reversible change in permeability of the blood–brain barrier to [^{14}C]sucrose. Brain Res. **377:** 286–291.
29. GRUBB, R. L. & M. E. RAICHLE. 1981. Intraventricular angiotensin II, increases brain vascular permeability. Brain Res. **210:** 426–430.
30. MAXWELL, K., H. V. VINTERS, J. A. BERLINER, J. V. BREADY & P. A. CANCILLA. 1986. Effect of inorganic lead on some functions of the cerebral microvessel endothelium. Toxicol. Appl. Pharmacol. **84:** 389–399.
31. BANKS, W. A. & A. J. KASTIN. 1983. Aluminum increases permeability of the blood–brain barrier to labelled DSIP and B-endorphin: Possible implications for senile and dialysis dementia. Lancet **ii:** 1227.
32. AUDUS, K. L. 1987. Aluminum effects on brain microvessel endothelial cell growth. Fed. Proc. **46:** 957.
33. SVED, A. F., I. M. GOLDBERG & J. D. FERNSTROM. 1980. Dietary protein intake influences the antihypertensive potency of methyldopa in spontaneously hypertensive rats. J. Pharmacol. Exp. Ther. **214:** 147–151.
34. BEALL, P. T., J. BOND, J. CASSIDY, K. ROSENZWEIG & F. H. CLARKE. 1985. Active transport of baclofen, a GABA agonist, by rat jejunum. Fed. Proc. **44:** 444.
35. PARDRIDGE, W. M., J. EISENBERG & J. YANG. 1985. Human blood–brain barrier insulin receptor. J. Neurochem. **44:** 1771–1778.
36. FRANK, H. J. L., W. M. PARDRIDGE, W. L. MORRIS, R. G. ROSENFIELD & T. B. CHOI. 1986. Binding and internalization of insulin and insulin-like growth factors by brain microvessels. Diabetes **35:** 651–661.
37. JEFFERIES, W. A., M. R. BRANDON, S. V. HUNT, A. F. WILLIAMS, K. C. GATTER & D. Y. MASON. 1984. Transferrin receptor on endothelium of brain capillaries. Nature **312:** 162–163.
38. FISHMAN, J. B., J. V. HANDRAHAN, J. CONNOR, B. F. DICKEY & R. E. FINE. 1985. Receptor-mediated transcytosis of transferrin across the blood–brain barrier. J. Cell Biol. **101:** 423a.
39. BANKS, W. A. & A. J. KASTIN. 1985. Peptides and the blood–brain barrier: Lipophilicity as a predictor of permeability. Brain Res. Bull. **15:** 287–292.
40. ERMISCH, A., H.-J. RUHLE, R. LANDGRAF & J. HESS. 1985. Blood–brain barrier and peptides. J. Cerebr. Blood Flow Metab. **5:** 350–357.

Obstacles to Polypeptide Delivery

L. A. STERNSON

Smith Kline & French Laboratories
Swedeland, Pennsylvania 19479

The ability of the pharmaceutical industry to develop peptides and proteins as drugs has increased markedly as such materials have become available in commercially viable quantities. Advances in chemical synthesis and recombinant DNA strategies, with attendant improvements in fermentation and purification technologies, now provide a means of producing rationally designed peptides and proteins (in addition to naturally occurring ones) in purified form and in large scale. Production efficiency is still generally poor and costs of goods high, but technological advances continue to drive costs down. Accordingly, the industry is now willing to invest in pharmaceutical development of products of biotechnology, viewing them as commercially profitable.

However, even if chemical availability can be made cost-effective, significant challenges to delivery of polypeptides will still limit their utilization as therapeutic agents. Many of the peptides being considered for development are autocrine or paracrine messengers (e.g., interleukin); others act within the central nervous system. After their administration into the blood stream, it is highly improbable that one will be able to direct such hormones to specific receptors on target cells in sufficient quantity to evoke the desired therapeutic response. Administration of such drugs via noninvasive routes creates additional obstacles to successful delivery. Barriers (*in vivo*) to the survival and transport of natural and foreign peptides and proteins have developed through evolution, further restricting the efficacious delivery of these peptides.

The simplest form of administration is by direct injection into the bloodstream, but even here one must consider properties of polypeptides that may impede their delivery, including (*a*) chemical, enzymatic and physical instability, resulting in limited formulation shelf life, short biological half-life of circulating drug, need for administration as a constant infusion and the attendant unacceptably high cost of therapy; (*b*) their potential for provoking an immunogenic response; and (*c*) their inability to be transported intact (as needed) from the vascular compartment to extravascular site(s) of action with efficiency suitable to support therapeutic needs. Site-specific modification of chemical structure has proved to be a powerful technique for reducing the fragility of many peptides and proteins, wherein sites of undesired instability are replaced by stabilizing residues without detrimentally altering biological activity. Structural alterations can also be introduced to alter transport (distribution) properties or to serve as targeting vectors.

Alternatively, peptides and proteins delivered directly into the bloodstream can be protected from harsh environmental factors by incorporation into polymeric microcapsules. Such systems are particularly useful for targeting drugs to cells of the reticuloendothelial system (RES). For other applications, rapid, undesired uptake by cells of the RES generally prevents drug-loaded microspheres from circulating long enough to elicit a therapeutic response. The inability of microcapsules to extravasate from the general circulation (and hence reach most cell types) further limits their value as intravenous drug carriers.

Polymeric microcapsules have also been successfully used as delivery systems for parenteral administration of peptides and proteins via nonintravenous routes. Such

19

carriers (in particular liposomes) have been recently used successfully as vehicles for vaccines. The antibody titer produced in response to liposome-encapsulated antigen has been consistently higher than the concentration secreted when free antigen was administered. This success has been attributed (a) to achieving a higher concentration of antigen bound to receptors on the surface of individual B cells, which results in a faster rate of proliferation of the plasma cells than is achieved when B cells encounter solitary antigens; and (b) to further stimulation of development of the plasma cell population resulting from activation of T-cell response triggered by the increased uptake of the encapsulated antigen by macrophages (relative to endocytosis of isolated antigens).

Although parenteral dosing may afford the opportunity for delivering certain polypeptides in clinical situations, noninvasive routes of delivery are desirable for many applications, and, from a commercial perspective, would significantly increase the monetary value of the drug product by increasing the feasibility for self-administration. The routes of administration pursued for peptides include the nasal, buccal, rectal, transdermal and the oral. In cases where systemic delivery via these routes has been achieved, the use of chemical absorption enhancers has generally been required to penetrate mucosal barriers.

Although oral delivery is the most attractive route, it is also the most difficult to achieve. The absorption efficiency of peptides is determined both by their resistance to hydrolysis, their ability to be transported intact across the gastrointestinal mucosa, and their propensity for avoiding capture by cells of the reticuloendothelial system. Blocking the N- and C-terminus of peptides with groups that are refractory to enzymatic hydrolysis can significantly retard peptide degradation. Modifying peptide polarity and hydrophobicity can facilitate membrane transport; however, the efficiency of absorption appears to vary inversely with the size and complexity of the peptide of interest. Peptides are subject to digestion both from luminal and membrane-associated mediators. The ability of substrate to be transported across the intestinal mucosa and to be taken up intact by the splanchnic blood supply may show region specificity. However, the likelihood of being able to efficiently target a therapeutically meaningful drug load to a specific region of the small bowel in a large population of patients presenting different pathophysiologies is extremely low. Some workers have suggested targeting peptidergic drugs (alone, chemically modified as a "pro-drug," or encapsulated in microparticulate carriers) to the gut-associated lymphoepithelial cells (M cells) covering Peyer's patches to deliver them to the general circulation via the lymphatic system, thus avoiding degradation through first-pass liver metabolism or biliary extraction. The effectiveness of this pathway for delivering peptides is severely compromised by (1) the limited efficiency and capacity of this absorption pathway; (2) the time to onset of pharmacologic response due to the kinetics of processing within lymphoid tissue and slow flow rate of lymph; and (3) the potential loss of drug to local lymphocytes and macrophages or through transport to mesenteric lymph nodes for processing there. Thus, biological barriers appear too formidable to support efficient peptide delivery via the oral route in all but those situations where coupling to active transport processes or masking of the normal peptide structure may permit absorption to occur. Yet antigen absorption from the GI tract and some isolated cases of oral delivery of peptides (e.g., polio vaccine, cyclosporin) have been shown to proceed with sufficient efficacy to serve a therapeutic function.

Difficulties in delivering peptides orally has stimulated interest in evaluating alternative noninvasive routes of administration. Modest success has been achieved by administering peptides rectally (in the form of an enema or suppository) or from the buccal cavity. In both cases, the harsh environment of the gut is avoided and the first-pass events are circumvented. However, an absorption enhancer, such as salicylate or a surfactant, is needed to deliver peptides/proteins across these mucosal tissues. These promotors provide little specificity with respect to the substances whose absorption they facilitate. Thus, a question arises as to the potential toxic liability associated with the use of such nondiscriminating, irritating substances as adjuvants (particularly on a chronic base) which must be resolved before this strategy can be widely tested clinically.

The nasal route has also been found to be a viable route of administration for peptides. As is the case with rectal and buccal delivery, nasal dosing avoids the hostile environment encountered after oral administration. Still, peptidase activity is present in the nasal cavity and can prove destructive to peptides containing sensitive amino acid sequences. The nasal mucosa is somewhat selective, so that the efficiency of transport is highly dependent on peptide structure and size. Whereas the nasal delivery of some peptides can be achieved from simple solutions, absorption of others requires the use of absorption enhancers (e.g., surfactants). Optimization of bioavailability after nasal instillation involves consideration of the (a) disposition of drug in the nasal cavity, (b) clearance from the nasal cavity and (c) rate of movement of drug into the nasal blood supply. The way in which drug is deposited inside the nasal cavity has a dramatic influence on the in vivo fate of the administered dose. Deposition should be avoided in both the poorly absorptive stratified epithelium of the anterior atrium and in the posterior nasopharyngeal region, which would lead to drug loss to the stomach by swallowing. The properties of the carrier vehicle and mode of application can be selected to target to the presumptively absorptive turbinate region. Once the drug is deposited onto the nasal turbinates, it must first diffuse across the mucus blanket before it encounters the nasal blood supply and can be absorbed systemically. If this is a rapid process, the clearance of vehicles from the nasal cavity becomes unimportant so long as the clearance takes longer than diffusion to the vascular bed. It is estimated that material that is entrapped on the mucus blanket is cleared from the nasal cavity within 15 minutes of deposition.

The blanket of nasal mucus is transported in a posterior direction by the synchronized beat of the cilia. At the pharynx, the mucus together with entrapped matter is swallowed. The rate of diffusion through the mucus blanket and clearance rates may be influenced by vehicle properties, particle size and surface charge, and "mucus modifier" (e.g., surfactants that may reduce the barrier resistance of the mucus blanket). Thus, formulation strategies may be developed to modulate absorption efficiency. The nasal route appears to be a viable means of systemically delivering many small peptides (MW <6000), although chronic nasal instillation may cause unacceptable local irritation. A further limitation of nasal administration is that it often results in irreproducible bioavailability, caused by inaccuracies in site-specific deposition and variability in nasal fluid composition, making it an undesirable route for delivery of potent peptides.

At present, our knowledge of physiology, biochemistry, and immunology is insufficient to meet the challenges of peptide/protein drug delivery. Furthermore, advances in drug analysis are needed to permit the monitoring of peptide/protein drugs with adequate selectivity and sensitivity to detect them at therapeutically relevant concentrations in biological matrices in order to evaluate drug delivery strategies and systems. However, advances in these areas continue to be made and thus bring us closer to realizing a rational approach to the delivery of peptides.

Molecular Modification of Lymphokines by *in Vitro* Mutagenesis

S. K. DOWER,[a] BRUCE MOSLEY, P. J. CONLON,
P. BENSON, C. GRUBIN, A. LARSEN, S. GILLIS,
AND D. COSMAN

Immunex Corporation
Seattle, Washington 98101

INTRODUCTION

The physiological functions of complex organisms are integrated by hormones, small molecules secreted into the blood or tissue fluids and carried to distant sites of action in the body. The action of such molecules on their target tissues is mediated by specific molecules, termed receptors. Since these natural signaling systems have a high degree of intrinsic specificity, they are attractive targets for the action of extrinsic pharmacologic agents. Conventional approaches to producing drugs have involved screening a large number of organic compounds for the ability to affect biological functions *in vivo* or *in vitro*. The availability of cDNA clones encoding a large number of polypeptide hormones provides the opportunity for a new approach to this problem, since it is now possible to construct any desired mutant of a cloned cDNA and express the mutant protein in unlimited quantities. Hence, the natural version of the hormone can be used as a starting point for the derivation of mutants with altered pharmacologic properties.

In the following report, we focus on the application of this approach to two polypeptide hormones that play a central role in the defense to disease and injury, the lymphokines interleukin-1α and interleukin-1β (IL-1α and IL-1β).[1-3] These two hormones are produced by activated macrophages and control a wide variety of processes associated with inflammatory responses, including fever, connective tissue and bone metabolism, lymphocyte activation, and acute-phase protein release by the liver.[3] Both forms of IL-1 are initially synthesized as M_r 30,000 polypeptides, subsequently processed, and the C-terminal portion secreted as M_r ca. 17,000 biologically active molecules.[4-7,10,11] Complementary DNA cloning has revealed that the two forms of IL-1 are distantly related proteins, being only 26% homologous at the primary sequence level.[7,12] It has also been demonstrated that the biological action of these two hormones is mediated by a specific cell surface receptor that binds the M_r 17,000 forms of both IL-1α and IL-1β.[8] This observation accounts for the fact that the two forms of IL-1 share the same spectrum of biological activities.[9]

In order to be able to construct and test a large number of mutants of both forms of IL-1 we have used *in vitro* transcription and translation to express the mutant proteins

---

[a]Address for correspondence: S. K. Dower, Immunex Corporation, 51 University Street, Seattle, Washington 98101.

in analytical quantities. The translation mixtures containing the mutant proteins were tested for the capacity to compete with ^{125}I-IL-1α for binding to the IL-1 receptor on murine T lymphoma cells and for biological activity in stimulation of IL-2 production by the same cells.

The first series of mutations we have explored are amino- and carboxyl-terminal deletions of the secreted form of both types of IL-1. The data show that as residues are deleted from the amino-terminal region of the proteins, biological and receptor binding activity decline in parallel, suggesting that loss of the former results from loss in the latter. By contrast, deletions of carboxyl-terminal residues produce some forms of IL-1 that show a more extensive loss of biological activity than receptor binding activity. With one caveat, these data indicate that some of these mutant IL-1 proteins can bind to the IL-1 receptor, but not deliver a signal to the cell. The results suggest that mutations in this region of the IL-1 molecules may yield antagonists of IL-1 action, which could be useful anti-inflammatory agents.

MATERIALS AND METHODS

Construction of SP6 Expression Vectors

SP6 vectors SP64 and SP65[13] were supplied by Promega Biotech. Appropriate restriction fragments for IL-1α and IL-1β were from cDNA clones previously described.[7] The construction of expression vectors for the full-length forms (β1-269 and α1-271) and the mature forms (β117-269 and α113-271) have been described elsewhere.[14] The construction of the truncated forms of IL-1 has been described in detail elsewhere.[28]

In Vitro *Transcription and Translation*

DNA was prepared by a standard alkaline lysis procedure[15] followed by purification over 0.5-ml Sephadex G-50 spun columns to remove small molecular weight contaminants. RNA transcription was done as described (Promega Biotech Riboprobe technical literature) with the modifications described previously.[14] Synthesized RNA was translated without further modification in a rabbit reticulocyte lysate translation system.[16,17] After translation, lysates were spun through Sephadex G-50 columns to remove small molecular weight contaminants responsible for high backgrounds in the receptor binding assay.

Protein Product Analysis

Aliquots (2 μl) of ^{35}S-labeled reticulocyte translation products were precipitated with trichloroacetic acid and from the amount of labeled methionine incorporated, the concentration of synthesized protein was determined. The M_r of the labeled translation product was also determined by analysis on a 15–20% exponential polyacrylamide gel.[18] This showed that >80% of the loaded counts were in the appropriately sized band.

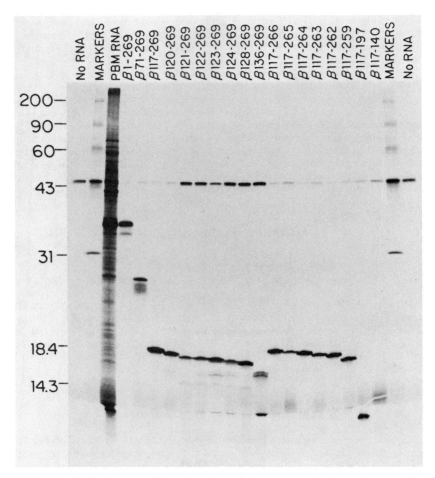

FIGURE 1A. SDS polyacrylamide gel analysis of *in vitro* translation products of IL-1β truncation series; each lane represents translated products from the construct indicated above. SDS-PAGE was performed as described in the MATERIALS AND METHODS section. PBM RNA was purified from human peripheral blood monocytes stimulated with LPS as described in March *et al.*[7] Indicated molecular weight standards are in kilodaltons.

Receptor Binding Assay

In vitro translated IL-1 proteins were tested for their ability to bind to receptors on EL-4 6.1 C10 cells by competition with ^{125}I-rIL-1α as described previously.[14]

Biological Assay

Biological activity was assayed by the capacity of IL-1 to stimulate IL-2 release from EL-4 6.1 C10 cells.[19] This assay is similar to that described previously using the LBRM-33-1A5 cell line.[14,20]

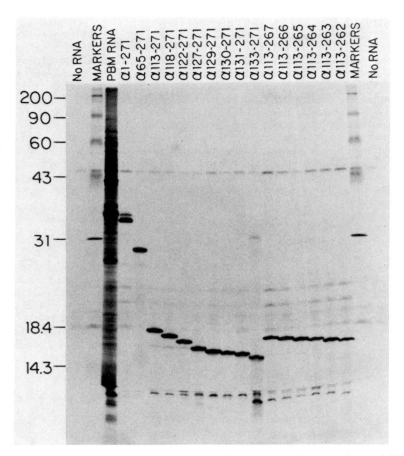

FIGURE 1B. SDS polyacrylamide gel analysis of *in vitro* translation products of IL-1α truncation series; each lane represents translated products from the construct indicated above. SDS-PAGE was performed as described in the MATERIALS AND METHODS section. PBM RNA was purified from human peripheral blood monocytes stimulated with LPS as described in March *et al.*[7] Indicated molecular weight standards are in kilodaltons.

RESULTS

Synthesis and Translation of IL-1 RNAs

We have previously reported an *in vitro* system that can be used to express biologically active IL-1 molecules.[14] Insertion of the IL-1 structural gene downstream of the SP6 RNA polymerase promotor in the SP65 vector allows synthesis of large amounts of pure IL-1 RNA. With no further processing of the RNA, translations are performed in a rabbit reticulocyte lysate system yielding between 10 and 40 ng of protein per microgram of RNA.

Cloning of the IL-1 full-length cDNAs into the SP65 vector required the use of synthetic oligonucleotides, the exact sequence of which has been published previously.[14] In the case of IL-1β, the oligonucleotide was initiated with an *Eco*RI site compatible with the polylinker region of SP65. This was followed by the natural sequence for IL-1β starting about 20 base pairs upstream of the initiation codon. The oligonucleotide was then extended to recreate the *Sst*I site at approximately amino acid 8. This oligonucleotide, with the *Sst*I/*Pst*I structural fragment of IL-1β was inserted into the *Eco*RI/*Pst*I vector fragment of SP65. The synthetic oligonucleotide for IL-1α was analogous to the IL-1β oligonucleotide extending from an *Eco*RI site upstream of the initiation codon to a *Bal*I site at amino acid 2 of the IL-1α gene. In this case, however, the sequence immediately upstream of the initiation codon was changed to conform with the consensus translational initiation sequence as published by M. Kozak.[21] This sequence allowed much higher translation rates than that of the natural IL-1α gene. The translational initiation sequence of the IL-1β gene conforms closely with the consensus sequence and high translation rates were achieved without modification.

Analysis of in Vitro Translated Protein Products

Because the IL-1 RNAs generated by SP6 polymerase were translated in an *in vitro* translation system where no processing of the polypeptide occurs, the presence of an initiator methionine is unavoidable. In some instances the methionine used as an initiator was already contained in the IL-1 sequence (α1-271, α127-271, β1-269, and β71-269). In other cases there is a Met-Gly sequence on the amino-terminus of the IL-1 construct (α65-271 and α118-271). All other constructs contain only a methionine on the amino terminus of the indicated polypeptide. FIGURE 1 shows SDS-PAGE analysis of these translation products.

Biological and Receptor Binding Activities

Each series of truncations was assayed between four and seven times for biological activity. The constructs were also assayed for receptor binding activity (FIGURE 2). The relative activity of the constructs, within each assay, was consistent. The data presented in TABLE 1 are representative of the amino-terminal truncations. Full-length IL-1β (β1-269) has no significant biological activity and no detectable receptor binding activity, which is consistent with earlier reports.[7,14] Biological activity was not seen until the amino terminus was positioned at amino acid 117 (β117-269). The further removal of three amino acids from the amino terminus reduced activity 4–5-fold, but the removal of Arg 120 reduced the specific activity more than 100-fold from that of the naturally secreted form (β117-269). Removal of the next 2–3 amino acids completely abolished biological activity. The receptor binding constants (K_A) parallel the biological activity with detectable binding only in the mature form and the β120-269 form of IL-1β (TABLE 1).

In contrast to the full-length IL-1β polypeptide, the full-length form of IL-1α (α1-271) has significant biological activity. High specific activities (within 10-fold of the mature form) were maintained through the amino-terminal truncation series up to and including the construct initiating at Met 127. The removal of Arg 128 caused a 100–200-fold drop in specific activity and a loss of essentially all biological activity. Receptor binding activity parallels biological activity, with binding detectable until Arg 128 is removed.

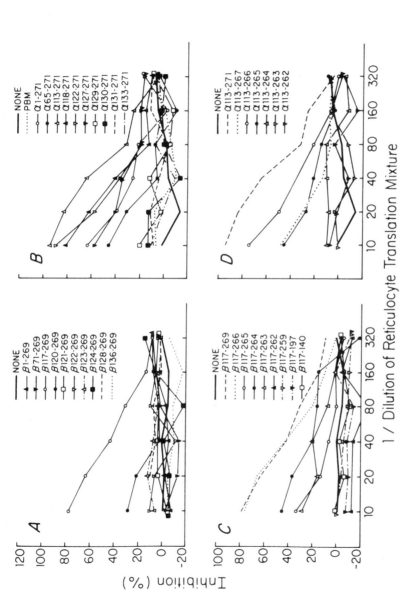

FIGURE 2. Inhibition of ^{125}I-rIL-1α binding to EL-4 6.1 C10 cells at 8°C by *in vitro* translated polypeptides. Assays were performed as described.[14] Control curves were generated using either a translation mixture in which no RNA (or PBM RNA) was included. (**A**) IL-1β amino-terminal truncations; (**B**) IL-1α amino-terminal truncations; (**C**) IL-1β carboxyl-terminal truncations; (**D**) IL-1α carboxyl-terminal truncations.

TABLE 1. Representative Data: Amino-Terminal Truncations

Construct	Protein Concentration (ng/ml)	Biological Activity (units/ml)	Specific Biological Activity (units/ng)	$K_A \times 10^{-9}$ (M^{-1})
		Assay 1		
No RNA		<50		
PBM RNA		14,234		
β1–269	323	4,308	13.3	<0.1
β71–269	368	5,938	16.1	<0.1
β117–269	442	4,099,577	9,275.0	2.9 ± 0.3
β120–269	248	1,188,642	4,792.9	0.57 ± 0.11
β121–269	272	29,107	107.0	<0.1
β122–269	140	14,326	102.3	<0.1
β123–269	165	1,255	7.6	<0.1
β124–269	519	3,001	5.8	<0.1
β128–269	57	<50	<0.5	<0.1
β136–269	100	<50	<0.5	<0.1
		Assay 2		
No RNA		<20		
PBM RNA		7,611		
α1–271	142	41,450	291.9	1.5 ± 0.3
α65–271	486	311,577	641.9	0.66 ± 0.15
α113–271	262	168,781	644.2	4.3 ± 0.9
α118–271	304	68,500	225.4	2.5 ± 0.3
α122–271	475	182,991	385.2	2.7 ± 0.5
α127–271	591	38,977	65.9	1.3 ± 0.2
α129–271	365	1,429	3.9	<0.1
α130–271	386	1,276	3.3	<0.1
α131–271	143	20	0.1	<0.1
α133–271	463	<20	<0.1	<0.1

Data for the carboxyl-terminal truncations are presented in TABLE 2. Removal of three amino acids from the carboxyl terminus of IL-1β had little effect on the specific activity (less than 10-fold). Removal of the next four amino acids sequentially reduced the biological activity of the resulting protein to less than detectable levels. For the IL-1α series, four amino acids could be removed without a significant loss of biological activity, but the sequential loss of the next three amino acids abolished any activity. Receptor binding ability partially parallels biological activity at the carboxyl-terminal end with receptor binding ability being lost over the same amino acid deletions as the biological activity. However, in this region, the receptor binding activity seems to be somewhat less sensitive to the deletions than the biological activity.

DISCUSSION

Through the use of *in vitro* transcription and translation systems we have generated various mutants of IL-1α and IL-1β. With this system we have determined the minimum polypeptide length of IL-1α and IL-1β required for biological activity and have shown that, in general, the IL-1 receptor binding capabilities of the polypeptides parallel this activity. This system has significant advantages over previously reported methods used to assess the minimum size for active IL-1.[22,23] Specifically we are able to generate much higher levels of IL-1 activity than reported for COS cell transfections[23] without background IL-1 biological activity. Furthermore, each IL-1 polypeptide can be visualized on a polyacrylamide gel and can be quantitated. Additionally, the IL-1 polypeptides can be assayed with only minimal further purification.

As previously reported, the initial transcript of the IL-1β gene is biologically inactive and shows no receptor binding.[14] However, after cleavage of the amino terminal 116 amino acids full biological activity is attained. The maximum size of biologically active IL-1β was not determined. Biological activity was markedly decreased with the removal of the arginine at position 120. Carboxyl-terminal truncations of IL-1β showed that the largely hydrophobic region near the carboxyl terminus of the mature protein is required for biological and receptor binding activity.

Truncations of IL-1α showed similar requirements for biological activity as for IL-1β. Activity was maintained for amino-terminal deletions until the arginine at position 128 was removed, while at the carboxyl terminus the hydrophobic region must be retained for biological activity and receptor binding.

The minimum polypeptide size for retention of full activity for IL-1β consists of 147 amino acids (120–266), and for IL-1α it is 140 amino acids (128–267). Both minimal IL-1 forms require an arginine at the amino terminus. It is striking that a basic amino acid is found at homologous positions in all IL-1 molecules yet characterized, namely, Lys 130 in murine IL-1α,[12] Arg 128 in rabbit IL-1α,[24] and Gln 117 in

TABLE 2. Representative Data: Carboxyl-Terminal Truncations

Construct	Protein Concentration (ng/ml)	Biological Activity (units/ml)	Specific Biological Activity (units/ng)	$K_A \times 10^{-9}$ (M^{-1})
		Assay 3		
No RNA		<20		
PBM RNA		1,510		
β117–269	183	85,828	469.0	2.9 ± 0.3
β117–266	319	115,523	362.1	1.5 ± 0.2
β117–265	108	3,268	30.2	0.67 ± 0.11
β117–264	177	2,383	13.5	0.96 ± 0.26
β117–263	185	428	2.3	0.41 ± 0.9
β117–262	165	<20	<0.1	<0.1
β117–259	62	<20	<0.1	<0.1
β117–197	136	<20	<0.1	<0.1
β117–140	9.3	<20	<0.1	<0.1
		Assay 4		
No RNA		<20		
PBM RNA		8,252		
α113–271	262	151,067	516.6	4.3 ± 0.09
α113–267	185	52,796	234.6	0.6 ± 0.12
α113–266	241	27,598	83.1	1.0 ± 0.1
α113–265	353	857	1.4	0.25 ± 0.03
α113–264	605	<20	<0.1	<0.1
α113–265	332	<20	<0.1	<0.1
α113–262	225	<20	<0.1	<0.1

bovine IL-1β (Maliszewski *et al.*, unpublished results). De Chiara *et al.*[22] reported that murine IL-1α starting at Leu 131 retained full biological activity, but the construction used to express this IL-1 analog fused a small peptide upstream of Leu 131 and thus reintroduced an arginine codon at the equivalent of amino acid 129. It thus seems likely that a basic amino acid in this region of IL-1 is essential for biological activity. This provides a structural explanation for earlier observations, from chemical modification studies, that one or more arginines are required for IL-1 biological activity.[25]

Our data are in disagreement with previous reports of biologically active subfragments of IL-1 of M_r 2,000–7,000.[23,26,27] It remains possible that smaller peptide fragments retain some biological activity below the level of detection in our assay. Such peptides however must have a specific activity at least 10,000-fold less than that of the mature form.

Finally, the carboxy-terminal truncation data for both forms of IL-1 suggest that some of the deleted mutants in this region may show a greater retention of receptor binding activity than capacity to transduce the signal leading to IL-2 release. A trivial explanation for this result is that these proteins are almost fully active but are less stable than wild-type IL-1. Since the binding assays were carried out for two hours at 8°C, while the biological assays were carried out for 48 hours at 37°C, such instability would be more likely to be revealed in the latter assay. Studies are currently under way to investigate whether these mutants bind to the receptor, but trigger cells inefficiently, and hence are potential IL-1 antagonists.

ACKNOWLEDGMENTS

We thank Suzanne Tyler and Jennifer Slack for excellent technical assistance, and Linda Troup for preparation of the manuscript.

REFERENCES

1. KAMPSCHMIDT, R. F. 1984. The numerous postulated biological manifestations of interleukin-1. J. Leuk. Biol. **36:** 341–355.
2. OPPENHEIM, J. J., E. J. KOVACS, K. MATSUSHIMA & S. F. DURUM. 1986. There is more than one interleukin-1. Immunol. Today **7:** 45–56.
3. DINARELLO, C. A. 1984. Interleukin-1 Rev. Infect. Dis. **6:** 51–95.
4. SCHMIDT, J. A. 1984. Purification and partial biochemical characterization of normal human interleukin-1. J. Exp. Med. **160:** 772–787.
5. CAMERON, P. M., G. A. LIMJUCO, J. CHIN, L. SILBERSTEIN & J. A. SCHMIDT. 1986. Purification of homogeneity and amino acid sequence analysis of two anionic species of human IL-1. J. Exp. Med. **164:** 237–250.
6. SAKLATVALA, J., S. J. SARSFIELD & Y. TOWNSEND. 1985. Pig interleukin-1: Purification of two distinct leukocyte proteins that cause cartilage resorption, lymphocyte activation and fever. J. Exp. Med. **162:**1208–1222.
7. MARCH, C. J., B. MOSLEY, A. LARSEN, D. P. CERRETI, G. BRAEDT, V. PRICE, S. GILLIS, C. S. HENNEY, S. KRONHEIM, K. GRABSTEIN, P. J. CONLON, T. P. HOPP & D. COSMAN. 1985. Cloning, sequence and expression of two distinct human interleukin-1 complementary DNAs. Nature **315:** 641–647.
8. DOWER, S. K., S. M. CALL, S. GILLIS & D. L. URDAL. 1986. Similarity between the interleukin-1 receptors on a murine T-lymphoma cell line and a murine fibroblast cell line. Proc. Natl. Acad. Sci. USA **83:** 1060–1064.
9. RUPP, E. A., P. M. CAMERON, C. S. RANAWAT, J. A. SCHMIDT & E. K. BAYNE. 1986. The specific bioactivities of monocyte derived interleukin-1α and interleukin-1β are similar to

each other on cultured murine thymocytes and on cultured human connective tissue cells. J. Clin. Invest. **78**: 836–839.

10. CAMERON, P., G. LIMJUCO, J. RODKEY, C. BENNETT & J. A. SCHMIDT. 1985. Amino acid sequence analysis of human interleukin-1 (IL-1): Evidence for biochemically distinct forms of IL-1. J. Exp. Med. **162**::790–801.
11. DEWHIRST, F. E., P. P. STASHENKO, J. E. MOLE & T. TSURUMACHI. 1985. Purification and partial sequence analysis of human osteoclast activating factor: Identity with interleukin-1β. J. Immunol. **135**: 2562–2574.
12. LOMEDICO, P. T., U. GUBLER, C. P. WELLMAN, M. DUKOVICH, J. G. GIRI, Y. E. PAN, K. COLLIER, R. SEMIONOW, A. O. CHUA & S. B. MIZEL. 1984. Cloning and expression of murine interleukin-1 cDNA in *Escherichia coli*. Nature **312**: 458–462.
13. MELTON, D. A., P. A. KREIG, M. R. REBAGLIATI, T. MANIATIS, K. ZINN & M. R. GREEN. 1984. Efficient *in vitro* synthesis of biologically active RNA and RNA hybridization probes from plasmids containing a bacteriophage SP6 promotor. Nucl. Acids Res. **12**: 7035–7056.
14. MOSLEY, B., D. L. URDAL, A. LARSEN, D. COSMAN, P. J. CONLON, S. GILLIS & S. K. DOWER. 1987. The IL-1 receptor binds the human IL-1α precursor but not the IL-1β precursor. J. Biol. Chem. **262**: 2941–2944.
15. MANIATIS, T., E. F. FRITSCH & J. SAMBROOK. 1982. Molecular Cloning: A Laboratory Manual. Cold Spring Harbor Laboratory. Cold Spring Harbor, NY.
16. PALMITER, R. D. 1973. Ovalbumin messenger ribonucleic acid translation. J. Biol. Chem. **248**: 2095–2106.
17. PELHAM, H. R. & R. J. JACKSON. 1976. An efficient mRNA-dependent translation system from reticulocyte lysates. Eur. J. Biochem. **67**:247–256.
18. SMITH, T. J. & J. E. BELL. 1986. An exponential gradient maker for use with minigel polyacrylamide electrophoresis systems. Anal. Biochem. **152**: 74–77.
19. LUSCHER, B., M. ROUSSEAU, R. LEES, H. R. MACDONALD & C. BRON. 1985. Cell surface glycoproteins involved in the stimulation of interleukin-1 dependent interleukin-2 production by a subline of EL-4 thymoma cells. J. Immunol. **135**: 3951–3957.
20. CONLON, P. J. 1983. A rapid biologic assay for the detection of interleukin-1. J. Immunol. **131**: 1280–1284.
21. KOZAK, M. 1984. Compilation and analysis of sequences upstream from the translational start site in eukaryotic mRNAs. Nucl. Acids Res. **12**: 857–872.
22. DECHIARA, T. M., D. YOUNG, R. SEMIONOW, A. S. STERN, C. BATULA-BERNARDO, C. FIEDLER-NAGY, K. L. KAFFKA, P. L. KILIAN, S. YAMAZAKI, S. B. MIZEL & P. T. LOMEDICO. 1986. Structure function analysis of murine interleukin-1: biologically active polypeptides are at least 127 amino acids long and are derived from the carboxyl-terminus of a 270 amino acid precursor. Proc. Natl. Acad. Sci. USA **83**: 8303–8307.
23. ROSENWASSER, L. J., A. C. WEBB, B. B. CLARK, S. IHRIE, L. CHANG, C. A. DINARELLO, L. GERKE, S. M. WOLFF, A. RICH & P. E. AURON. 1986. Expression of biologically active human interleukin-1 subpeptides by transfected simian COS cells. Proc. Natl. Acad. Sci. USA **83**: 5243–5246.
24. FURUTANI, Y., M. NOTAKE, M. YAMAYOSHI, J. YAMAGISHI, H. NOMURA, M. OHUE, R. FURUTA, T. FUKUI, M. YAMADA & S. NAKAMURA. 1985. Cloning and characterization of the cDNAs for human and rabbit interleukin-1 precursor. Nucl. Acids Res. **13**: 5869–5882.
25. GILLIS, S. & S. B. MIZEL. 1981. A T-cell lymphoma model for the analysis of interleukin-1 mediated T-cell activation. Proc. Natl. Acad. Sci. USA **78**: 1133–1137.
26. KIMBALL, E. S., S. F. PICKERAL, J. J. OPPENHEIM & J. L. ROSSIO. 1984. Interleukin-1 activity in normal human urine. J. Immunol. **133**: 256–260.
27. DINARELLO, C. A., G. H. CLOWES, A. H. GORTON, C. A. SARAVIS & S. M. WOLFF. 1984. Cleavage of human interleukin-1: Isolation of a peptide fragment from plasma of febrile humans and activated monocytes. J. Immunol. **133**: 1332–1338.
28. MOSLEY, B., S. K. DOWER, S. GILLIS & D. COSMAN. 1987. Determination of the minimal polypeptide length for active human IL-1α and IL-1β. Proc. Natl. Acad. Sci. USA **84**: 4572–4576.

Transdermal Iontophoretic Delivery of Therapeutic Peptides/Proteins

I: Insulin

Y. W. CHIEN, O. SIDDIQUI, Y. SUN, W. M. SHI,
AND J. C. LIU

Controlled Drug-Delivery Research Center
Rutgers, The State University of New Jersey
College of Pharmacy, Busch Campus
Piscataway, New Jersey 08855-0789

Peptides/proteins are biopolymers with both physiological and therapeutic importance. Many of these biopolymers not only are the essential nutrients of human body, but can also be used to treat various diseases. Each of the peptide and protein molecules consists of a unique genetically defined sequence of α-amino acids connected together by peptide linkage to form a specific molecular configuration, which often determines its physiological functions and therapeutic activities. The peptides and proteins are known to serve as hormones, enzymes, antigens, antibodies, or structural elements, and are involved in metabolic processes, immunogenetic defense mechanisms, cell growth, and other biological activities.[1-3]

Since the inception of genetic engineering, numbers of new therapeutically important peptides/proteins are being produced commercially. These biopolymers are comparatively easier and cheaper than those obtained through natural sources. As a result of such progress, the therapeutic applications of peptides/proteins have received increasing attention in recent years. A number of peptides and proteins have been approved by the regulatory authorities for medical uses, as in treatment of endocrine disorders, cardiovascular diseases, cancers, viral infections, or in preventive medicine, as in active and passive immunization (TABLE 1). These therapeutically active peptides/proteins have emerged as a very important class of therapeutic agents. They are very potent and often require only a daily dose of micrograms or less for medication.

Numerous studies have been initiated to investigate potential techniques for the delivery of therapeutically important peptides/proteins. Unfortunately, peptides/proteins are easily metabolized by proteolytic enzymes in the gastrointestinal tract and are subjected to an extensive hepatic first-pass elimination when taken orally; consequently, they are usually orally inactive and often require parenteral administration to be therapeutically effective. Additionally, peptides/proteins are inherently short-acting in their biological activities and require frequent injections, often several times a day, to maintain a therapeutically effective level. This treatment regimen has often subjected patients not only to constant pain but also to health hazard. These problems often prevent many patients from accepting rigid treatment regimens. Over the years, much effort has been made to find a viable route, other than through parenteral injections, for effective administration of peptide/protein drugs with fewer side effects and better patient compliance.[4-13] Although peptide/protein drugs are highly potent, there are a number of potential problems associated with their delivery through routes other than the parenteral; these problems include the extremely short biological half-life, and low chemical and enzymatic stabilities as well as large

32

TABLE 1. Peptide/Protein Drugs Currently Approved for Therapeutic, Preventive, and Other Applications

Category	Peptide/Protein	Biomedical Applications
Antibodies	(1) Anti-Rh globulin	Prevention of Rh isoimmunization
	(2) Antivenins	Treatment of snakebite
	(3) "General" immune globulin	Immunodeficiency
	(4) "Specific" immune globulins	Passive immunization to rabies, tetanus, hepatitis B and pertussis
Antigens	Vaccines	Active immunization against viral diseases, e.g., smallpox, mumps, poliomyelitis, hepatitis B, etc.
Enzymes	(1) Asparaginase	Leukemia
	(2) Chymopapain	Herniated lumbar disc
	(3) Collagenase	Topical debridement
	(4) Hyaluronidase	Enhancement of SQ absorption
	(5) Pancreatic enzymes (amylase, β-galactosidase, trypsin, etc.)	Digestive supplement
	(6) Plasminogen activators	Thrombolysis in MI and other thromboses
	(7) Thrombin	Topical hemostasis
	(8) Trypsin	Digestive supplement or topical debridement
Hormones	(1) Insulin	Diabetes mellitus
	(2) Oxytocin	Maintenance of labor
	(3) Vasopressin	Diabetes insipidus
	(4) Human growth hormone	Hypopituitary dwarfism
	(5) Gonadotropins (hCG, LH, FSH, etc.)	Induction of ovulation, spermatogenesis and cryptorchidism
Immune Factors	Interferon-α	Anticancer (hairy cell leukemia) Antiviral
Miscellaneous	(1) Aspartame	Sugar supplement
	(2) Collagen	Dermal reconstruction
	(3) Cyclosporin	Antibiotic
	(4) Factor VIII	
	(5) Factor IX complex	Hemophilia
	(6) Protein hydrolysate	Nutrient
	(7) Serum albumin	Plasma extender

molecular size. These problems have limited the successful development of a viable dosage form for effective administration of peptide/protein drugs through nonparenteral routes.

Transdermal controlled delivery of drugs has gained increasing recognition in recent years.[14-18] Since gastrointestinal degradation and hepatic first-pass metabolism would be avoided by a transdermal drug delivery and because it would promote better patient compliance,[19-25] it can be considered as a potential route for the delivery of peptide/protein drugs. A review of the literature suggests an additional advantage: the skin lacks proteolytic enzymes,[26] which are responsible for the enzymatic degradation of peptides/proteins. All these factors have made the skin an appealing site for the administration of therapeutically important peptides and proteins.

In this laboratory, for many years we have studied transdermal controlled delivery as a noninvasive means for drug administration.[25,27-35] Thus we found it interesting to extend our present transdermal research program to investigate the possibility of systemic delivery of peptide/protein drugs through the skin.

The majority of drugs that have been successfully delivered through intact skin are lipophilic and are of small molecular size, while the therapeutically active peptides/ proteins are mostly hydrophilic in nature and often rather large in molecular size. Therefore, in theory the transdermal delivery of such macromolecules is often extremely difficult, if not impossible, in the absence of a facilitated skin transport. So, to successfully deliver a peptide or a protein drug across the intact skin to attain a therapeutically effective level, it is essential to develop a valid enhancing technique to facilitate the transdermal permeation of hydrophilic peptides/proteins through the rate-limiting barrier of lipophilic stratum corneum and the diffusional resistance across the skin tissues.

TRANSDERMAL FACILITATED DELIVERY OF PEPTIDE/PROTEIN DRUGS BY IONTOPHORESIS

Iontophoresis is a process that induces an increased migration of ions or ionic substances in an electrolyte medium with the flow of electric current.[36] It has been

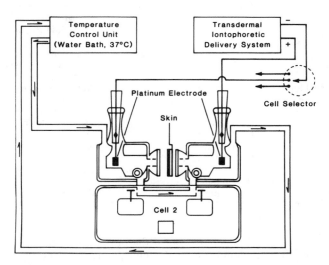

FIGURE 1. Experimental setup for the *in vitro* permeation kinetics studies with application of direct current or pulse current iontophoresis generated from the Transdermal Iontophoretic Delivery System.

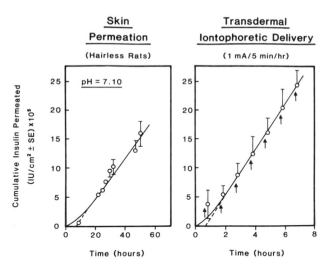

FIGURE 2. *In vitro* skin permeation profiles of insulin, from donor solution at pH 7.10 across hairless rats, and the enhancement of skin permeation by DC iontophoresis at current intensity of 1 mA applied for 5 min on the hour for 7 hr.

explored as a potential technique to facilitate the membrane transport of charged molecules on the basis of their ionic characteristics.[37-44] Iontophoresis with DC mode has recently been proved to be a safe and useful technique to facilitate the penetration of charged anti-inflammatory drugs into cutaneous tissues for localized effects.[45] Peptide/protein drugs can be rendered to carry a charge by the control of the solution's pH and thus may penetrate through the skin, as ionic substances, with the assistance of iontophoresis.

In addition, electric current may also alter the molecular arrangement of skin components, which could yield some changes in skin permeability. The "flip-flop gating mechanism"[46] could be an operating model in the voltage-dependent pore formation in the stratum corneum, which is rich in alpha-helical polypeptides. As an electrical potential is applied across a biological membrane, such as the skin, the flip-flop of polypeptide helices may occur to form a parallel arrangement in response to the application of voltage. Pores are thus opened as a result of the repulsion between neighboring dipoles, and water molecules and ions will flow in the pore channels to neutralize the dipole moments. This phenomenon should lead to an increase in skin permeability.

Feasibility of skin permeation of thyrotropin-releasing hormone (TRH), a small peptide molecule, by iontophoresis was investigated under *in vitro* conditions.[47] The results indicated that the total skin permeation flux of TRH, which has three amino acid residues, is contributed from a passive diffusion due to the concentration gradient, an electric term driven by applied current, and an electrically induced convective term which may be affected by ionic strength.

The transdermal delivery of insulin, a protein drug, was recently studied by Stephen *et al.*[48] They reported that a highly ionized monomeric form of insulin can be delivered through the pig skin, in the presence of iontophoresis, to produce systemic effects.

FUNCTIONS AND DELIVERY OF INSULIN

Insulin, a protein hormone containing 51 amino acid residues, has a molecular weight of approximately 6,000 and an extremely short biological half-life of less than 30 minutes. In healthy humans, it is secreted by beta cells in the Langerhans islet of the pancreas in response to an increase in blood glucose level to facilitate the process of glucose utilization for either energy or storage.[49]

In patients with diabetes mellitus, however, the capacity of the pancreas to supply insulin in response to the increase in blood glucose level is impaired. For the control of diabetes mellitus, insulin must be supplied externally by subcutaneous injection at a dose of 10–20 units three to four times a day.[49]

IN VITRO SKIN PERMEATION OF INSULIN

Experiments were conducted in a modified V-C skin permeation cell (FIGURE 1) to study the feasibility of facilitating the transdermal delivery of insulin across the freshly excised abdominal skin of hairless rats by applying iontophoresis with a direct current

TABLE 2. Apparent Skin Permeability Coefficients of Insulin in Hairless Rats[a]

Donor Solution pH	Permeability Coefficient[b] (cm/hr ± SE) × 10^7	
	No TIDD	With TIDD[c]
3.7	6.50 (±1.42)	242.59 (±18.43)
5.2	10.02 (±1.94)	120.07 (±22.86)
7.1	7.43 (±0.54)	70.76 (±8.56)

[a]5.2 IU/ml (with 0.3 μCi ^{125}I-labeled insulin) in donor solution.
[b]Triplicate determinations.
[c]Application of Transdermal Iontophoretic Drug Delivery System (TIDD) at 1 mA for 5 min on the hour for 7 hours.

at 1 mA for 5 min on the hour for 7 hr. The results demonstrated that the skin permeation rate of insulin thus applied is enhanced substantially as compared to that achieved by passive diffusion alone, i.e., without iontophoresis application (FIGURE 2). The degree of enhancement in the iontophoresis-facilitated skin permeation rate is pH dependent (TABLE 2). The results suggest that the lower the pH of the donor drug solution, the greater the degree of enhancement in the apparent permeability coefficient of insulin molecules.

The observations outlined above can be explained by the fact that a peptide/protein drug like insulin can be rendered as positively or negatively charged molecules by controlling the pH of the drug solution below or above the isoelectric point (pH_{iso}) of the drug.[50] The solubility and the charge density of peptide/protein molecules increase when the solution pH is made higher or lower than its isoelectric point as a result of protonation or dissociation of the peptide/protein molecule. It has also been reported that insulin molecules become aggregated as pH increases,[50] which may explain why iontophoresis yielded a 37.3-fold increase in skin permeability coefficient for insulin at pH 3.7, which is 1.7 pH units below its pH_{iso} ($\approx$5.4), but only a 9.5-fold increase at pH 7.1, which is 1.7 pH unit above its pH_{iso}.

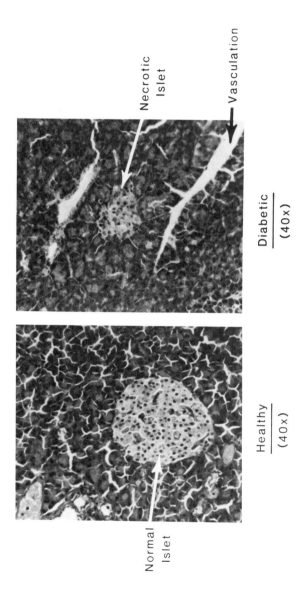

FIGURE 3. By single intraperitoneal injection of streptozotocin, the beta cells in the hairless rat's pancreas appeared to be extensively damaged and a necrotic islet of Langerhans was observed microscopically.

IN VIVO TRANSDERMAL DELIVERY OF INSULIN

To study the pharmacodynamic responses after the transdermal iontophoretic delivery of insulin, in terms of effective control of blood glucose level, a diabetic animal model was developed by intraperitoneal injection of streptozotocin to hairless rats.[51] The beta cells appeared to be extensively damaged: the Langerhans islet necrotized (FIGURE 3) after a single injection of streptozotocin and the blood glucose level was found to increase, within 24 hours after the streptozotocin administration, from a normoglycemic level of around 80 mg/dL to more than 200 mg/dL, which remained fairly stable for 3–4 days (FIGURE 4). The hyperglycemic state was found to be unaffected by fasting, anesthesia, and iontophoresis treatment with placebo formulation, i.e., no insulin in the reservoir electrode (FIGURE 5).

By consecutive daily injection of streptozotocin, another diabetic animal model (New Zealand white rabbits) was also successfully developed (FIGURE 4). Because of its large size in comparison with rats, the diabetic rabbit was used as the animal model for studying simultaneously the pharmacokinetics and pharmacodynamics of insulin and their relationship.

TRANSDERMAL DELIVERY OF INSULIN IN DIABETIC HAIRLESS RATS

The Transdermal Periodic Iontotherapeutic System (TPIS) developed in this laboratory was first applied to studying the transdermal iontophoretic delivery of insulin in the diabetic hairless rat. Transdermal iontophoretic drug delivery with simple DC mode was initiated by applying the insulin-containing reservoir electrode, which contains insulin formulations at various pHs, and the receptor electrode to the skin surface on the abdominal region of a diabetic rat (FIGURE 6). The results demonstrated that the blood glucose levels in the treated diabetic rats were rapidly reduced after the application of iontophoresis at 4 mA (current density = 0.67 mA/cm^2) for 80 min.[51] A pronounced reduction in blood glucose level was observed

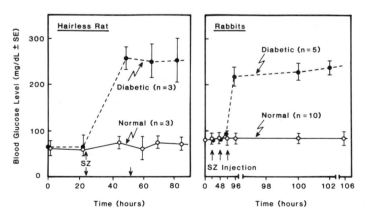

FIGURE 4. Successful induction of stable hyperglycemic levels in hairless rats and rabbits, as the animal model for diabetes studies, by streptozotocin (SZ) injections.

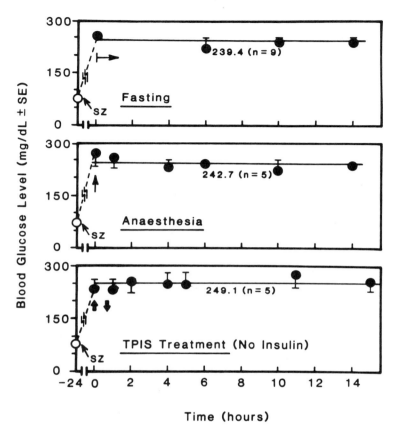

FIGURE 5. Hyperglycemia in the diabetic hairless rats is stable for at least 14 hr and its stability is unaffected by fasting, anesthesia, or transdermal periodic iontotherapeutic system (TPIS) treatment with no insulin in the drug reservoir electrode.

when the insulin formulation used had a solution pH at 3.68 (FIGURE 7), while the blood glucose level in the untreated diabetic controls remained at hyperglycemic state over the course of experiment. A reservoir effect was also evident, as the normogly-cemic level was maintained for more than 2–3 hours, even after the completion of the treatment (80 min). The reduction of blood glucose level in diabetic rats in response to the transdermal iontophoretic delivery of insulin appears to be dependent upon the pH of insulin solution (FIGURE 8), with the maximum effect (a 71.2% reduction in blood glucose level) achieved at pH 3.68.[51] This observation could be attributed to the acidic nature of the solution, in which insulin molecules (with isoelectric point at pH 5.4) exist predominantly as positively charged ions and are likely to be less aggregated.[50]

As observed in the *in vitro* studies, the *in vivo* data on the reduction of blood glucose level also indicated that when the pH of the solution is higher than the isoelectric point of insulin ($pH_{iso} \simeq 5.4$), the efficacy of normalizing the blood glucose level in the diabetic animal is reduced: a normoglycemic effect of 54.5% was achieved at pH 7.1, which is 1.7 pH units above the pH_{iso}, and an effect of 37.5% was obtained at pH 8.0, which is 2.6 pH units above the pH_{iso}. This observation again could be attributed to the possible effect of molecular aggregation of insulin at pH higher than pH_{iso} as reported previously.[50]

THEORETICAL CONSIDERATIONS IN TRANSDERMAL PERIODIC IONTOPHORETIC DELIVERY OF MACROMOLECULES

The skin is known to produce a large impedance to charged molecules as they are driven through the skin by an applied electrical field. The electrical properties of the skin are known to be dominated by the least conductive stratum corneum. The stratum corneum consists of multilayers of horny cells that have lost their nuclei and are formed and continuously replenished by the slow upward migration of cells produced by the basal cell layer of stratum germinativum. These cells have a water content of only 20% as compared to the normal physiological level of 70% and are electrically insulated. Skin is breached by hair follicles and sweat ducts, which could provide a potential pathway for shunt-diffusion across the skin. This shunt pathway may be significant for ionic penetrants, which show an extremely poor skin permeation through the transcellular route.[52] Under the influence of electric current, ionic species or charged molecules are driven across the skin, possibly through the shunt pathways or intercellular spacings in the stratum corneum, since the skin is likely to be perturbed during iontophoresis, which may remove or disrupt the intercellular lipids, resulting in the formation of artificial "shunts."

The stratum corneum shows two important electrical features: first, it is polarized by the electrical field, and second, its impedance changes with the frequency of the applied electrical field. These properties can be viewed as an electrical equivalent circuit (FIGURE 9). In this equivalent circuit, a parallel combination of R_{sc} and C_{sc} is in series with R_{vs}. R_{vs} denotes the pure resistance, which originates from the viable skin tissues, to the current of charged molecules and does not change with the frequency. The parallel combination of R_{sc} and C_{sc} represent, respectively, the resistor and the

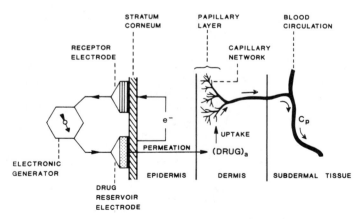

FIGURE 6. Diagrammatic illustration of the transdermal iontophoretic delivery of drugs across live animal's skin for systemic administration.

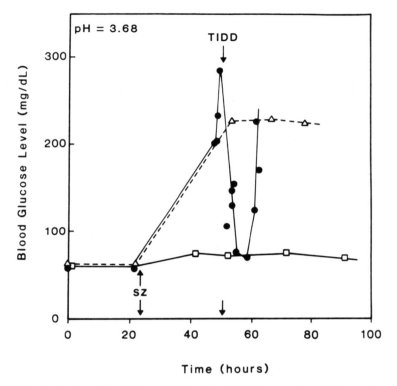

FIGURE 7. Reduction of blood glucose level in diabetic hairless rats from the hyperglycemic to normoglycemic level as a result of the transdermal iontophoretic delivery of insulin, at pH 3.68, by application of DC at current intensity of 4 mA for 80 min.

capacitor of the capacitive impedance of the stratum corneum. This impedance is a function of the frequency and is known to decrease with the increases in frequency.[53]

When an electrical field with DC mode is applied to facilitate the skin permeation of ionic molecules, an electrochemical polarization may occur in the skin. This polarization often operates against the applied electrical field, which greatly decreases the magnitude of effective current across the skin. The polarization of the stratum corneum is similar to the charging of the capacitor C_{sc} in the electric equivalent circuit (FIGURE 9) by the input current. Therefore, the effective current through the skin decays exponentially when a constant DC voltage is applied continuously (FIGURE 10). Consequently, the efficiency of transdermal iontophoretic delivery is reduced with the application time of DC iontophoresis.

To avoid the counterproductive polarization, the current should be applied in a periodic manner, which is called pulse DC. The pulse DC is a DC voltage that is turned on and off alternatively in a periodic fashion (FIGURE 10). In the state of "on," charged molecules are forced to diffuse into the skin and polarization is soon produced. On the other hand, in the state of "off," external stimulation is not present and depolarization occurs in the skin, similar to the discharging of the current from the capacitor C_{sc}

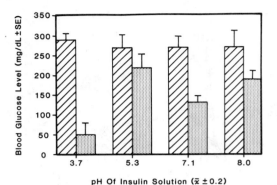

FIGURE 8. pH-dependence of the hypoglycemic effect of insulin delivered transdermally by DC iontophoresis at current intensity of 4 mA for 80 min.

(FIGURES 9 and 10). By proper selection of frequency, every new cycle could start with no residual polarization from the previous cycle (FIGURE 10).

The energy required to drive a charge peptide/protein molecule, such as insulin, through the skin can be expressed by:

$$E_s = IVt = I^2 R_T t \tag{1}$$

where E_s is the energy required to deliver a charged molecule with a current intensity of I under a voltage of V for a duration of t. Higher efficiency of transdermal iontophoretic delivery can be achieved for the skin with low impedance (i.e., less polarization effect), which may be accomplished by controlling the frequency and the on/off ratio of applied voltage at such pattern that polarization is not allowed to occur. Therefore, it is essential to select an optimum combination of frequency and on/off ratio (Eq. 2) to provide the best facilitating effect on the transdermal iontophoretic delivery of peptide/protein drugs. Frequency is related to on/off ratio (FIGURE 11) by the following relation:

$$\text{Frequency} = \frac{\text{Duration of "off" state}}{(\text{on/off}) + 1} \tag{2}$$

FIGURE 9. Diagrammatic illustration of the analogous equivalent circuit of skin impedance. R_{vs}, the resistance generated from the deep tissues of the skin, forms a series with a parallel combination of R_{sc}, the resistance, and C_{sc}, the capacitance from the stratum corneum.

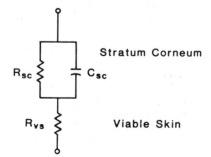

FIGURE 10. Current profiles across the skin barrier as a function of the applied electrical field: Periodic versus continuous application. Use of periodic waveform minimizes the production of polarization and allows the skin to depolarize during the "off" state so that the intensity of effective current across the skin will not decay exponentially as a function of treatment duration.

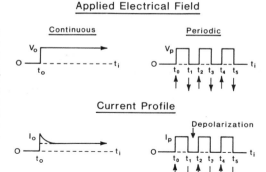

Additionally, the skin tolerance could also be improved, since only lower current density is required when a pulse DC iontophoresis is applied.

The higher effectiveness of pulse DC iontophoresis can also be attributed to the change occurring in the instant momentum and entropy.[54] This is most important when one is dealing with a charged molecule as large as the peptide/protein drug, since the back flow in the pores created by the large dimension of macromolecules is expected to be higher.

The experimental results outlined in FIGURE 12 show the effect of the mode of current delivery on the efficiency of transdermally delivered insulin in controlling the blood glucose levels, in which direct current is applied to the diabetic hairless rats from the TPIS's controlling module using either the conventional DC mode or the periodic wave mode with the same current density and for the same duration. The results demonstrated that blood glucose levels are much more effectively reduced when pulse DC is applied as compared to the conventional DC mode. It was possible to effectively reduce the blood glucose levels with pulse DC for a duration of at least 12 hours before the levels went back to the original hyperglycemic state (which is defined as 100%). The percent of change in blood glucose level (BGL) in the diabetic animals is calculated from the following relationship:

$$\% \text{ Change in BGL} = \frac{(BGL)_t}{(BGL)_i} \times 100\% \tag{3}$$

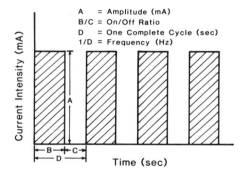

A = Amplitude (mA)
B/C = On/Off Ratio
D = One Complete Cycle (sec)
1/D = Frequency (Hz)

FIGURE 11. Diagrammatic illustration of the direct current (DC) profiles delivered in square waveform at periodic manner.

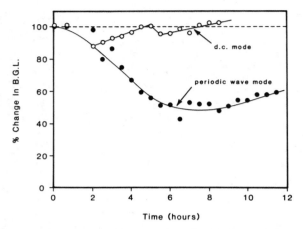

FIGURE 12. Effect of delivery mode of current from transdermal periodic iontotherapeutic system (TPIS) on the magnitude and the duration of percentage reduction in blood glucose level (BGL) from hyperglycemic state (100 percent) in the diabetic hairless rat.

The results in FIGURE 12 suggest that the pulse DC iontophoresis is much more efficient in facilitating the transdermal delivery of macromolecular insulin than the conventional direct current method.[55]

Current has four features: intensity, frequency, on/off ratio, and waveforms (FIGURE 11). They need to be characterized in order to optimize the facilitating effect on the transdermal delivery of peptide/protein molecules. Current intensity controls the amount and rate of charged peptide molecules penetrating through the skin

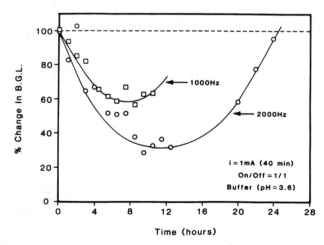

FIGURE 13. Effect of the frequency of periodic current delivered by the transdermal periodic iontotherapeutic system (TPIS) on the magnitude and the duration of percentage reduction in blood glucose level (BGL) from hyperglycemic state (100 percent) in the diabetic hairless rat.

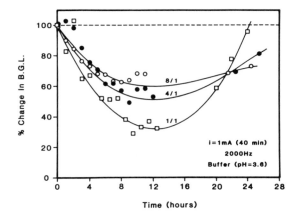

FIGURE 14. Effect of the on/off ratio of periodic current delivered by transdermal periodic iontotherapeutic system (TPIS) on the magnitude and duration of percentage reduction in blood glucose level (BGL) from hyperglycemic state (100 percent) in the diabetic hairless rat.

(Faraday's Law). However, the establishment of a quantitative correlation between the theoretical predictions and the experimental observations is extremely difficult, if not impossible, due to the fact that the skin is not a homogeneous membrane. The data generated so far have demonstrated that the control of blood glucose levels in diabetic rats is dependent upon the frequency (FIGURE 13), the on/off ratio (FIGURE 14), and the waveform (FIGURE 15) of the input current as well as the duration of TPIS application (FIGURE 16). More systematic investigations are currently under way to gain a better understanding of the roles that each system parameter might play, the

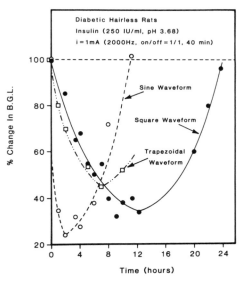

FIGURE 15. Effect of the waveform of periodic current delivered by transdermal periodic iontotherapeutic system (TPIS) on the magnitude and duration of percentage reduction in blood glucose level (BGL) from hyperglycemic state (100 percent) in diabetic hairless rat.

relationship among these parameters, and their optimum combinations for a regulated transdermal iontophoretic delivery of peptide/protein drugs.

TRANSDERMAL DELIVERY OF INSULIN IN DIABETIC RABBITS

For studying the relationship between the plasma profiles of insulin, after transdermal iontophoretic delivery, and its pharmacodynamic responses, an animal that is larger than the hairless rat, like New Zealand white rabbits, was selected as the animal model. As shown in FIGURE 4, diabetes was successfully induced in rabbits by daily intravenous injection of streptozotocin for three consecutive days. A stable hyperglycemic level was also achieved, as in hairless rats, with blood glucose level increasing from the normoglycemic level of approximately 80 mg/dL to a sustained level of greater than 200 mg/dL.

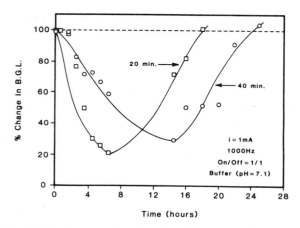

FIGURE 16. Effect of the treatment duration of periodic current delivered by transdermal periodic iontotherapeutic system (TPIS) on the magnitude and duration of percentage reduction in blood glucose level (BGL) from hyperglycemic state (100 percent) in the diabetic hairless rat.

The feasibility of using this diabetic rabbit model to study the relationship of pharmacodynamic responses, in terms of the percentage of reduction in blood glucose levels, to the plasma profiles of insulin delivered transdermally was demonstrated experimentally by assaying simultaneously blood glucose levels and plasma immunoreactive insulin concentrations. The results are compared with parenteral administrations in FIGURES 17–19.

The data in FIGURE 17 demonstrate that by transdermal iontophoretic delivery using the conventional DC mode (TIDD, at 4 mA for 80 min), the plasma profile of immunoreactive insulin, as determined by radioimmunoassay, yield the peak level within 1–2 hours. Even though the peak plasma concentration of immunoreactive insulin achieved by the transdermal iontophoretic delivery of insulin was only approximately 1/38th of that obtained by intravenous administration (0.63 mIU/ml versus 24 mIU/ml), the transdermal iontophoretic delivery was essentially as effective as the intravenous delivery in reducing the blood glucose levels in the diabetic rabbits.

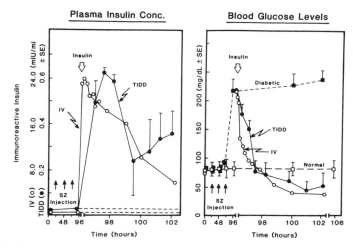

FIGURE 17. Comparative plasma profiles of immunoreactive insulin from the transdermal delivery of insulin by TPIS using direct current alone (TIDD) and intravenous administration (IV) as well as the corresponding reduction in blood glucose levels in diabetic rabbits. Equivalent efficacy was achieved by TIDD with significantly lower plasma insulin concentration, which may be attributed to the continuous delivery of short-acting insulin by TPIS.

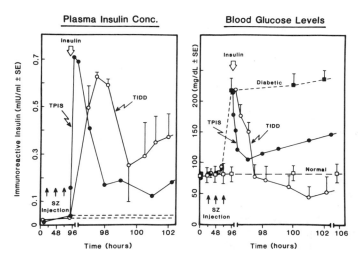

FIGURE 18. Comparative plasma profiles of immunoreactive insulin from the transdermal delivery of insulin by TPIS and the corresponding reduction in blood glucose levels in diabetic rabbits: Transdermal iontophoretic delivery of insulin using periodic waveform (TPIS) versus direct current only (TIDD). Apparently, TPIS produces a faster transdermal absorption of insulin into the systemic circulation and a better control of blood glucose levels in the diabetic animal than does TIDD.

This efficacy may be attributed to the continuous administration of short-acting insulin by transdermal iontophoretic delivery.

The *in vivo* studies conducted in diabetic hairless rats suggested that the efficiency of transdermal iontophoretic delivery of insulin can be improved by using periodic waveform (FIGURE 12). The results carried out in the diabetic rabbits further demonstrated that by delivering insulin using pulse DC (TPIS, with square waveform at current intensity of 1 mA, frequency of 2,000 Hz, and on/off ratio of 1:1 for a duration of 40 min), the peak plasma level (0.72 mIU/ml) of immunoreactive insulin was reached within 60 min (FIGURE 18). On the other hand, by using the conventional DC (TIDD) at current intensity of 4 mA for a treatment duration of 80 min, which is eight times greater than the conditions used in the pulse DC, the peak plasma level (0.63 mIU/ml) of immunoreactive insulin was achieved within 1–2 hours. Both the

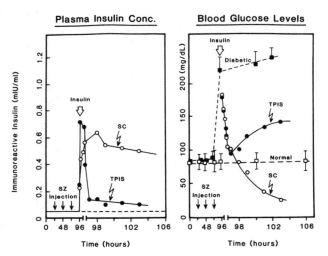

FIGURE 19. Comparative plasma profiles of immunoreactive insulin from the transdermal delivery of insulin by TPIS and from the conventional subcutaneous injection (SC) as well as the corresponding reduction in blood glucose levels in diabetic rabbits. The results indicate that TPIS produces a faster appearance of immunoreactive insulin in the plasma, but for a shorter duration, than does the subcutaneous administration of insulin. TPIS also gives better control of blood glucose level in the diabetic animal.

plasma insulin concentration profiles and the blood glucose level profiles demonstrated that TIDD is slower in onset, but achieves a longer duration of action than TPIS, which could be the result of longer treatment duration used in TIDD (80 min versus 40 min for TPIS). Further investigation is currently under way to compare TPIS versus TIDD using the same current intensity and treatment duration.

The plasma profile of immunoreactive insulin resulting from the transdermal iontophoretic delivery of insulin using pulse DC and its effect on the time course for the reduction in blood glucose levels were also compared with results achieved by the conventional subcutaneous administration of insulin in the diabetic rabbits (FIGURE 19). Results suggested that the insulin delivered transdermally by TPIS produces a rapid appearance of immunoreactive insulin in the plasma, which reaches the peak level of 0.72 mIU/ml within 10 min and lasts for only 30 min. On the other hand, the subcutaneously administered insulin produced a slow appearance of immunoreactive insulin in the plasma, which reached the peak concentration of 0.64 mIU/ml within 2 hours and lasted for longer than 8 hours. However, both routes of administration were equally effective in reducing blood glucose levels, except that TPIS maintained the reduced blood glucose level for approximately 1 hour, whereas the blood glucose level continued to drop below the normoglycemic level in response to subcutaneous insulin. The results suggest that the blood glucose level can be more easily controlled at a normoglycemic state by periodic applications of TPIS as needed or at appropriate internals than it can be by subcutaneous administration. Studies are currently being carried out to investigate this possibility.

In summary, a macromolecular drug such as insulin can be successfully delivered through the intact skin by iontophoresis. Using diabetic hairless rats and diabetic rabbits, we quantitated by radioimmunoassay the systemic bioavailability of insulin by transdermal iontophoretic delivery; the bioavailability correlated well with the pharmacodynamic responses as determined by glucose level measurement. Comparative studies with the intravenous and subcutaneous administration of insulin demonstrated that the insulin delivered transdermally by a specially designed transdermal periodic iontotherapeutic system has achieved a therapeutically effective concentration that efficiently controls blood glucose levels in diabetic animals. The results further documented that the transdermal iontophoretic delivery of insulin can be more efficiently accomplished by using the pulse rather than the conventional DC.

ACKNOWLEDGMENT

We wish to express our appreciation to Ms. M. Boslet for her able assistance in preparing this manuscript.

REFERENCES

1. HEY, D. H. & D. I. JOHN. 1973. Amino Acids, Peptides and Related Compounds. Organic Chemistry. Series 1, Vol 6, Chapt. 1, 2, 3, and 5. University Park Press. Baltimore, MD.
2. DENCE, J. B. 1980. Steriods and Peptides: Selected Chemical Aspects for Biology, Biochemistry and Medicine, Chapt. 4. Wiley. New York, NY.
3. MATTHEWS, D. M. 1975. Intestinal absorption of peptides. Physiol. Rev. **55:** 537.
4. SIDDIQUI, O. & Y. W. CHIEN. 1987. Non-parenteral administration of peptides and protein drugs. *In* CRC Critical Reviews in Therapeutic Drug Carrier Systems. 3(3): 195–208.
5. EARLE, M. P. 1971. Isr. J. Med. Sci. **8:** 899.
6. WALTON, R. P. & C. F. LACEY. 1938. J. Pharmacol Exp. Ther. **54:** 61.
7. ICHIKAWA, K., I. OHATA, M. MITOMI, S. KAWAMURA, H. MAENO & H. KAWATA. 1980. J. Pharm. Pharmacol. **32:** 314.
8. YAMASKI, Y., M. SCHICHIRI & R. KAWAMARI. 1981. Diabetes Care **4:** 454.
9. LEE, S. W. & J. J. SCIARRA. 1976. J. Pharm. Sci. **65:** 567.
10. WIGLEY, F. M., J. H. LONDONO & S. H. WOOD. 1971. Diabetes **20:** 552.
11. GORDON, G. S., A. C. MOSES, R. D. SILVER, J. S. FLIER & M. C. CAREY. 1985. Proc. Natl. Acad. Sci. USA **82:** 7419.
12. KARI, B. 1986. Diabetes **35:** 217.
13. NISHIHATA, T., S. KIM, S. MORISHITA, A. KAMADA, N. YATA & T. HIGUCHI. 1983. J. Pharm. Sci. **72:** 280.
14. ———1982. Industrial Pharmaceutical R & D Symposium on Transdermal Controlled Release Medication. Rutgers College of Pharmacy, Piscataway, New Jersey, January 14 and 15, 1982. (Proceedings published in Drug Develop. & Ind. Pharm. 9(4): 497–744 [1983].)

15. ———World Congress of Clinical Pharmacology Symposium on Transdermal Delivery of Cardiovascular Drugs, Washington, DC, August 5, 1983. (Proceedings published in Am. Heart J. **108**(1): 195–236 [1984].)

16. ———1985 International Pharmaceutical R & D Symposium on Advances in Transdermal Controlled Drug Administration for Systemic Medication, Rutgers College of Pharmacy, Piscataway, New Jersey, June 20 and 21, 1985.

17. ———Symposium on Problems and Possibilites for Transdermal Drug Delivery, The Schools of Medicine and Pharmacy, University of California, San Francisco, California, February 2–3, 1985.

18. ———1986 Neu-Ulm Conference on Transdermal Drug Delivery Systems, University of Ulm, West Germany, December 1–3, 1986.

19. CHIEN, Y. W. 1983. Logics of transdermal controlled drug administration. Drug Devel. Ind. Pharm. **9:** 497.

20. CHIEN, Y. W. 1987. Transdermal Controlled Systemic Medications. Marcel Dekker. New York, NY.

21. CHIEN, Y. W. Transdermal delivery systems—their mechanisms, origin and future in medicine. Presented at the 11th Annual A. R. Granito Memorial Lecture. December 10, 1985, Saddle Brook, New Jersey.

22. CHIEN, Y. W. 1987. Transdermal therapeutic systems. *In* Controlled Drug Delivery: Fundamentals and Application, 2nd ed. J. R. Robinson & V.H. L. Lee, Eds., Marcel Dekker. New York, NY.

23. CHIEN, Y. W. 1986. New Frontiers, in transdermal drug delivery. *In* Proceedings of the 11th Conference on Pharmaceutical Technology.: 1–56. Academy of Pharmaceutical Science and Technology of Japan. Shirakabako, Nagano Prefecture, Japan.

24. KYDONIEUS, A. F. & B. BERNER. 1987. Transdermal Delivery of Drugs. CRC Press. Boca Raton, FL.

25. CHIEN, Y. W. & C. S. LEE. 1987. Transdermal drug delivery system with enhanced skin permeability. *In* Proceedings of American Chemical Society's Symposium Recent Advances in Controlled Release Technology. P. I. Lee, Ed. American Chemical Society. Washington, DC.

26. PANNATIER, P. J., B. TESTA & J. C. ETTER. 1978. The skin as a drug-metabolizing organ. Drug Metab. Rev. **8:** 319.

27. CHIEN, Y. W. 1984. Navel absorption: Transdermal bioavailability of testosterone. J. Pharm. Sci. **73:** 283.

28. CHIEN, Y. W. 1984. Long-term controlled navel administration of testosterone. J. Pharm. Sci. **73:** 1064.

29. KESHARY, P. R. & Y. W. CHIEN. 1984. Mechanisms of transdermal controlled nitroglycerin administration (II): Assessment of rate-controlling step. Drug Devel. Ind. Pharm. **10:** 1663–1699.

30. KESHARY, P. R., Y. C. HUANG & Y. W. CHIEN. 1985. Mechanisms of transdermal controlled nitroglycerin administration (III): Control of skin permeation and optimization. Drug Devel. Ind. Pharm. **11:** 1213–1253.

31. CHIEN, Y. W. & K. H. VALIA. 1984. Development of a dynamic skin permeation system for long-term permeation studies. Drug Devel. Ind. Pharm. **10:** 575–599.

32. VALIA, K. H., Y. W. CHIEN & E. C. SHINAL. 1984. Long-term skin permeation kinetics of estradiol (I): Effect of drug solubilizer—polyethylene glycol 400. Drug Devel. Ind. Pharm. **10:** 951–981.

33. VALIA, K. H. & Y. W. CHIEN. 1984. Long-term skin permeation kinetics of estradiol (II): Kinetics of skin uptake, binding and metabolism. Drug Devel. Ind. Pharm. **10:** 991–1015.

34. VALIA, K. H., K. TOJO & Y. W. CHIEN. 1985. Long-term skin permeation kinetics of estradiol (III): Kinetic analyses of the simultaneous skin permeation and bioconversion of estradiol esters. Drug Devel. Ind. Pharm. **11:** 1133–1173.

35. CHIEN, Y. W., K. H. VALIA & U. B. DOSHI. 1985. Long-term skin permeation kinetics of estradiol (V): Development and evaluation of transdermal bioactivated hormone delivery system. Drug Devel. Ind. Pharm. **11:** 1195–1212.

36. HARRIS, R. 1967. Iontophoresis. *In* Therapeutic Electricity and Ultraviolet Radiation, 2nd edit. Chapt. 4. S. Licht, Ed. John Wiley. New York, NY.

37. COMEAU, M., R. BRUMMETT & J. VERNON. 1983. Arch. Otolaryngol. **98:** 114.
38. ECHOLS, D. F., C. H. NORRIS & H. G. TALB. 1975. Arch. Otolaryngol. **101:** 418.
39. SIDDIQUI, O., M. S. ROBERTS & A. E. POLACK. 1985. J. Pharm. Pharmacol. **37:** 732.
40. VON SALLMAN, L. 1942. Am. J. Ophthal. **25:** 1292.
41. BERTOLUCCI, L. E. 1982. J. Orthopaed. Sport Phys. Ther. **4:** 103.
42. GANGAROSA, L. P., N. H. PARK & J. M. HILL. 1977. Proc. Soc. Exp. Biol. Med. **154:** 439.
43. MARCHAND, J. E. & N. HAGINO. 1982. Exp. Neurol. **78:** 790.
44. OKABE, K., H. YAMAGUCHI & Y. KAWAI. 1986. J. Controlled Rel. **4:** 79.
45. HILL, J. M., L. P. GANGAROSA & N. H. PARK. 1977. Ann. N. Y. Acad. Sci. **248:** 604.
46. JUNG, G., E. KATZ, H. SCHMITT, K.-P. VOGES, G. MENESTRINA & G. BOHEIM. 1983. Conformational requirements for the potential dependent pore formation of the peptide antibiotics alamethicin, suzukacillin and trichotoxin. *In* Physical Chemistry of Transmembrane Ion Motion. G. Spach, Ed. Elsevier. New York, NY.
47. BURNETTE, R. R. & D. MARRERO. 1986. J. Pharm. Sci. **75:** 738.
48. STEPHEN, R. L., T. J. PETELENZ & S. C. JACOBSEN. 1984. Biomed. Biochim. Acta **43:** 553.
49. OSOL, A. 1980. Remington's Pharmaceutical Sciences, Chapter 51. Mack. Easton, PA.
50. KLOSTERMEYER, H. and R. E. HUMBEL. 1966. Angew. Chem. (Internat. Ed.) **5:** 807.
51. SIDDIQUI, O., Y. SUN, J. C. LIU & Y. W. CHIEN. 1987. Facilitated transdermal transport of insulin. J. Pharm. Sci. **76:** 341–345.
52. CHIEN, Y. W. 1982. Novel Drug Delivery Systems, Chapt. 5. Marcel Dekker. New York, NY.
53. YAMATOTO, T. & Y. YAMAMOTO. 1976. Med. Biol. Eng. Comp. **14:** 151.
54. ZUKAS, J. A., T. NICHOLAS, H. F SWIFT, L. B. GRESZCZUK & D. R. CURRAN. 1982. Impact Dynamics. John Wiley. New York, NY.
55. LIU, J. C., Y. SUN, O. SIDDIQUI & Y. W. CHIEN. 1987. Blood glucose control in diabetic rats by transdermal iontophoretic delivery of insulin. Int. J. Pharm. Submitted for publication.

Analytical Methodology to Support the Pharmaceutical Development of Peptides and Proteins

LARRY A. STERNSON

Smith Kline & French Laboratories
Philadelphia, Pennsylvania 19101

Peptides represent a chemical class of compounds whose development as therapeutic agents has been made possible by advances in chemical synthesis and recombinant technology. The physical and chemical fragility of polypeptide-like drugs and the ambiguity of the relationship between their "purity" and biological activity place severe demands on methodology suitable for their analysis from a variety of complex matrices, including fermentation broths, pharmaceutical formulations, and biological fluids. The quality and power of these analytical methods will, in large part, define the limitations of our ability to characterize, evaluate, and understand approaches for their delivery.

The development of analytical methodology to support drug development activities is particularly challenging. Peptides and proteins of therapeutic interest are generally potent molecules requiring methods that are very sensitive (capable of detecting sub-ng/ml quantities of analytes). Additionally, the striking similarity in structure between analyte, degradation products, impurities and matrix components places severe demands for selectivity on analytical methodology. Analysis is further complicated by the inherent instability of peptides. The most prevalent degradation pathway involves hydrolysis of amide linkages, but oxidation, racemization, and other modifications of amino acid side chains are also frequently encountered. Larger oligomers are subject to unfolding and other conformational perturbations in addition to chemical degradation. Aggregation or adsorption of sample material onto container surfaces can also result in an apparent loss of analyte. While adherence to container surfaces does not present a significant problem in analyzing microgram or greater amounts of material, the loss from adsorption can become significant in samples containing trace levels of such analytes. Attempts to circumvent surface adsorption by chemically coating glassware, using "nonadsorptive" containers or by the addition of competing adsorptive amines to the test solution have been less than satisfactory.

The chemical complexity of peptides/proteins places overwhelming demands on an analytical method that is expected to assess the structural integrity (or "purity") of the entire analyte and be correlatable with biological activity. Thus, for many applications, panels of methods must be employed to respond to different aspects or segments of the structure of the oligomeric analyte. Four general categories of methods have been developed for peptide/protein analysis: bioassays, binding (immunologic or receptor) assays, enzyme methods and physical chemical approaches. This article will touch on the first three types of methods, but will focus on advances in procedures having a physicochemical basis. Attention to physicochemical methods is prompted by the uncertainty inherent in the other types of analytical procedures, i.e., undetected, nonanticipated impurities and degradates in samples may affect the analytical response, resulting in significant inaccuracies in determination of analyte concentration.

BIOASSAYS

Bioassays measure biological response and therefore may provide the truest indication of drug potency. Since biological inactivation of polypeptides is often subtle and may not be readily detected by chemical/instrumental methods of analysis, FDA-approved peptidergic drugs uniformly use animal bioassays to assess potency. Their widespread use is not by choice, but is precipitated by inadequacies in current technology. There are a number of significant drawbacks to the routine use of bioassays. In general, the procedures are cumbersome, costly, time-consuming and labor-intensive. Variability within laboratory animals, coupled with interferences from other substances in the test samples often give rise to poor assay reproducibilities (>20%) and inaccuracies. The magnitude of some of these problems can be reduced by using in vitro or cytochemical bioassays, which are carried out with isolated tissues or cultured cells rather than with whole animals. However, this simplification may also compromise the value of the assay, since such procedures measure a secondary or biochemical phenomenon, rather than biological function. Bioassays are impractical for many drug development tasks in which large numbers of experimental variables are to be evaluated and optimized; however, because of the inadequacies of current technology, they remain a necessary component in analyzing peptides and proteins.

BINDING ASSAYS

The association of an antibody or a cellular receptor with its complementary drug substrate can be exploited to determine very low concentrations of the drug in a variety of complex matrices.

Immunochemical techniques are of particular value in monitoring antigens/haptens present in submicromolar concentrations in biological fluids. The specificity of immunoassays is determined by the cross reactivity of the antibody component, i.e., affinity of the analyte for the antibody relative to other species present in the sample. Sensitivity is also dependent on the antigen-antibody binding constant and on the instrumental sensitivity of the "reporter" group. Four types of reporter groups have been used: radiolabels, fluorescent moieties, enzyme conjugates, and spin labels. Recently, visible immunodiagnostic assays have been developed[1] in which an antibody-coated dipstick is placed in a sample and then incubated with latex microspheres covalently linked to the antibody. When these submicron-sized particles attach to the dipstick they form a "sandwich," and an optical phenomenon called Mie scattering occurs, causing the stick to change color [color intensity can be related to antigen concentration]. Immunoassays are usually competitive, but direct (immunoradiometric) methods have also been described. The methods can be heterogeneous (requiring separation of bound from free labeled antigen or homogeneous (eliminating need for separating free from bound fractions).

Applicability of immunochemical techniques for monitoring larger molecules, such as peptides and proteins, is somewhat compromised by the antibody's ability to only recognize a relatively small portion of a macromolecular antigen. Thus, assays involving a single antibody may not be purity-indicating. Further limitations to their general usage in peptide analysis include specificity uncertainties, antibody inhomogeneity, and their insensitivity to conformational perturbations.

The value of and confidence in immunoassays increase when (a) they are used in combination with other analytical techniques that provide added assurance of specificity (e.g., chromatography); (b) panels of antibodies are employed that recognize the entire structure of the analyte [and antibodies are raised that recognize conformationally dependent epitopes that correlate with biological activity]; or (c) monoclonal antibodies are employed as reagents. Hybridoma technology now offers the opportunity for obtaining monoclonal antibodies that adhere to the same rigorous standards of purity and homogeneity that have been established for more traditional analytical reagents. Their inherent selectivity and sensitivity make immunoassays valuable approaches to peptide quantification, despite their limitations.

Radioreceptor assay (RRA) determines analyte concentration on the basis of its binding with receptors on cell membranes or within their interior. A competitive radioassay technique is employed, applying the same principle upon which radioimmunoassays (RIA) are based. RRAs offer the advantage of generally correlating very well with *in vitro* bioassays although correlations with *in vivo* bioassays have been poorer. This is to be expected since antibody binding affinity need not coincide with biological response, while *in vitro* bioassay results are strongly influenced by the affinity of the analyte for its receptor. Correlations between RRAs and *in vivo* bioassays are less favorable because of the influence of distribution and disposition phenomena on biological response. RRAs may thus have important application in clinical analysis of drugs in cases where determination by RIA is at variance with clinical observations. Limitations of radioreceptor assays include: perturbation in receptor binding affinity of analyte upon radiolabeling, heterogeneity and variablity within and among cell receptor preparations, and alteration in binding affinity caused by other components in the test mixture.

ENZYME ASSAYS

Drug molecules that are enzymes or that influence enzyme activity can be quantitated by methodology based on kinetic measurement of enzyme activity. Enzyme assays are of inherently high specificity, are suitable for automation, and can often be made very sensitive. Sensitivity, limited only by background signal, is provided by monitoring a cofactor or product of the enzymatic reaction produced under kinetic control. The generation of many product molecules per molecule of reactant amplifies the analytical signal, providing the basis for achieving high sensitivity. This amplification concept has been further extended[2] by the introduction of "enzyme cycling" assays. Such procedures have claimed amplification factors of 400,000,000 and the ability to measure 10^{-18} moles of certain cellular metabolites. The possibility of creating geometric amplification cycles (which would further increase the amplification magnitude) has been proposed,[3] but has not been fully developed.

The most serious concern regarding enzyme assays lies with the possible influence on enzyme activity exerted by other species in the sample. Even slight alterations in enzyme kinetics produced by impurities, degradates, or matrix components could be greatly magnified by the amplification factor and cause large inaccuracies in the analysis. Furthermore, if a macromolecular drug degrades at a site remote from its catalytic or binding sites, enzyme assays may be unable to sense the structural change. Thus, enzyme assays are also plagued with uncertainties as to the effect of sample components on accuracy of analyses, as well as by the size and complexity of the analyte.

PHYSICOCHEMICAL/INSTRUMENTATION-BASED ASSAYS

Traditional "small" drug molecules have routinely been analyzed by physicochemical methods. Such methods can conveniently be divided into four stages: (1) gross

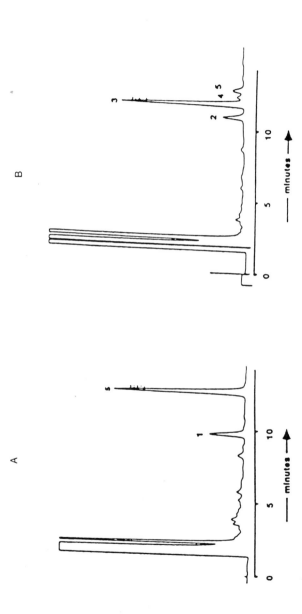

FIGURE 1. Reaction mixture of LDH (231–242) in the presence of protein carboxymethyl-transferase after (**A**) 2 hr and (**B**) 24 hr incubation. Separations were carried out on a 4.6 mm × 100 mm Aquapore RP-300 column used with a 4.6 mm × 30 mm guard cartridge. *Eluent*: **A**,0.1% TFA; **B**, 90% ACN in 0.1% TFA (12 to 21 percent B in 14 min). *Flow rate*: 2 ml/min; *Detector*: UV, 254 mm. *Peaks*: 1, L-iso ASP; 2, L-imide + L-iso-ASP methyl ester; 3, L-ASP; 4, D-iso-ASP; 5, D-ASP.

separation of analytes from the matrix; (2) high-efficiency separation of compounds of interest from their degradation products and from endogenous components; (3) detection; and (4) signal-processing and data manipulation. The size, complexity, and fragility of peptides and proteins has severely limited the application of this classical approach to peptides and proteins. Physicochemical methods are now employed to determine (*a*) total protein concentration, (*b*) amino acid composition and sequence, and (*c*) conformation of single component samples. These methods are useful for analysis from simple, well-defined systems, or in situations where specificity is not demanded. However, to support drug delivery efforts, methods must be capable of monitoring these analytes in complex matrices, e.g., pharmaceutical formulations, biological fluids. In many instances, it is not only the drug that must be monitored, but also its degradates or "metabolites." The opportunity for simultaneously and selectively determining the concentration of drug and its degradates is not available through bioassay, immunoassay, or enzyme assay; combination of physicochemical and instrumental techniques, however, can potentially be employed to obtain such information. For such applications, the availability of powerful separation techniques capable of resolving proteinaceous components within mixtures is necessary.

Separation of peptides and proteins has been achieved by electrophoretic and a variety of chromatographic techniques, including paper chromatography, thin-layer (TLC), gas-liquid (GLC), and column liquid chromatography. The first two chromatographic techniques, although valuable for qualitative identification, are of limited value in quantitative trace analysis of peptides. GLC can only be used to analyze peptides containing a few residues because of their thermal lability and the nonvolatility of the larger oligomers. Over the past decade, high-performance liquid chromatography (HPLC) has emerged as a powerful and versatile technique for separating peptidergic solutes. The key advantages of HPLC are speed, simplicity, and intact recovery of eluted components to allow low-level detection; moreover, unlike most other peptide separation methods, HPLC procedures can be automated. The successful application of HPLC to peptide analysis has been due in large part to significant technical improvements leading to the availability of inert, pressure-resistant stationary phases. Reversed-phase (and the companion technique, hydrophobic interaction HPLC), ion-exchange, and size-exclusion modes of separation have all been successfully applied to peptide/protein separations. The varied uses of HPLC for peptide analysis have been the subject of numerous articles; the interested reader is referred to recent reviews[4,5] for an introduction to the theoretical and practical considerations involved.

Of the liquid chromatographic approaches, reversed-phase HPLC (RPLC) and hydrophobic interaction chromatography offer particularly powerful resolving capabilities for polypeptides. The major determinant of retention behavior of small peptides (i.e., those containing 20 or fewer residues) in these chromatographic modes is the hydrophobicity of the component amino acids.[6] Additionally, there are silanophilic (electrostatic) and size-exclusion contributions to the retention mechanism. Prediction of retention becomes more complicated for peptides larger than 20 residues due to the existence of long-range intramolecular interactions between various amino acids brought about by folding. While very polar peptides can be eluted with a purely aqueous solvent system, in most cases an organic modifier is added to the mobile phase. Column selectivity can be further enhanced by addition of an ion-pairing agent to the mobile phase. An example of the selectivity achievable with RPLC[7] is the recent separation of an LDH-related peptide from the corresponding isoaspartate peptide, its D-isoAsp peptide diasteriomer, and its methylated and cyclic imide analogs. Baseline resolution (FIG. 1) allowed the authors[7] to study the kinetics of protein carboxymethyltransferase reactions and competing racemization side reactions, monitoring substrate disappearance and appearance of all pertinent reaction products in a single chromato-graphic system, with total analysis time of <20 min.

Ion-exchange and size-exclusion chromatography[8] have also been applied to peptide/protein analysis. However, their usage has been hindered by a lack of stationary phases with suitable stability, loading capability and/or chromatographic efficiency (due to slow rates on-column mass exchange). In some instances, ion-exchange HPLC and RPLC have been shown to be complementary,[9] i.e., peptides that cannot be well resolved by one method may be resolved by the other.

Peptide and protein separations have also been successfully accomplished by electrophoretic methods. The major limitations of such methods in support of drug development activities include their unsuitability for automation, difficulties in sample recovery, limited resolution capabilities, and poor sensitivity and imprecision inherent in making quantitative measurements from electrophoretic gels or plates. Resolution capabilities approaching that achieved with modern HPLC have been realized using an adaptation of conventional zone electrophoresis—capillary zone electrophoresis.[10] Although this technique offers significantly greater resolution capability, it shares the other limitations of traditional zone electrophoresis. An indication of the high separation efficiency that can be achieved with capillary zone electrophoresis is given in FIGURE 2. Other modes of electrophoresis, e.g., isotachophoresis[11] and isoelectric focusing[12] have also been applied to peptide/protein analysis. Thus, a variety of separation techniques have been developed that are capable of separating peptidergic drugs from complex matrices, although research to develop more powerful techniques for the resolution of such solutes is needed.

Of additional concern in the development of analytical methodology suitable for supporting drug delivery activities is achieving adequate sensitivity. For drugs such as peptides and proteins, which are generally potent and short-lived in the body, exquisitely low levels of detection (pg/ml) must be achieved. Several approaches have been developed to achieve the necessary sensitivity. Instrumental techniques are preferred, but the appropriate detection devices must usually be interfaced with a module that separates the components in the sample to be analyzed. Techniques such as absorption and emission spectrophotometry, amperometry, radioactive monitoring, and mass spectrometry provide the potential for low-level detectability, but only for a limited population of molecules that incorporate specific structural features that yield maximal response from such transducers. Peptides and proteins normally do not possess the structural attributes allowing their direct detection by these techniques at submicromolar levels. Thus, to detect and quantitate trace levels of peptides, an indirect approach is needed, where something other than the actual analyte is detected and related to drug concentration after resolution of sample components. Examples of this approach include (1) chemical derivatization of analyte (either prior to or after the high-resolution separation step) and (2) immunochemical or enzyme surveillance of chromatographically or electrophoretically developed bands. Immunochemical tech-niques have been reviewed earlier and will not be discussed again here.

Chemical derivatization approaches have been used to enhance detectability with limited success. These approaches have primarily focused on conversion of peptides to fluorescent derivatives during the analysis sequence. Current fluorescence detector technology, using either conventional or laser sources, offers the potential for detection at subpicogram levels, for compounds that strongly absorb ultraviolet light and emit radiation efficiently. Ideally, the derivatization reagent itself should not fluoresce (at least in the region in which the derivative emits light) so that background signals are minimized, thereby lowering potential detection limits. Such "fluorogenic" reagents have been developed for derivatization of peptides and proteins. The most common of these can be applied either pre- or post-column and include fluorescamine,[13] dansyl chloride,[14] 7-fluoro-4-nitro-2,1,3-benzoxadiole[15] (NBDF), and o-phthalaldehyde[16] (OPA).

Of these reagents, OPA offers advantages not available with the others: (a) reaction is instantaneous; (b) derivatization can be carried out in totally aqueous environments; (c) reaction byproducts are not fluorescent; (d) reagents are inexpensive; and (e) detection can be achieved either spectrofluorimetrically or amperometri-

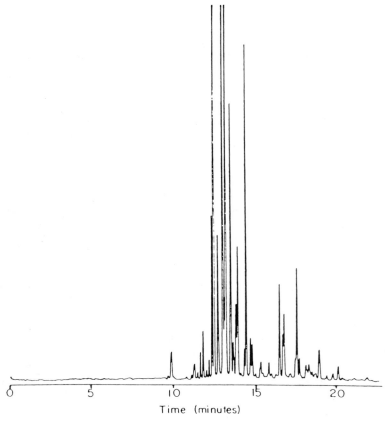

Time (minutes)

FIGURE 2. Separation of fluorescamine-labeled peptides obtained from a tryptic digest of reduced and carboxymethylated egg white lysozyme by capillary zone electrophoresis.[23]

cally (i.e., electrochemical detection[17]). However, there are some distinct limitations to its use: (1) a thiol is required as a coreactant; its strong objectionable odor and toxicity require the reaction to be carried out in a fume hood (such cabinets are often not available in clinical laboratories); and (2) the fluorescent product is chemically unstable,[18] requiring rapid analysis after the derivative is formed. For derivatization of peptides, OPA reacts to form products that lack intense fluorescence, and accordingly this reagent has only been used successfully for derivatizing lysine-containing peptides (and single amino acids), where reaction to form fluorescent products occurs at the ε-amino functionality. Recently, after elucidation of the mechanism of the OPA reaction,[19] Sternson and co-workers[20] have designed, synthesized, and evaluated several analogs of OPA that produce more stable products (than those produced with OPA) and react with a broader spectrum of peptides (i.e., not only with Lys residues).

The first of these analogs, o-acetylbenzaldehyde, **1b**, confers a 150 percent improvement in the stability of the resulting fluorescent isoindole derivative, **2b** (in comparison with the OPA derivative, **2a**) without altering the reactivity profile of the reagent or the fluorescent intensity of the product.[20] Blocking the 1-position of the isoindole with an alkyl group (e.g., methyl) significantly reduced the proclivity for rapid autoxidation of the isoindole (which is initiated by hydrogen abstraction at C-1 in the OPA analog) to a series of nonfluorescent heterocyclic products.[21] Although

| **1a** | R = H | **2a** | R = H |
| **1b** | R = CH$_3$ | **2b** | R = CH$_3$ |

3   4

stability was enhanced, this analog (and other o-alkyl and -aryl keto benzaldehydes) fails to form fluorescent products with peptides.

To further improve the sensitivity achievable by derivatization with OPA, the corresponding naphthalene derivative, naphthalene 2-3-dicarboxaldehyde (NDA), **3**, was prepared.[22] This reagent failed to produce stable fluorescent products in the presence of thiols, but when cyanide was substituted as nucleophile, fluorescent benzisoindoles, **4**, were formed from reaction with amino acids that showed no degradation over a 24-hr period. This improvement in fluorophore stability over that achievable with OPA (half-life ≈ 1 hr) greatly increases the value and flexibility of aromatic dialdehydes as analytical reagents. As predicted, the increase in planar surface area and extended electronic conjugation found in **4** (over that found in **2** and related bicyclic products) and the increase in quantum efficiency from 0.11 (for **2**) to

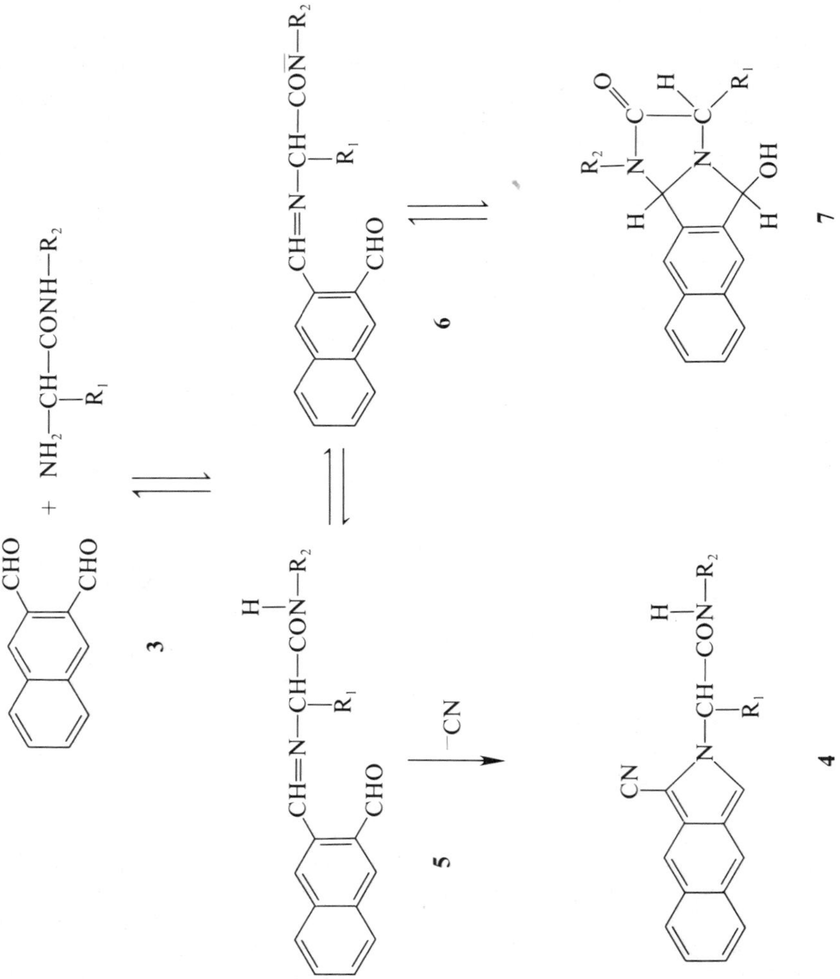

CHO
CHO
3
+ NH2—CH—CONH—R2
R1
CH=N—CH—CON—R2
H
R1
CHO
5
−CN
CN
N—CH—CON—R2
H
R1
4
CH=N—CH—CON—R2
R1
CHO
6
R2
N
C
O
H
C
R1
N
H
H
OH
7

0.71 (for **4**) provides the basis for the significant improvement in sensitivity that is realized with NDA.

However, at the pH usually chosen for the OPA reaction (pH 9–10), peptides failed to generate fluorescent products with NDA/cyanide. A pH-rate profile of reaction of NDA/cyanide with alanine, dialanine, and trialanine (FIG. 3a) reveals that the optimal pH for reaction with peptides is 7.0 (optimal pH is 9 for amino acids) and that this pH correlates with maximal chemical yield of the respective benzisoindole derivative (FIG. 3b). Further investigation[24] of the reaction suggested that the inability to form fluorescent products with peptides was due to a side reaction, which could be minimized by carrying out the reaction at reduced pH (7.0) and by increasing cyanide concentration. Under these conditions, after initial formation of Schiff base, **5**, reaction with cyanide and subsequent cyclization yields the fluorescent isoindole, **4**. At pH 9 or 10, ionization of the peptide amide nitrogen produces a nucleophilic species, **6**, which participates in a preferential intramolecular cyclization to yield a nonfluorescent imidazol-4-one derivative, **7**. Thus, by optimizing pH (to suppress ionization of the amide nitrogen) and maintaining a high cyanide concentration (to trap the Schiff

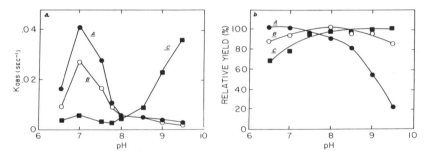

FIGURE 3. (a) pH rate profile and (b) pH chemical yield plots on the cyano benzimidazole derivatives of trialanine (A), dialanine (B) and alanine (C). For each profile, derivatization was carried out with DA (2×10^{-6} M), sodium cyanide (1×10^{-3} M), and the amine (1×10^{-3} M).

base, eliminating its ability to form imidazolone), NDA/cyanide is an effective fluorogenic derivatizing reagent for peptides.

This reagent has now been successfully applied[24] to the analysis of leu-enkephalin from plasma. Plasma samples were deproteinized with perchloric acid and then subjected to solid-phase extraction on a octylsilane (C_8)-bonded silica gel cartridge. The eluted enkephalins were derivatized with NDA/cyanide and the reaction mixture was subjected to RPLC on an octadecylsilane (C_{18}) column. Monitoring of the column effluent by conventional fluorimetry afforded a detection limit of 50 pmol/ml of plasma. Significant improvements in the detection limits may be achieved by injecting a larger fraction of the derivatized solution on-column and/or by extracting a larger volume of plasma. By utilizing a laser source tuned to the absorption maximum of the benzisoindole, a further increase in sensitivity of approximately two orders of magnitude is anticipated. A chromatogram of a plasma sample containing 250 pmol of leu-enkephalin (with leu-enkephalinamide added as an internal standard) is shown in FIGURE 4. Analysis time is short (8 min) and amenable to automation, and the chromatographic system is sufficiently efficient to allow concurrent monitoring of leu-enkephalin degradates.

The OPA-NDA example illustrates the improvements in analytical capabilities that can be made by rational design of derivatizing reagents utilizing established chemical principles and by taking advantage of established detector technology. However, further improvements in derivatization technology are needed to provide the selectivity and sensitivity that will be required to evaluate peptide drugs. Means of extending derivatization technology to larger peptides and proteins are also necessary.

CONCLUSION

The design and evaluation of improved drug delivery strategies is critical to the development of peptides and proteins as drugs. Analytical methodology which offers

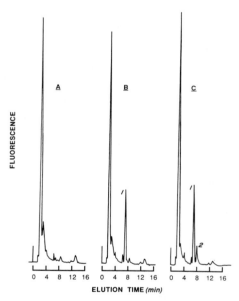

FIGURE 4. Chromatograms of (*A*) a plasma blank and (*B, C*) spiked plasma samples with leu-enkephalinamide (peak 1, 1 nmol/ml) and leu-enkephalin (peak 2, 0.25 nmol/ml).

reliability, selectivity, and sensitivity in monitoring "drug" and drug degradates is essential to meeting this objective. At present, analytical technology is inadequate to meet anticipated needs, in large part because of the size, complexity, and fragility of polypeptide drugs. These complexities will likely require that future analytical strategies include components of each of the types of methods described in this article, as well as others that are not enumerated or are yet to be discovered. It is unlikely that one analytical test will be sufficient to characterize the integrity of a peptide present in a complex matrix. Rather, it is likely that batteries of tests will be needed to account for all aspects of the structural integrity of peptide analytes that contribute to their biological activity.

REFERENCES

1. KLAUSNER, A. 1987. Biotechnology **5:** 8–10.
2. LOWRY, O. H. & J. V. PASSONNEAU. 1972. A Flexible System of Enzymatic Analysis. Academic Press. New York, NY.
3. STERNSON, L. A. & T. MALEFYT. 1985. Analytical aspects of drug delivery: An important and often overlooked problem. *In* Directed Drug Delivery. R. T. Borchardt, A. J. Repta & V. J. Stella, Eds.: 291–307. Humana Press. Clifton, NJ.
4. KRUMMEN, K. 1980. J. Liq. Chromatogr. **3:** 1243–1254.
5. HEARN, M. T. W. 1983. HPLC of peptides. *In* HPLC: Advances & Perspectives, Vol. 3 (C. Horvath, Ed.: 88–155. Academic Press. New York, NY.
6. MEEK, J. L. & Z. L. ROSETTI. 1981. J. Chromatogr. **211:** 15–28.
7. JOHNSON, B. A. , E. D. MURRAY, JR., S. CLARKE, D. B. GLASS & D. W. ASWAD. J. Biol. Chem. (In press.)
8. REGNIER, F. E. 1983. Science **222:** 245–252.
9. DIZDAROGLO, M. 1985. J. Chromatogr. **334:** 49–69.
10. JORGENSON, J. W. & K. D. LUKACS, 1983. Science **222:** 266–272.
11. EVARAERTS, F. M. & F. E. P. MIKKERS. 1980. Isotachophoresis: A general introduction. *In* Biochemical and Biological Applications of Isotachophoresis. C. Schots, Ed. Elsevier. Amsterdam.
12. RIGHETTI, P., E. GIANAZZA & A. B. BOSISIO. 1979. Biochemical and clinical applications of isoelectric focusing. *In* Recent Developments in Chromatography and Electrophoresis. A. Frigerio & L. Renoz, Eds. Elsevier. Amsterdam.
13. RUBENSTEIN, M., S. CHEN-KIANG, S. STEIN & S. UDENFRIEND. 1979. Anal. Biochem. **95:** 117–121.
14. DEJONG, C., G. J. HUGHES, E. VAN WIERINGEN & K. J. WILSON. 1982. J. Chromatogr. **241:** 345–359.
15. WATANABE, Y. & K. IMAI. 1981. Anal. Biochem. **116:** 471–472.
16. BENSON, J. R. & P. E. HARE. 1975. Proc. Natl. Acad. Sci. USA **72:** 619–622.
17. ALLISON, L. A., G. S. MAYER & R. E. SHOUP. 1984. Anal. Chem. **56:** 1089–1096.
18. BONNETT, R. & S. A. NORTH. 1981. Adv. Heterocycl. Chem. **29:** 395–397.
19. STERNSON, L. A., J. F. STOUBAUGH & A. J. REPTA. 1985. Anal. Biochem. **144:** 233–246.
20. WONG, O. S., L. A. STERNSON & R. L. SCHOWEN. 1985. J. Am. Chem. Soc. **107:** 6421–6422.
21. STOBAUGH, J. F., A. J. REPTA, & L. A. STERNSON. 1984. J. Org. Chem. **49:** 4306–4308.
22. DEMONTIGNY, P., J. F. STOBAUGH & L. A. STERNSON. 1987. Anal. Chem. **59:** 1096–1101.
23. JORGENSON, J. W. & K. D. LUKACS. 1981. J. High Resol. Chromatogr. Comm. **4:** 230–231.
24. STOBAUGH, J. F., P. DEMONTIGNY & L. A. STERNSON. Manuscript in preparation.

Targeting of Liposomes to Tumor Cells
in Vivo[a]

D. PAPAHADJOPOULOS[b,c] AND A. GABIZON[b]

[b]Cancer Research Institute and
[c]Department of Pharmacology
University of California, San Francisco
San Francisco, California 94143

This presentation marks the tenth year since the New York Academy of Sciences organized the first conference on liposomes.[1] Since then, several important developments have taken place. The most significant is the advent of clinical trials utilizing liposomes as drug carriers, and that these trials have already produced encouraging results.[2,3] These and other trials that have started recently have relied on earlier data obtained with animals[4–7] which indicated two important characteristics of liposomes: one, that they concentrate drugs in cells of the reticuloendothelial system (RES) of liver and spleen; and two, that they reduce drug uptake in heart, kidney, and the gastrointestinal tract. The first observation has resulted in the use of encapsulated antiparasitic drugs to fight infections where the microorganisms reside within the RES cells[8–11] as well as in the encapsulation of macrophage-activating factors which may be useful for both antitumor and antiviral effects.[12–14] The second observation has led to the use of liposome-associated doxorubicin, an antitumor agent, which substantially reduced cardiotoxicity[15–18]; and of liposome-associated amphotericin B, an antifungal agent, which yielded an impressive reduction in renal and other toxicities.[19–21]

The studies conducted so far indicate that liposomes can affect the therapeutic index either by localizing a particular drug within the RES or by avoiding certain tissues which are normally sensitive to the drug. Specific targeting of liposomes to particular tissues outside the RES would be of obvious advantage in numerous pathologic situations such as cancer, where existing drugs lack pharmacologic specificity.[6] There have been some reports of enhanced uptake of liposomes by cells other than those of the RES on the basis of either alterations of the liposome size[23–25] or the addition of specific carbohydrate groups on the liposome surface.[26–29] However, some of these observations have been of limited therapeutic value,[30] and in many cases they have relied on prior blockade of the RES by other liposomes.[31,32]

Targeting of liposomes to a variety of tissues would therefore require the ability to avoid uptake by cells of the RES. Obviously, it would also be required that the liposomes have accessibility to the target cells[33] in the various tissues. Considering the relative permeability of the vascular endothelium in various tissues it appears that a minimal-size liposome with a diameter of 300–1000 Å may have a reasonable chance to extravasate through sinusoidal or fenestrated endothelia as in liver and spleen, or in tissues with impaired endothelia such as in some primary and metastatic tumors and areas of inflammation or injury.[34,35] By contrast, liposomes will be unlikely to extravasate in tissues with "tight" continuous endothelia, unless they are able to transverse the endothelial layer by the transcellular vesicular transport. The evidence

[a]This investigation was supported by Grant CA 35340 from the National Cancer Institute.

64

so far indicates that there is indeed very little extravasation in such tissues.[33] In such situations targeting could still be possible if liposomes were injected within a specific anatomic compartment such as the subarachnoidal space,[36] or the peritoneal cavity.[37]

The clearance rate of nontargeted liposomes and their uptake by the RES and various other tissues have been studied extensively.[38–42] The accumulated experience can be summarized as follows: Blood half-lives ($T_{1/2}$) can vary widely from a few minutes to many hours (up to 20 hr) depending on the dosage, particle diameter, surface charge, and bilayer fluidity. The longest $T_{1/2}$ values have been obtained with the smallest (200–300-Å diameter) liposomes composed of solid-phase neutral lipids.[38,42] The dosage effect seems to be an important variable, probably relating to the saturation of the RES.[31] Some of the reported effects on size could be due to dosage effects if one considers that, on an equal lipid weight basis, small unilamellar vesicles (SUV) would have a much larger total surface area and particle numbers compared with those of large multilamellar vesicles (MLV)[43] and could therefore be removed with different $T_{1/2}$ on the basis of different saturation levels.

The development of two key methodologies was an important element of our strategy for achieving targeting of liposomes to various cells within the vasculature. The first one was the extrusion method, which made it possible to prepare liposomes of varying particle size and reasonably homogeneous size distribution.[44–46] The second one relates to various conjugation methods[47–52] allowing for the efficient covalent attachment of proteins such as antibodies on the liposome surface. *In vitro* investigations of the cellular uptake of liposomes prepared by such methods delineated the following important parameters: (1) Liposomes are taken into cells via "coated pit" endocytosis, and their contents accumulate in a low-pH intracellular compartment.[53] (2) There is a "size effect," which allows smaller liposomes to enter into the cellular interior, while larger liposomes remain attached to the external surface.[53–55] (3) The presence of covalently attached IgG enhances liposome uptake by target cells that express the appropriate antigen[48,51] and can result in much higher cytotoxicity for an encapsulated drug[56,57] if the uptake is accompanied by internalization.[58,59] (4) Encapsulation of weakly acidic molecules can result in higher cytoplasmic release, when the pK of the molecule is such that acidification within the endocytic or lysosomal compartment enhances their membrane permeability.[60,61] This can produce diffuse cytoplasmic fluorescence with carboxyfluorescein[53] and enhanced cytotoxicity with γ-aspartate methotrexate.[60,61] (5) Use of pH-sensitive liposomes, which fuse and release their contents when the pH is reduced from 7.4 to 6.0,[62,63,64] enhances cytoplasmic delivery of molecules normally accumulating within the lysosomal vacuoles.[65,66]

In our first studies attempting to target liposomes to cells of the lymphoid tissue, we used SUV composed of distearoyl phosphatidylcholine (DSPC) and cholesterol, since these were reported to have the longest $T_{1/2}$ after intravenous injection in mice.[38] However, the conjugation of IgG was found to have a profound shortening effect on the $T_{1/2}$, resulting in a 30-fold reduction of the liposome blood pool.[74] The magnitude of this effect appears to correlate with the ratio of protein to phospholipid, and several mechanisms may be responsible for this. The liposomes may be recognized to some extent by the Fc receptor of the liver Kupffer cells, since the conjugation method employed results in random positioning of the conjugated IgG molecule and therefore may allow interaction with Fc receptors. This has been shown to be the case with some cells *in vitro*.[68] It is also possible that the conjugated protein is recognized nonspecifically or via some unreacted thiol groups, since conjugation of an irrelevant protein, albumin, resulted also in a short $T_{1/2}$.[74] A third possibility is that conjugation of protein enhances the aggregation of liposomes, thus resulting in their fast removal by the liver.

In spite of their fast clearance from the circulation, such antibody-conjugated liposomes were found to accumulate in 2–3-fold higher amounts in lymph nodes of Thy 1.1-positive AKR/J mice when the targeting IgG was an anti-Thy 1.1 antibody and the label was a nitriloacetic acid -[111]indium complex.[74] The significance of these results was strengthened by parallel studies in our laboratory using a lipid marker and large unilamellar vesicles which also pointed at a targeting effect on lymph nodes in the same antibody-animal model.[67] These studies provided a preliminary indication of targeting *in vivo*, although the high uptake by the liver was still unacceptable.

At this point it was obvious that we needed to develop a different type of liposome that would circulate in blood for much longer periods of time even when conjugated to antibodies. The hope was that we could imitate the circulating erythrocytes and produce a coating that would not be recognized by the RES. The work of S. Davis and colleagues had already shown that polymeric glycols could prolong the $T_{1/2}$ of polystyrene particles.[69] We needed an equivalent solution with more biodegradable materials such as glycolipids. A significant hint came from the work of T. Allen, who was spending a sabbatical year in our laboratory at that time. This work, in collaboration with J. Ryan, indicated that gangliosides in combination with cholesterol, could improve the stability of liposomes composed of egg phosphatidylcholine (PC) in the presence of plasma *in vitro*.[70] Since then, *in vivo* experiments of T. Allen *et al.* (personal communication) have indicated substantial reduction of liver uptake with ganglioside-containing liposome formulations.

In the following sections we shall summarize some of the highlights of our recent work on tissue distribution of various liposomes with and without antibody conjugation and its impact on targeting to tumors *in vivo*. These observations are covered in detail elsewhere.[75]

EXPERIMENTAL DESIGN

The results reported below were obtained with formulations based on a mixture of PC and cholesterol (2/1) containing 10 percent of various glycolipids or negatively charged phospholipids. We wish to point out some new methodologic points that became important ingredients of our experimental approach. These include the use of deferoxamine-[67]gallium (DF-^{67}Ga) complex as a tracer of liposome contents and the use of an extrusion step to turn polydisperse MLV preparations into homogeneous vesicle populations of approximately 100 nm in diameter.

Once released from liposomes, DF-^{67}Ga complexes are cleared at a very fast rate by the kidneys.[71] The high affinity of this complex prevents the translocation of ^{67}Ga to transferrin or other plasma proteins.[72] These features of the DF-^{67}Ga complex, together with its usefulness as a gamma-emitter for imaging, make it a reliable *in vivo* marker for liposomes.

For optimization of liposome size, we aimed at a size range that could offer a reasonable chance of extravasation. DF-containing MLV were extruded three consecutive times through 0.08-μm polycarbonate double membranes using a high-pressure device. The diameter of the extruded vesicles was in the range of 80 to 120 nm as measured by dynamic laser scattering. We chose not to use small sonicated liposomes because of their extremely reduced payload and their potential instability due to the strong curvature resulting in elastically stressed bilayers.[73]

Liposomes were conjugated with antibodies (monoclonal IgG$_1$, MRCOX7 anti-Thy 1.1) after procedures described previously,[49] with an additional step of re-

TABLE 1. Tissue Disposition of Unconjugated Liposomes in Normal Mice[a]

| Liposome Composition | Percentage of Recovered Dose per Organ | | | | Total Body Recovery (% of Injected Dose) |
	Liver and Spleen	Carcass and Skin	Blood	Rest[b]	
PG-PC-Chol	71.5	21.5	5.8	1.2	76.1
PI-PC-Chol	37.6	25.3	29.4	7.8	49.0
Sulf-PC-Chol	32.7	30.3	33.6	3.4	61.0
GM1-PC-Chol	34.0	21.2	33.3	11.5	63.2

[a]Intravenous injection of 1 μmol phospholipid per mouse (female Swiss Webster) and sacrifice 4 hours after injection.
[b]Includes kidneys, gut, lungs and heart.

extrusion after conjugation to ensure no change in size and to eliminate any aggregates.

Loading of vesicles with ^{67}Ga was carried out one day before injection into animals. For chelation of ^{67}Ga by DF, a lipophilic 8-hydroxyquinoline-^{67}Ga complex was previously formed. This complex, when coincubated with liposomes, crosses the bilayer, allowing for the transfer of ^{67}Ga to DF. The encapsulation efficiency of ^{67}Ga was approximately 70 percent. Tissue distribution experiments were done in mice with a dose of 1 μmol of phospholipid per animal injected intravenously.

TISSUE DISPOSITION IN NORMAL MICE

TABLE 1 summarizes the tissue disposition of four different liposome preparations, all with the same particle size distribution, 4 hours after injection into normal Swiss Webster mice. Blood content varied from 5.8 percent to 33.3 percent of the total recovered dose at that time, depending on lipid composition. The liposomes containing phosphatidylglycerol (PG) showed the lowest blood and highest liver and spleen accumulation. This is in accordance with previous observations[38,41] indicating that the presence of negative charge increased drastically the uptake by liver Kupffer cells. The results obtained with liposomes containing phosphatidylinositol (PI) show a much higher liposome concentration in blood (i.e., longer $T_{1/2}$) and therefore indicate that the surface charge is not the only important factor in determining liposome $T_{1/2}$ in

TABLE 2. In Vitro Binding of Antibody-Targeted Liposomes to Tumor Cells[a]

| Liposome Composition | Cell Type | |
| | AKR/SL2 (Thy 1.1) | J-6456 (Thy 1.2) |
	(nmoles phospholipid/10^7 cells $\pm$ SD)	
AntiThy 1.1-GM1-PC-Chol	9.1 $\pm$ 1.0	4.4 $\pm$ 0.6
GM1-PC-Chol	2.2 $\pm$ 0.7	4.0 $\pm$ 1.1

[a]Cell concentration: 10^7/ml in RPMI-1640 medium with 5 percent fetal calf serum. Liposome concentration: 100 nmol phospholipid/ml. Antibody class: monoclonal IgG$_1$. Incubation: 4°C, 1 hour.

TABLE 3. Tissue Disposition of Antibody-Conjugated Liposomes in Normal Mice[a]

Liposome Composition	Percentage of Recovered Dose per Organ				Total Body Recovery (% of Injected Dose)
	Liver and Spleen	Carcass and Skin	Blood	Rest[b]	
GM1-PC-Chol	34.0	21.2	33.3	11.5	63.2
Ab-GM1-PC-Chol	41.1	30.0	24.6	4.4	72.0
Ab-PG-PC-Chol	70.6	19.7	3.9	5.8	81.0

[a]Intravenous injection of 1 μmol phospholipid per mouse (female Swiss Webster) and sacrifice 4 hours after injection.
[b]Includes kidneys, gut, lungs and heart.

plasma. The results obtained with liposomes containing the two glycolipids, sulfatides (Sulf) and monosialoganglioside (GM_1), show similar tissue disposition and the most favorable blood-to-liver ratios. We have chosen to study in more detail the properties of the GM_1-containing liposomes and compare them with those of PG-containing liposomes, the latter formulations having been used for clinical applications.[2,3] A similar concentration of negatively charged lipid (10 percent) was present in both types of liposomes.

The results obtained with glycolipid-containing liposomes were encouraging for further targeting studies, since long circulation time should theoretically increase the probability of contact and possibly binding to target cells. It was therefore important to find out whether such relatively long $T_{1/2}$ could be obtained even when IgG was covalently bound to the liposome surface. The targeting antibody used in these experiments was an IgG_1 anti-Thy 1.1, used previously.[6,7] For the present studies, we conjugated the antibody to liposomes with final yields in the range of 50 to 100 μg protein per μmol phospholipid. *In vitro* assays indicated that antibody conjugation resulted in a four-fold increased binding to specific target cells in the cold (4°C). No increase in binding was observed when tumor cells expressing the Thy 1.2 antigen were used in TABLE 2.

To investigate the effect of antibody conjugation on the clearance rate of GM_1 liposomes, we injected them into normal Swiss Webster mice intravenously, under conditions identical to those used in TABLE 1. Some of the results are summarized in TABLE 3, which compares the levels in blood and other tissues 4 hours after injection.

TABLE 4. Blood and Liver Levels of Antibody-Conjugated Liposomes[a]

Liposome Composition	Area under the Curve (Concentration versus Time) (μmol $\times$ hr/g tissue)	
	Liver	Blood
PG-PC-Chol	3.86	0.55
Ab-PG-PC-Chol	4.68	0.37
GM1-PC-Chol	1.39	1.69
Ab-GM1-PC-Chol	2.93	1.83

[a]Calculated from three time points along the first 24 hr after intravenous injection of liposomes (1 μmol phospholipid/mouse). Each time point was obtained from the mean of three female Swiss Webster mice.

The antibody-conjugated GM_1 liposomes remained in blood at 24.6 percent of recovered dose, only slightly less than the unconjugated GM_1 liposomes (33.3 percent) and at a level much higher than that obtained when the antibody was conjugated to PG liposomes (3.9 percent). A more detailed account of the blood and liver levels of antibody-conjugated liposomes is given in TABLE 4, which lists the integrated areas under the curve during the first 24 hours after injection. It indicates a clear difference in favor of the GM_1 liposomes with a significantly enhanced residence time in blood and much smaller accumulation in the liver.

TISSUE DISPOSITION IN TUMOR-BEARING MICE

The above results strengthened the prospect of targeting with the antibody-conjugated GM_1 liposomes to tumors. The next series of experiments were therefore performed in AKR/J mice injected with 10^6 AKR/SL2 tumor cells intramuscularly in the hind leg. TABLE 5 summarizes the results obtained with three types of liposomes by comparing the percent injected dose found in liver, tumor and body average 24 hours after injection. While all three liposomes showed approximately the same value for body average, the tumor uptake was higher with the antibody-GM_1 liposomes (5.1) compared to GM_1 liposomes (3.7), a difference that is statistically significant ($p < 0.0015$). Both values were above the body average, and much higher than the value obtained with antibody-PG-liposomes (1.4). The accumulation in the liver was

TABLE 5. Tissue Disposition of Liposomes in Tumor-Bearing Mice[a]

| | Percentage of Injected Dose/g Tissue | | |
Liposome Composition	Liver	Tumor[b]	Body Average
Anti-Thy 1.1-GM1-PC-Chol	12.0 ± 0.2	5.1 ± 0.2	2.1 ± 0.1
GM1-PC-Chol	9.9 ± 1.1	3.7 ± 0.4	1.9 ± 0.1
Anti-Thy 1.1-PG-PC-Chol	15.8 ± 2.0	1.4 ± 0.2	2.1 ± 0.3

[a]Intravenous injection of 1 μmol phospholipid per mouse (male AKR/J bearing the SL2, Thy 1.1+ lymphoma in the hind leg) and sacrifice 24 hr after injection.
[b]Statistical analysis of differences in tumor dose (t test): GM_1-PC-Chol versus anti-Thy 1.1-GM_1-PC-Chol, $p < 0.0015$; anti-Thy 1.1-PG-PC-Chol versus Anti-Thy 1.1-GM_1-PC-Chol, $p < 0.0001$.

highest with antibody-PG liposomes and slightly larger with antibody-targeted as compared to plain GM_1 liposomes.

A more detailed examination ot the amount of antibody-GM_1 liposomes accumulated in various tissues at different times over 24 hours indicates that of all the organs examined, the tumor showed the most significant increase (five-fold) of the percent injected dose per gram of tissue between 4 and 24 hours (FIG. 1). This finding is similar to what has been observed with accumulation of free antitumor antibodies in implanted tumors.[73] At forty-eight hours after injection of antibody-conjugated GM_1 liposomes the implanted tumor is still containing a very high dose (6 percent of the recovered dose per gram of tissue) second only to liver and spleen (16 percent), and higher than carcass (1 percent), other tissues (3 percent) or the body average (1.7 percent).

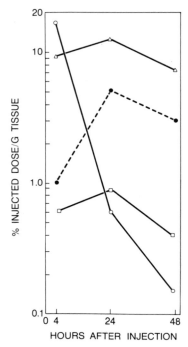

FIGURE 1. Distribution of Ab (Anti-Thy 1.1)-targeted GM₁ liposomes in tumor-bearing mice (male AKR/J, bearing the Thy 1.1+, SL2 lymphoma in the hind leg). O, blood; △, liver; ●, tumor; □, carcass.

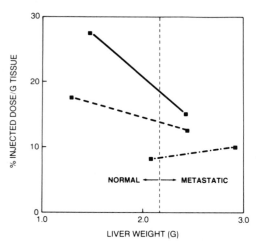

FIGURE 2. Liver uptake of liposomes in normal and tumor-bearing mice sacrificed 24 hours after injection. Mice and tumors were as in FIGURE 1. ■——■, Ab (anti-Thy 1.1)-PG liposomes; ■--■, Ab (anti-Thy 1.1)-GM₁ liposomes; ■-•-•-■ plain GM₁ liposomes.

Due to the fact that the AKR/SL2 tumor metastasizes heavily to the liver, it is difficult to determine the respective contribution of normal liver cells and liver-residing tumor cells in the uptake of liposomes. To gain some insight into this problem by analysis of the present data, we have plotted in FIGURE 2 the percent of the injected dose per gram of liver against the liver weight for three types of liposomes. In this tumor model the increase in liver weight is due to the presence of metastatic tumor cells. Hence, when the percent of injected dose per gram tissue remains unchanged, in spite of the fact that a significant fraction of liver tissue is taken up by tumor, we may infer that liposomes have as good accessibility to tumor cells as to normal liver cells. FIGURE 2 shows that the decrease in percent of injected dose per gram with increasing liver weight, as indicated by a negative slope, was largest with the antibody-conjugated PG liposomes, intermediate with the antibody-GM_1 liposomes, and nil with the unconjugated GM_1 liposomes. These findings support the possibility of an equal penetration to tumor areas and normal tissue of the liver by the long-half-life glycolipid-containing liposomes. Obviously before any firm conclusion can be reached, a more direct assessment of the relative amounts accumulating in the different cells within the liver is needed.

An additional point to be made here is that the biodistribution of these GM_1-containing antibody-conjugated liposomes can be further optimized by eliminating the Fc portion of the IgG and by conjugating only the Fab fragments on the liposome surface.[49] It is expected that this will further diminish the uptake of such liposomes by normal liver cells expressing the Fc receptor, while it will not affect their specific recognition by the target tumor cells.[49] Experiments are presently in progress to test this hypothesis.

CONCLUDING REMARKS

We have presented evidence that the clearance rate of liposomes can be controlled by the presence of specific glycolipids and phospholipids. Furthermore, we have demonstrated that such liposomes can have a reasonably long $T_{1/2}$ in blood even after conjugation of IgG on their surface. We were also able to show that tumor cells growing either intramuscularly or after metastasizing to the liver are accessible to small liposomes ($\sim$100 nm in diameter) with long $T_{1/2}$. The presence of a targeting antibody on the liposomes' surface further increases their ability to accumulate in specific tumors. Although the system is not optimized as yet, the results are very encouraging, and therefore enhance the prospect for targeting liposomes to specific cells within the vasculature or within tissues with fenestrated or "leaky" endothelium.

REFERENCES

1. PAPAHADJOPOULOS, D. Ed. 1978. Ann. N.Y. Acad. Sci. Vol. 308.
2. LOPEZ-BERESTEIN, G., V. FAINSTEIN, R. HOPFER, K. MEHTA, M. P. SULLIVAN, M. KEATING, M. G. ROSENBLUM, R. MEHTA, M. LUNA, E. M. HERSH, J. REUBEN, R. J. JULIANO & G. P. BODEY. 1985. J. Inf. Dis. 151: 704–712.
3. GABIZON, A., T. PERETZ, R. BEN-YOSEF, R. CATANE, S. BIRAN & Y. BARENHOLZ. 1986. Proc. Am. Soc. Clin. Oncol. 5: 43.
4. GREGORIADIS, G. 1981. Lancet 2: 241–246.
5. JULIANO, R. L. 1981. Trends Pharmacol. Sci. 2: 39–41.
6. MAYHEW, E. & D. PAPAHADJOPOULOS. 1983. In Liposomes. M. J. Ostro, Ed.: 289–341. Marcel Dekker, Inc. New York.

7. POZNANSKY, M. J. & R. L. JULIANO. 1984. Pharmacol. Rev. **36:** 277–336.
8. BLACK, C. D. V., C. J. WATSON & R. J. WARD. 1977. Tr. Royal Soc. Trop. Med. Hyg. **71:** 550–552.
9. NEW, R. R. C., M. L. CHANCE, S. C. THOMAS & W. PETERS. 1978. Nature (London) **272:** 55–56.
10. ALVING, C. R., E. A. STECK, W. L. CHAPMAN, V. B. WAITS, L. D. HENDRICKS, G. M. SWARTZ & W. L. HANSON. 1978. Proc. Natl. Acad. Sci. USA **75:** 2959–2963.
11. NEW, R. R. C., M. L. CHANCE & S. HEATH. 1981. J. Antimicrobial Chemother. **8:** 371–381
12. FIDLER, I. J. & G. POSTE. 1982. Springer Semin. Immunopathol. **5:** 161–174.
13. FIDLER, I. J., S. SONE, W. E. FOGLER & Z. L. BARNES. 1981. Proc. Natl. Acad Sci. USA **78:** 1680–1684.
14. KOFF, W. C., S. D. SHOWALTER, D. HOUNPAR & I. J. FIDLER. 1985. Science **228:** 495–497.
15. RAHMAN, A., A. KESSLER, N. MORE, B. SIKIC, G. ROWDEN, R. WOOLLEY & P. S. SCHEIN. 1980. Cancer Res. **40:** 1532–1537.
16. FORSSEN, E. A. & Z. A. TOKES. 1981. Proc. Natl. Acad. Sci. USA **78:** 1873–1877.
17. OLSON, F., E. MAYHEW, D. MASLOW, Y. RUSTUM & F. SZOKA. 1982. Eur. J. Cancer Clin. Oncol. **18:** 167–176.
18. GABIZON, A., A. DAGAN, D. GOREN, Y. BARENHOLZ & Z. FUKS. 1982. Cancer Res. **42:** 4734–4739.
19. GRAYBILL, J. R., P. C. CRAVEN, R. L. TAYLOR, D. M. WILLIAMS & W. E. MAGEE. 1982. Br. J. Infect. Dis. **145:** 748–752.
20. LOPEZ-BERESTEIN, G., R. MEHTA, R. L. HOPFER, K. MILLS, L. KASI, K. MEHTA, V. FAINSTEIN, M. LUNA, E. M. HERSH & R. JULIANO. 1983. J. Infect. Dis. **147:** 939–945.
21. MEHTA, R., G. LOPEZ-BERESTEIN, R. L. HOPFER, K. MILLS & R. L. JULIANO. 1984. Biochim. Biophys. Acta **770:** 230–234.
22. TREMBLAY, C., M. BARZA, C. FIORE & F. SZOKA. 1984. Antimicrob. Agents Chemother. **26:**170–183.
23. HUNT, C. A., Y. M. RUSTUM, E. MAYHEW & D. PAPAHADJOPOULOS. 1979. Drug Metab. Disposition **7:**124–128.
24. FIDLER, I. J., A. RAZ, W. E. FOGLER, R. KIRSH, P. BUGALSKI & G. POSTE. 1980. Cancer Res. **40:** 4460–4466.
25. JULIANO, R. L. & D. LAYTON. 1980. *In* Drug Delivery Systems: Characteristics and Biomedical Applications. R. L. Juliano, Ed.: 189–236. Oxford University Press. Oxford, England.
26. CERNY, E. A., Y. E. RAHMAN, K. R. PATEL, E. H. LAU & B. J. WRIGHT. 1982. Life Sci. **31:** 2061–2071.
27. SZOKA, F. C. & E. MAYHEW. 1983. Biochem. Biophys. Res. Comm. **110:** 140–146.
28. SORIANO, R., J. DIJKSTRA, A. LEGRAND, H. SPANJER, D. LONDOS-GAGLIARDI, F. ROERDINK, G. SCHERPHOF & C. NICOLAU. 1983. Proc. Natl. Acad. Sci. USA **80:** 7128–7131.
29. WU, M. S., J. C. ROBBINS, R. L. BUGIANESI, M. M. PONPIPOM & T. Y. SHEN. 1981. Biochim. Biophys. Acta **674:** 19–29.
30. DEBS, R. J., W. BLUMENFELD, E. N. BRUNETTE, R. M. STRAUBINGER, A. B. MONTGOMERY, E. LIN, N. AGABIAN & D. PAPAHADJOPOULOS. 1987. Antimicrob. Agents Chemother. **31:** 37–41.
31. ABRA, R. M. & C. A. HUNT. 1982. Res. Commun. Chem. Pathol. Pharmacol. **36:** 17–31.
32. PROFFIT, R., L. E. WILLIAMS, C. A. PRESANT, G. W. TIN, J. A. ULIANA, R. C. GAMBLE & J. D. BALDESCHWIELER. 1983. Science **220:** 502–505.
33. POSTE, G. 1983. Biol. Cell **47:** 19–36.
34. PETERSON, H. I. 1979. *In* Tumor Blood Circulation: Angiogenesis, Vascular Morphology and Blood Flow of Experimental and Human Tumors. H. I. Peterson, Ed.: 77–85. CRC Press. Boca Raton, FL.
35. DVORAK, H. F. 1986. N. Engl. J. Med. **315:** 1650–1659.
36. KIMELBERG, H. K., T. F. TRACY, R. E. WATSON, D. KUNG, F. L. REISS & R. S. BOURKE. 1978. Cancer Res. **38:** 706–712.
37. MYERS, C. 1984. Sem. Oncol. **11:** 251–257.

38. GREGORIADIS, G. & J. SENIOR. 1986. *In* Targeting of Drugs with Synthetic Systems. G. Gregoriadis, J. Senior & G. Poste, Eds.: 193–192. Plenum Press. New York, NY.
39. PATEL, H. & B. RYMAN. 1981. *In* Liposomes: From Physical Structure to Therapeutic Application. C. G. Knight, Ed.: 409–441. Elsevier-North Holland. Amsterdam.
40. YATVIN, M. D. & P. I. LELKES. 1982. Med. Phys. **9:** 149–175.
41. SCHERPHOF, G., F. ROERDINK, J. DIKSTRA, H. ELLENS, R. DEZANGER & E. WISSE. 1983. Biol. Cell **47:** 47–58.
42. HWANG, K. J., K.-F. LUK & P. L. BEAUMIER. 1980. Proc. Natl. Acad. Sci. USA **77:** 4030–4034.
43. PIDGEON, C. & C. A. HUNT. 1981. J. Pharmacol. Sci. **70:** 173–176.
44. OLSON, F., C. A. HUNT, F. C. SZOKA, W. J. VAIL & D. PAPAHADJOPOULOS. 1979. Biochim. Biophys. Acta **557:** 9–23.
45. SZOKA, F. C., F. OLSON, T. HEATH, W. VAIL, E. MAYHEW & D. PAPAHADJOPOULOS. 1980. Biochim. Biophys. Acta **601:** 559–571.
46. HOPE, M. J., M. B. BALLY, G. WEBB & P. R. CULLIS. 1985. Biochim. Biophys. Acta **812:** 55–65.
47. HEATH, T. D., R. FRALEY & D. PAPAHADJOPOULOS. 1980. Science **210:** 539–541.
48. MARTIN, F., W. HUBBELL & D. PAPAHADJOPOULOS, 1981. Biochemistry **20:** 4229–4238.
49. MARTIN, F. & D. PAPAHADJOPOULOS. 1982. J. Biol. Chem. **257:** 286–288.
50. HUANG, A., L. HUANG & S. J. KENNEL. 1980. J. Biol. Chem. **255:** 8015–8018.
51. LESERMAN, L. D., J. BARBET, F. M. KOURILSKY & J. N. WEINSTEIN. 1980. Nature (London) **288:** 602–604.
52. SINHA, D. & F. KARUSH. 1982. Biochim. Biophys. Acta **684:** 187–194.
53. STRAUBINGER, R., K. HONG, D. S. FRIEND & D. PAPAHADJOPOULOS. 1983. Cell **32:** 1069–1079.
54. MACHY, P. & L. D. LESERMAN. 1983. Biochim. Biophys. Acta **730:** 313–320.
55. MATTHAY, K. K., T. D. HEATH & D. PAPAHADJOPOULOS. 1984. Cancer Res. **44:** 1880–1886.
56. HEATH, T. D., J. A. MONTGOMERY, J. R. PIPER & D. PAPAHADJOPOULOS. 1983. Proc. Natl. Acad. Sci. USA **80:** 1377–1381.
57. LESERMAN, L. D., P. MACHY & J. BARBET. 1981. Nature (London) **293:** 226–228.
58. MACHY, P., J. BARBET & L. D. LESERMAN. 1982. Proc. Natl. Acad. Sci. USA **79:** 4148–4152.
59. BERINSTEIN, N., K. K. MATTHAY, D. PAPAHADJOPOULOS, R. LEVY & B. I. SIKIC. 1987. Cancer Res. (In press.)
60. TRUNEH, A., Z. MISHAL, J. BARBET, P. MACHY & L. LESERMAN. 1983. Biochem. J. **214:** 189–194.
61. HEATH, T. D., N. G. LOPEZ, W. H. STERN & D. PAPAHADJOPOULOS. 1985. FEBS Lett. **187:** 73–75.
62. DUZGUNES, N., R. M. STRAUBINGER, P. A. BALDWIN, D. S. FRIEND & D. PAPAHADJOPOULOS. 1985. Biochemistry **24:** 3091–3098.
63. CONNOR, J., M. B. YATVIN & L. HUANG. 1984. Proc. Natl. Acad. Sci. USA **81:** 1715–1718.
64. ELLENS, H., J. BENTZ & F. SZOKA. 1984. Biochemistry **23:** 1532–1538.
65. STRAUBINGER, R. M., N. DUZGUNES & D. PAPAHADJOPOULOS. 1985. FEBS Lett. **179:** 148–154.
66. CONNOR, J. & L. HUANG. 1985. J. Cell Biol **101:** 582–589.
67. DEBS, R. J., T. D. HEATH & D. PAPAHADJOPOULOS. 1987. Biochim. Biophys. Acta. **901:** 183–190.
68. BRAGMAN, K., T. D. HEATH & D. PAPAHADJOPOULOS. 1984. J. Natl. Cancer Inst. **73:** 127–131.
69. DAVIS, S. S., S. J. DOUGLAS, L. ILLUM, P. D. E. JONES, E. MAK & R. H. MULLER. 1986. *In* Targeting of Drugs with Synthetic Systems. G. Gregoriadis, J. Senior & G. Poste, Eds.: 123–146. Plenum Press. New York, NY.
70. ALLEN, T. M., J. L. RYAN & D. PAPAHADJOPOULOS. 1985. Biochim. Biophys. Acta **818:** 205–210.

71. YOKOYAMA, A., Y. OHMOMO, K. HORIUSHI, H. SAJI, H. TANAKA, K. YAMAMOTO, Y. ISHII & K. TORIZUKA. 1982. J. Nucl. Med. **23:** 903–914.
72. WEINER, R. E., M. L. THAKUR, M. GOODMAN & P. B. HOFFER. 1979. *In* Radiopharmaceuticals II. V. J. Sodd, D. R. Hogland, D. R. Allen, R. D. Ice & J. A. Sorensen, Eds.: 331–340. The Society of Nuclear Medicine. New York, NY.
73. WETTERAU, J. R. & A. JONAS. 1982. J. Biol. Chem. **257:** 10961–10966.
74. ABAI, A., T. HEATH & D. PAPAHADJOPOULOS. In preparation.
75. GABIZON, A., J. HUBERTY, R. S. STRAUBINGER, D. PRICE & D. PAPAHADJOPOULOS. In preparation.

Lipid Emulsions as Drug Delivery Systems

STANLEY S. DAVIS, CLIVE WASHINGTON,
AND PHILIP WEST

Pharmacy Department
University of Nottingham
Nottingham, United Kingdom

LISBETH ILLUM

Department of Pharmaceutics
Royal Danish School of Pharmacy
Copenhagen, Denmark

GARRY LIVERSIDGE, LARRY STERNSON,
AND RICHARD KIRSH

Smith Kline and French Laboratories
Philadelphia, Pennsylvania 19101

INTRODUCTION

Colloidal Carriers

Colloidal carriers used for the delivery of drugs take a variety of forms to include those that are solid-like in nature, such as microspheres and nanoparticles, and liquids in the form of emulsions, or vesicles (better known as liposomes). Natural colloidal particles (lipoproteins and chylomicrons present in circulating blood, for example) have also been investigated as potential carrier systems. The recent literature covering these different systems can be found in various detailed papers, review articles, and monographs.[1-4] This article will consider recent studies on the use of lipid emulsions as drug delivery systems and will concentrate on the intravenous route of administration. The earlier literature has been reviewed by Davis and others.[2]

Emulsions as Drug Delivery Systems

An emulsion can be defined as a mixture of two (or more) immiscible phases with a third component (emulsifier) used to stabilize the dispersed droplets. Emulsions used in pharmacy and medicine can be of different types to include oil-in-water (o/w) and water-in-oil (w/o) systems as defined by the nature of the dispersed and continuous phases. More complex systems like multiple emulsions, that are formed by the re-emulsification of o/w or w/o systems (for example, water-in-oil-in water (w/o/w)) also exist. Thermodynamically stable systems, known as microemulsions, that basically comprise swollen micelles containing solubilized drug, have also been described. Microemulsion systems are transparent but on dilution they can form conventional emulsion systems. Consequently, they are sometimes referred to self-emulsifying systems.[5] The choice of the emulsion system to be used for drug delivery is normally dictated by the route of administration desired, the drug to be delivered, and the effect required (e.g. simple delivery, controlled or sustained release, or a more ambitious

75

objective in the form of drug targeting). Clearly the intended use can have an important bearing on the nature of the constituent components of the system. Hence, the toxicological considerations relevant to, say, topical use will be very different to those for parenteral use. Davis et al.[2] have discussed these aspects in detail.

PARENTERAL EMULSIONS

Emulsions can be administered by almost all available routes including topical, parenteral, oral, and even aerosolization to the lungs.[6] The formulated systems can contain drugs, vaccines, or diagnostic agents, or the disperse phase of the emulsion can by itself be clinically beneficial as in the case of fat emulsions for clinical nutrition. In some applications, suitable emulsions can be used to transport gases, in particular oxygen.

The purpose of this paper is to consider the applicability of emulsions as drug delivery systems for parenteral administration with special reference to intravenous (i.v.) applications. Thus, while w/o systems and even w/o/w systems can be given by intramuscular (i.m.) injection, only o/w (and perhaps a few suitable microemulsion systems) can sensibly be given intravenously.

Lymphotropic Emulsions

Important contributions on the use of emulsions as lymphotropic agents have been presented in recent years by Japanese workers.[7-9] The emulsions investigated were the w/o and w/o/w type (with some containing microspheres of gelatin) and were given by intramuscular, intraperitoneal, subcutaneous, and intralesional injection. The drugs studied included mitomycin C (and its lipophilic prodrug esters), bleomycin, and 5-fluorouracil. It was suggested that the emulsions could find their way to the regional lymph nodes, thereby providing a greatly enhanced uptake of the drug at these sites as would be beneficial in cancer chemotherapy. The possibility of transferring the emulsion particles to the regional lymphatics has also been invoked as an important stage in the role of emulsions (w/o and w/o/w) as adjuvants for vaccines.[2] Interestingly, liposomes are now also being advocated as adjuvants[10] but few studies have compared the two different colloidal systems. In the field of drug delivery, Sasaki et al.[11] have examined the i.m. administration of mitomycin C prodrugs in lipid emulsions and in liposomes. Both colloids were similar in providing a sustained release effect as compared to saline solution controls.

Oil-in-water emulsions

Emulsions that are made of an oil dispersed in an aqueous phase with a suitable emulsifying agent have an important place in drug delivery, as well as for parenteral nutrition, oxygen transport, and diagnostic imaging.[2] In some instances, systems that were originally developed for non-pharmacological applications have been found to have interesting uses in drug delivery. For example, perfluorochemical emulsions, which have been studied extensively as potential red blood cell substitutes because of their ability to transport oxygen and carbon dioxide, are now being proposed as combined oxygen and drug carriers for use in cancer chemotherapy.[12] Konno et al.[13] have demonstrated that the radiodiagnostic emulsion known as Ethiodol (iodinated poppy-seed oil) could be used to deliver the lipophilic anticancer agent SMANCS (poly(styrene-maleic acid) conjugated neocarzinostatin). Following intra-arterial administration via the hepatic artery, a marked anti-tumor effect on unresectable hepatoma was observed. Both Ethiodal and the drug accumulated more selectively in the tumor than in other tissues and it was claimed that their activity persisted for more than 3 weeks. The fat emulsion system Intralipid (formulated from soybean oil and stabilized by fractionated egg-lecithin) and various copies thereof, has been used successfully as a carrier for a variety of lipophilic drugs.[2] This is a logical approach since Intralipid is intended as a copy of the natural fat particle system present in the circulation, the chylomicra, which carry endogenous and exogenous lipophiles. The Intralipid system has been mixed with various drugs in order to improve drug stability and reduce adverse reactions and side effects. The drugs have included valinomycin, CCNU, and hexamethylmelamine (HMM).[14-16] Wickes and Howell[16] have shown that the pharmacokinetics of HMM can be changed markedly when given by the intraperitoneal route in an emulsion formulation, as compared to a saline control (clearance half-lives were 25 and 2 minutes, respectively). As will be discussed in detail below, modifications of the Intralipid system have now been developed *de novo* for the delivery of a wide variety of pharmacological agents. Some putative drug targeting systems have even been described.

Intravenous Lipid Emulsions

As mentioned above, there is presently interest in the use of lipid emulsions for drug delivery. These o/w systems are based largely on vegetable oils (10–20% vol/vol) stabilized by phosphatides (1–2% w/vol) and they therefore have certain similarities to liposomes. In contrast to the latter, fat emulsions are easy to manufacture using proven technology and furthermore they have good long-term stability (typically 2 years at 4°C). The oil phase acts as a solubilizer of lipophiles and it can also serve to stabilize drugs that are unstable in an aqueous environment.[15] Fat emulsions are well tolerated by the body since they resemble chylomicra and a lower incidence of side effects has been observed as compared to equivalent systems based on organic solvents and surface active agents (e.g. Cremophor), due to the fact that there can be no precipitation of the drug upon administration. This precipitation effect can lead to pain on injection and thrombophlebitis. In addition, lipid emulsions do not lead to anaphylactoid reactions which have been reported for Cremophor formulations.[17] In some cases an alteration in the pharmacokinetics and body distribution of the incorporated drug have been described, thereby opening up the possibilities of targeting drugs to specific sites. The disadvantages of fat emulsions include the fact that water-soluble components cannot be entrapped unless lipophilic prodrugs are prepared, and that the incorporated drug may alter the stability of the emulsion as well as its surface characteristics. Surface character can well be important in determining the fate of the system, particularly in terms of its capture by the defense system of the body, the reticuloendothelial system (RES).

The oil droplets in formulated fat emulsions intended for drug delivery are typically of about 250 nm in average size. The chosen emulsifier is selected on the basis of toxicological considerations ("GRAS" status) and the intended destination of the system in the body. In some instances, by changing surface character (as well as particle size) it is possible to control the interaction of the systems with elements of the RES. The drug to be delivered can be dissolved or suspended in the oil phase or adsorbed (attached) or intercalated in the interfacial region. An attachment mechanism has been proposed for o/w emulsion systems prepared from myocobacterial cell wall skeletons and trehalose dimycolate. These emulsions have been used clinically to achieve tumor regression and systemic immunity.[18]

Custom-made fat emulsions containing drugs have been developed largely by workers in the Swedish (e.g., Kabi) and Japanese (e.g., Green Cross) pharmaceutical industries. The various systems developed by Kabi have largely resulted from the pioneering studies of Jeppsson and others on barbituric acids[19] and have led to the introduction of two i.v. emulsion products, namely a diazepam emulsion (Diazemuls) and very recently the i.v. anesthetic di-isopropylphenol (Propofol).[20,21] In both cases the intention has been to produce a delivery system that avoids the problems inherent in delivering lipid-soluble materials using solvents and surface active agents. As desired, the pharmacokinetics of the drugs were unaltered, even though they were incorporated in an emulsion vehicle. The Green Cross team has developed a number of emulsion systems (termed lipid microspheres) for the administration of prostaglandin E_1 (PGE_1), steroids and prodrugs of non-steroidal anti-inflammatory drugs.[22-26] (Other similar formulations have been produced for the i.p. administration of anti-tumor drugs[27] and even for aerosolization of PGE_1[6]). In some instances the emulsions were developed as simple vehicles for easy administration, while in other cases the emulsion systems resulted in a change in the pharmacokinetics of the drug and the resultant clinical effect. Kimura et al.,[28] also from Japan, have reported the use of lipid emulsions for the delivery of the lipophilic enzyme coenzyme Q10, and how the nature of the emulsifying agent can alter the plasma concentration versus time profile and apparently direct a very significant proportion of the administered dose to the spleen (20% calculated from the data provided by the authors on the assumption that the rat has an average weight of 250 g and a spleen of weighing 0.8 g). There is some evidence in the published literature to suggest that emulsions may be taken up selectively by certain tissues (for example, the myocardium[2]). However, recent claims for targeting (sic) to inflamed sites, when less than 1% of the administered dose is delivered selectively, would seem to be inappropriate.[24] One always needs to consider where the remainder of the drug has ended up and the possibility for unwanted adverse reactions due to fortuitous targeting. The toxic ablation of the RES is a distinct possibility when dealing with colloidal carriers for cytotoxic agents.[29]

Two other aspects relevant to the use of o/w emulsions for intravenous administration are worth mentioning before dealing with some of our own data to include a case history. The active targeting of emulsions to the lungs has been reported by Akimoto et al.[30] using magnetic emulsions formulated from ethyl oleate–based magnetic fluids. The incorporated drugs were nitrosoureas. The magnetic system was capable of directing more of the drug to the lung, when an external magnet was applied, than were the cases when the drug was given in aqueous solution or as an emulsion without an applied magnetic field. Interesting as such results might be, an alternate and simpler strategy would be the use of emulsion droplets that were large enough to form temporary emboli in the lung capillaries.

The second aspect concerns the use of low density lipoprotein (LDL) as a drug carrier. The uptake of LDL by a receptor-mediated process has been well described and it is known that certain tissues, particularly tumors, have a higher affinity for LDL than normal tissues because of their need for cholesterol. Various groups have attempted to exploit this fact to deliver lipophilic prodrugs of anticancer agents to tumors.[4,31] The results so far presented have described the use of reconstituted LDL particles. It would be of considerable advantage to have available LDL analogs and some efforts are being made in this direction using microemulsions produced from egg phosphatides and cholesterol oleate.[32,33] Clearly in such work it will be necessary to have, not only a particle of the same size and apparent constitution as LDL, but also one that bears the correct recognition signal for uptake by the intended cells (apolipoprotein B). The future availability of apolipoproteins through recombinant DNA technology could be the next important step forward.

Having reviewed the general field of lipid emulsions for drug delivery, with special emphasis on the i.v. route, we will now consider the factors that determine the fate of an administered emulsion system and how evaluation can be conducted *in vivo* using the rabbit as an animal model. Finally, a case history dealing with a new emulsion formulation for the drug amphotericin B will be presented.

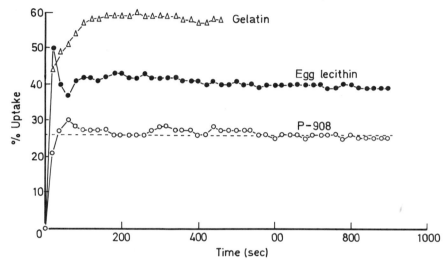

FIGURE 1. The effect of the nature of the emulsifying agent and added gelatin on the liver (and spleen) levels of fat emulsions administered by i.v. injection to the rabbit. Mean data, $N = 3$, s.e.m. from 1–2%. Legend: (O) 2% poloxamine 908 as emulsifying agent (27%), (●) 1.2% egg lecithin as emulsifying agent (34%), and (△) Lecithin stabilized emulsion with 0.3% added gelatin (47%). (Figures in parentheses represent liver values after 6 hours.) Dotted line represents the liver "blood-pool."

INTRAVENOUS ADMINISTRATION OF RADIOLABELED EMULSIONS AND THE ROLE OF THE EMULSIFYING AGENT

Background

Previous studies have demonstrated that the fate of colloidal particles injected i.v. is determined not only by their size but also by their surface characteristics.[34] For example, using the block copolymers of the poloxamer and poloxamine series, it has been possible to direct small particles to the bone marrow or to retain particles in the systemic circulation for long periods of time. This work was conducted largely with model particles made from polystyrene and it was therefore appropriate to repeat such investigations using biodegradable materials. Here we report studies using radiolabeled emulsions that demonstrate that the block copolymer poloxamine 980 is also able to retain a fat emulsion in the systemic circulation. These studies will be described in more detail elsewhere.[35]

Methods

Preparation of emulsions

Soybean oil was labeled with iodine-123 (using sodium iodide from Harwell) according to the method of Lubran and Pearson.[36] This method involves the covalent attachment of iodine across the double bond of unsaturated components in the oil. The labeled oil was mixed with a further portion of unlabeled oil and then emulsified using an ultrasonic probe (Dawe Soniprobe) (10 min) using either 2% w/vol poloxamine 908 (BASF) or egg lecithin (Lipoid E80) as stabilizers. The final oil phase volume was 10%. The particle size of the droplets, as determined by photon correlation spectroscopy (PCS) (Malvern), was of the order of 250 nm, a size similar to that found for Intralipid 10%. One sample of the egg lecithin stabilized system was mixed with gelatin (Sigma) at a level of 0.3% w/vol according to the procedure of Tonaki et al.[37] In this process some of the gelatin is either adsorbed to the surface of the droplets or forms a mixed interfacial film. In doing so, it will potentiate the uptake of the opsonic factor fibronectin, when the emulsion is injected into the systemic circulation.

In one experiment a model compound that can be easily labeled with a gamma emitter, lasolocid (Sigma), was incorporated into the emulsion system at a concentration of 1.0 mg/ml. The chosen label was indium-111. This could be imaged concurrently with iodine-123 so that the fate of both the emulsion and the model drug could be ascertained.

Experimental Procedure

Animals

Female new Zealand white rabbits (three per group) of an approximate weight of 2 kg were injected via the marginal ear vein using 1 ml samples of the emulsion systems. The administered activity was about 8 MBq for iodine-123 and about 1.5 MBq for indium-111. The animals were imaged using a gamma camera (GEC Maxicamera, 40 cm field of view) tuned to the relevant photopeaks of the two radionuclides. Dynamic images were recorded every 20 seconds over a period of 15 minutes. Static images of 1 minute duration were then recorded at suitable intervals over a 6 hour period. Scintigraphic data were stored on computer for analysis. The activity in the liver (and also the underlying spleen) were measured by creating a region of interest and applying the necessary corrections for ratio-decay and background activity. In the dual isotope study a correction was made for the "scatter-down" of the indium-111 activity into the lower photopeak of iodine-123. Blood samples were removed at selected times from the contralateral ear to that used for administration and the samples diluted and counted in a conventional gamma counter (Ortec).

Results

The recorded levels of activity for the labeled emulsion in the liver (and spleen) region were dependent on the nature of the emulsifying agent (and additive) used (FIG. 1). Emulsification with poloxamine 908 provided a liver uptake value of approximately 25% of administered dose, while the emulsions stabilized with egg lecithin were taken up by the liver to a higher extent (40%). The emulsions containing added gelatin were taken up to a value of about 60%.

The activity recorded in the liver of an animal, following the administration of a colloidal delivery system, as measured using the technique of gamma scintigraphy, will include activity resulting from not only the uptake of those particles by the various cells of the liver (usually the Kupffer cells representing part of the RES) but also circulating particles within the liver "blood pool." In the rabbit this "blood pool" represents about 25% of the administered dose of an unsequestered radiolabeled material.[38] Thus, in the studies with emulsions stabilized using poloxamine 908, it can be concluded that the block copolymer effectively prevents uptake of the emulsion by the liver (and spleen). The corresponding data obtained with egg lecithin systems show that a proportion of the emulsion is taken up by the liver, most probably by the Kupffer cells and hepatocytes, which are known to have a role in the metabolism of triglycerides. Such a process of uptake may well be mediated by the adsorption of apolipoproteins (e.g. apo CII and CIII).[2] As expected, added gelatin encourages the uptake of particles by the

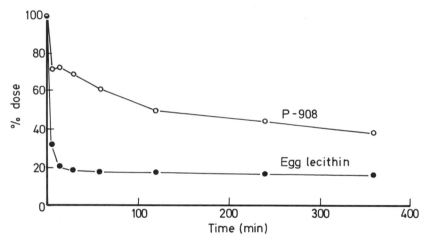

FIGURE 2. The effect of the nature of the emulsifying agent on the blood clearance of fat emulsions administered by i.v. injection to rabbit. Mean data, $N = 3$, s.e.m. from 4–6%. Legend: (O) 2% poloxamine 908 as emulsifying agent and (●) 1.2% egg lecithin as emulsifying agent.

liver, most probably through the adsorption of fibronectin and subsequent removal by the Kupffer cells.[39]

The measured blood level data available for the poloxamine 908 and egg lecithin systems reflect the liver uptake situation. The emulsions stabilized by egg lecithin are cleared much more quickly than the counterparts stabilized by poloxamine 908 (FIG. 2). (The initial rapid fall in blood level for both systems can be attributed to the presence of small quantities of free iodine-123, while the apparent plateau levels at longer times represent iodinated species released by metabolism of the emulsions.[40] Correcting the data for the initial level of free iodine, a first-order kinetic analysis could be performed. This indicated that the half-lives for clearance for the egg lecithin and poloxamine 908 systems were about 5 and 208 minutes, respectively. These values are in accord with the studies of Jeppsson and Rossner[41] who reported data on the blood clearance of fat emulsions stabilized by egg lecithin and the block copolymer poloxamer 338.

The investigations conducted using labeled oil and labeled model drug showed that the liver profiles for the two components were similar and that the "drug" was retained within the emulsion during the time course of the experiment (6 hours) (FIG. 3).

Conclusions

The results confirm the earlier studies using model particles, that the uptake of colloidal particles by the cells of the RES residing in the liver can be prevented by using a block copolymer of the poloxamine series. An emulsion system with a long circulation life-time (and for that matter other biodegradable colloids), could find use as a delivery system for the administration of lipid soluble drugs to include anti-infectives,

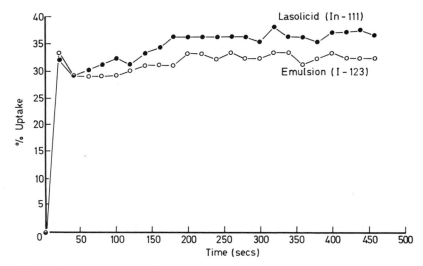

FIGURE 3. The liver (and spleen) levels of a fat emulsion stabilized by egg lecithin and a solute dissolved in the oil phase (Lasolocid) as determined in the rabbit using the technique of gamma scintigraphy with two isotopes. Mean data, $N = 3$, s.e.m. from 1–2%. Legend. (O) Emulsion (iodine-123 label) and (●) Lasolocid (indium-111 label).

anticancer agents, antithrombotics etc. The attachment of a suitable "homing" ligand, such as a monoclonal antibody, a sugar residue, or a apolipoprotein could provide a means for the selective delivery of these colloids to designated sites within the vascular compartment.[34] The use of these emulsion systems for delivery to the lymphatic system is under consideration.

AN EMULSION FORMULATION OF AMPHOTERICIN B

Background

Amphotericin B (AmB) is the drug of choice for the treatment of disseminated mycoses.[42] It belongs to the group of polyene antibiotics that cause cell lysis by formation of pores in membranes. Amphotericin shows selective cytotoxicity to fungal cells, which is believed to be due to its stronger binding affinity for the sterol within the fungal membrane (ergosterol), than the primary mammalian membrane sterol, cholesterol. However, toxicity to mammalian cells is still present. When used in therapeutic concentrations (0.25–1.0 mg/kg) AmB displays numerous side effects, primarily nephrotoxicity and damage to the CNS, which may be irreversible at high doses. The patient also experiences chills, fever, and nausea although these become less severe as treatment progresses.[42] Recently AmB has been formulated entrapped in liposomes.[42,43] This preparation has been found to retain the antifungal potency in mice as well as in limited trials in patients. Furthermore no lysis of human red blood cells was found *in vitro* at drug concentrations of 100 μg/ml. In contrast "free" AmB (Fungizone, Squibb; a solubilized formulation containing deoxycholate) caused detectable lysis above concentrations of 6 μg/ml. The LD 50 of AmB in mice was 1.2 mg/kg when given in the form of Fungizone, whereas the LD 50 of the liposomal system was 20 mg/kg. The liposomal material did not cause symptomatic malaise in humans at the normal therapeutic level of 0.5 mg/kg, thereby representing a significant increase in the therapeutic range.[43] Unfortunately, problems associated with the production of liposomes in bulk and their stability may well preclude the development of a successful commercial product. We have therefore investigated the possibility of delivering AmB in an emulsion formulation. This can be accomplished with conventional technology and the system developed has been found to retain the benefits of the liposomal material in terms of reduced toxicity.

Methods

Emulsion Formulation

AmB is soluble only in DMSO and strongly hydroxylic solvents, such as methanol, which is the only solvent that can be removed easily during processing. The AmB (Sigma) was dissolved in methanol and then the emulsifer (egg lecithin, Lipoid E80) dissolved in water, was added. The methanol was evaporated thoroughly leaving a crude solubilized preparation. The oil phase (soybean oil, final volume fraction 20%) was then added and the system emulsified using a sonic probe. It is suggested that the AmB is held (intercalated) in the interfacial film of phosphatide since it is insoluble in both oil and water. The stability of the drug in the emulsion formulation was measured in terms of both shelf storage and sterilization conditions. Drug release *in vitro* was followed using a UV spectroscopic method since the drug has an intense structured spectrum and free drug content can be easily deconvoluted from droplet scatter. Full details of the preparation and evaluation of these emulsion systems will be presented elsewhere.[44]

Lysis of Human Erythrocytes

The method of Mehta *et al.* was employed.[45] Blood was donated from healthy males in the age range 19–26 years. It was centrifuged to sediment the erythrocytes, which were washed twice with isotonic saline. The final washing showed no detectable absorbance due to hemoglobin. Washed erythrocytes were suspended in isotonic saline to an absorbance of 2.0 at a wavelength of 550 nm. The AmB formulation was added to produce final AmB concentrations in the range 0–32 μg/ml. These were mixed on a vortex mixer and incubated for 20 minutes at 37°C. The tubes were then centrifuged for 10 minutes at 3,000g and the clear supernatant assayed for hemoglobin at 550 nm. The mixtures containing the emulsion formulation were too turbid for absorbance measurements even after prolonged centrifugation, and so their absorbance was estimated by reference to a set of standards made by adding a soybean oil emulsion (Intralipid) to solutions of hemoglobin (Sigma) of known absorbance.

Animal Studies

Webster-derived CD-1 male mice (25 g) from Charles River Laboratories were injected i.v. with approximately 1.2×10^6 colony forming units of *Candida albicans* 3153A in saline for the establishment of experimental candidosis. This represented eight times the LD 50 and at this inoculum level 100% of the untreated animals died from a disseminated infection between 15–20 days post-inoculation. Infected animals were treated with either emulsion formulation, Fungizone, or virulence control formulation consisting of blank emulsion. Random groups of 10 infected mice were used for each drug level or for control. The preparations of AmB were given as a single injection i.v. 48 hours after infection. At this time fungal lesions were present in the kidneys, liver, and brain of infected animals. Fungizone was administered in doses up to 4.0 mg/kg. Emulsion-associated AmB was administered in doses up to 9.0 mg/kg. Survivors were recorded daily. The maximum tolerated dose (MTD) for Fungizone injected i.v. was 1.0 mg/kg in the infected mice. Emulsion associated AmB was tolerated at the highest dose administered (9.0 mg/kg).

Results

Lysis of Human Erythrocytes

The lysis of erythrocytes by the three formulations comprising Fungizone, AmB emulsion and AmB in methanol, as measured by the release of hemoglobin is shown in FIGURE 4. Both Fungizone and the methanolic solution of AmB caused cell lysis at AmB concentrations above 2 μg/ml. Lysis was total for both formulations at concentrations above 12 μg/ml, since no intact cells could be sedimented from these systems by centrifugation. Methanol alone (2%) did not cause detectable lysis. The cells incubated with the emulsion formulation showed no detectable hemoglobin release.

Treatment of Established Murine Candidosis

The effect of different formulations and concentrations of AmB on the survival of mice bearing established candidosis is shown in FIGURE 5. Eighteen days post infection with *C. albicans* 3153A, and eight days after the control animals had died, the ED 50 values for Fungizone and the emulsion formulation were 0.78 mg/kg and less than 0.5 mg/kg, respectively, with 80% of the mice treated with the emulsion system surviving compared to the loss of all control animals 10 days after infection. Equally important, the reduced toxicity of the emulsion formulation (MTD > 8 mg/kg) allowed the use of much higher doses of AmB such that at doses of 8 mg/kg all animals survived for 35 days as compared with only 60% survival during similar therapy with the much lower tolerated dose of Fungizone.

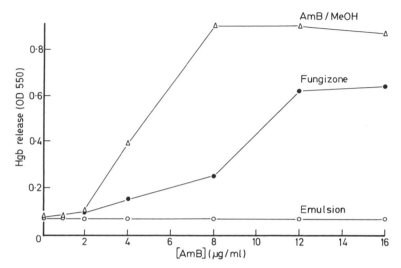

FIGURE 4. The lysis of human erythrocytes by amphotericin B formulations, the effect of amphotericin B concentration. Hemoglobin release determined at a wavelength of 550 nm. Legend: (△) Methanolic solution, (●) Fungizone, and (○) Emulsion.

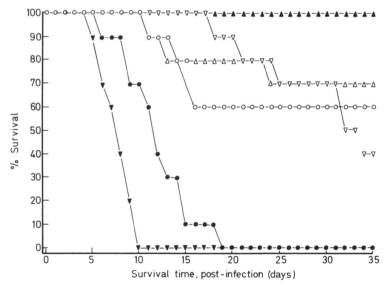

FIGURE 5. The influence of amphotericin B formulations on the survival time of mice infected with *Candida albicans*. Legend: (●) Fungizone (AmB 0.5 mg/kg), (○) Fungizone (AmB 1.0 mg/kg), (△) Emulsion (AmB 0.5 mg/kg), (▽) Emulsion (AmB 1.0 mg/kg), (▲) Emulsion (AmB 8.0 mg/kg), and (▼) Emulsion control.

Conclusions

The lack of erythrocyte lysis *in vitro* by the AmB emulsion systems suggests that the new formulation is less toxic to mammalian cells than is Fungizone. Furthermore, the encouraging results obtained *in vivo* demonstrate that the emulsion formulation can provide higher doses of AmB than can Fungizone with pronounced therapeutic benefit. The results obtained so far with the new emulsion formulation suggest that the increased therapeutic range is similar to that achieved using liposomal formulations. The emulsion has the important additional advantages of being easy to prepare industrially and should be available in a final form for direct administration to the patient without the need for extemperaneous procedures.

REFERENCES

1. DAVIS, S. S., L. ILLUM, J. G. MCVIE & E. TOMLINSON, Eds. 1984. Microspheres and Drug Therapy, Pharmaceutical, Immunological and Medical Aspects. Elsevier. Amsterdam.
2. DAVIS, S. S., J. HADGRAFT & K. J. PALIN. 1985. Pharmaceutical emulsions. *In* Encyclopedia of Emulsion Technology. P. Becher, Ed. 3: 159–238. Dekker. New York.
3. GREGORIADIS, G., J. SENIOR, B. WOLFF & C. KIRBY. 1984. Fate of liposomes *in vivo*. Control leading to targeting. *In* Receptor Mediated Targeting of Drugs. G. Gregoriadis, G. Poste, J. Senior & A. Trouet, Eds.: 243–266. Plenum Press. New York.
4. MASQUELIER, M., S. VITOLS & C. PETERSON. 1986. Low density lipoprotein as a carrier of antitumoral drugs: *in vivo* fate of drug-human low density lipoprotein complexes in mice. Cancer Res. 46: 3842–3847.
5. POUTON, C. W. 1985. Self-emulsifying drug delivery systems: assessment of the efficiency of emulsification. Int. J. Pharmaceut. 27: 335–348.
6. MIZUSHIMA, Y., K. HOSHI, H. AIHARA & M. KURACHI. 1983. Inhibition of bronchoconstriction by aerosol of a lipid emulsion containing prostaglandin E_1. J. Pharm. Pharmacol. 35: 397.
7. SASAKI, H., Y. TAKAKURA, M. HASHIDA, T. KIMURA & H. SEZAKI. 1984. Antitumor activity of lipophilic prodrugs of mitomycin C entrapped in liposome or o/w emulsion. J. Pharm. Dyn. 7: 120–130.
8. TANIGAWA, N., T. KANAZAWA, K. SATOMURA, Y. HIKASA, M. HASHIDA, S. MURANISHI & H. SEZAKI. 1981. Experimental study on lymphatic vascular changes in the development of cancer. Lymphology 4: 149–154.
9. TAKAHASHI, T. 1986. Emulsion and activated carbon in cancer chemotherapy. CRC Crit. Rev. Therapeutic Drug Carrier Systems 2: 245–274.
10. VAN ROOIJEN, N. & R. VAN NIEUWMEGEN. 1982. Immunoadjuvant properties of liposomes. *In* Targeting of Drugs. G. Gregoriadis, J. Senior & A. Trouet, Eds.: 301–326. Plenum Press. New York.
11. SASAKI, H., T. KATUTANI, M. HASHIDA & H. SEZAKI. 1985. Absorption characteristics of the lipophilic prodrug of mitomycin C from injected liposomes or an emulsion. J. Pharm. Pharmacol. 37: 461–465.
12. KLUBES, P., S. HIRAGA, R. L. CYSYK & R. G. BLASBERG. 1985. Attempts to increase blood flow in the rat solid Walker 256 tumor by the use of the perfluorochemical emulsion Fluosol DA (F-DA). Proc. Ann. Meet. Am. Assoc. Cancer Res. 26: 321.
13. KONNO, T., H. MAEDA, K. IWAI, S. TASHIRO, S. MAKI, T. MORINAGA, M. MOCHINAGA, T. HIRAOKA & I. YOKOYAMA. 1983. Effect of arterial administration of high molecular weight anticancer agent SMANCS with lipid lymphographic agent on hepatoma: a preliminary report. Eur. J. Cancer Clin. Oncol. 19: 1053–1065.
14. LITTERST, C. L., E. G. MIMNAUGH, A. C. COWLES, T. E. GRAM & A. M. GUARINO. 1974. Distribution of ^{14}C-lomustine (^{14}C-CCNU)-derived radioactivity following intravenous administration of three potential clinical formulations to rabbits. J. Pharm. Sci. 63: 1718–1721.
15. REPTA, A. J. 1981. Formulation of investigational anticancer drugs. *In* Topics in Pharmaceutical Sciences. D. D. Breimer & P. Speiser, Eds.: 131–151. Elsevier. Amsterdam.

16. WICKES, A. D. & S. B. HOWELL. 1985. Pharmacokinetics of hexamethylmelamine administered via the Ip route in an oil emulsion vehicle. Cancer Treatment Rep. **69:** 657–662.
17. GLEN, J. B. & S. C. HUNTER. 1984. Pharmacology of an emulsion formulation of ICI 35868. Br. J. Anaesth. **56:** 617–625.
18. VOSIKA, G., C. GIDDINGS & G. R. GRAY. 1984. Phase I study of intravenous mycobacterial cell wall skeleton and trehalose dimycolate attached to oil droplets. J. Biol. Response Modifiers **3:** 620–626.
19. JEPPSSON, R. 1972. Effect of barbituric acids using an emulsion form injected intravenously. Acta Pharm. Suec. **9:** 81–90.
20. VON DARDEL, O., C. MEBIUS, T. MOSSBERG & B. SVENSSON. 1983. Fat emulsion as a vehicle for diazepam. A study of 9492 patients. Br. J. Anaesth. **55:** 41–47.
21. CUMMINGS, G. C. & A. A. SPENCE. 1985. Comparison of propofol in emulsion with althesin for induction of anaesthesia. Br. J. Anaesth. **57:** 234.
22. MIZUSHIMA, Y., K. YANAGAWA & K. HOSHI. 1983. Prostaglandin E₁ is more effective, when incorporated in lipid microspheres, for treatment of peripheral vascular diseases in man. J. Pharm. Pharmacol. **35:** 666–667.
23. MIZUSHIMA, Y. 1985. Lipid microspheres as novel drug carriers. Drugs Exptl. Clin. Res. **9:** 595–600.
24. MIZUSHIMA, Y., T. HAMANO & K. YOKOYAMA. 1982. Use of a lipid emulsion as a novel carrier for corticosteroids. J. Pharm. Pharmacol. **34:** 49–50.
25. MIZUSHIMA, Y., Y. WADA, Y. ETOH & K. WATANABE. 1983. Anti-inflammatory effects of indomethacin ester incorporated in a lipid microsphere. J. Pharm. Pharmacol. **35:** 398–399.
26. SHOJI, Y., Y. MIZUSHIMA, A. YANAGAWA, T. SHIBA, H. TAKEI, M. FUJI & M. AMINO. 1986. Enhancement of anti-inflammatory effects of biphenylylacetic acid by its incorporation into lipid microspheres. J. Pharm. Pharmacol. **38:** 118–121.
27. MIZUSHIMA, Y., Y. SHOJI, T. KATO, M. FUKUSHIMA & S. KUROZUMI. 1986. Use of lipid microspheres as a drug carrier for antitumour drugs. J. Pharm. Pharmacol. **38:** 132–134.
28. KIMURA, A., H. YAMAGUCHI, K. WATANABE, M. YAYASHI & S. AWAZU. 1986. Factors influencing the tissue distribution of coenzyme Q₁₀ intravenously administered in an emulsion to rats: emulsifying agents and lipoprotein lipase activity. J. Pharm. Pharmacol. **38:** 659–662.
29. POSTE, G. & R. KIRSH. 1984. Site specific (targeted) drug delivery in cancer therapy. Biotechnology **1:** 869–878.
30. AKIMOTO, M., K. SUGIBAYASHI & Y. MORIMOTO. 1985. Application of magnetic emulsions for sustained release and targeting of drugs in cancer chemotherapy. J. Controlled Rel. **1:** 205–215.
31. GAL, D., M. OHASHI, P. C. MCDONALD, H. J. BUCHSBAUM & E. R. SIMPSON. 1981. Low density lipoprotein as a potential vehicle for chemotherapeutic agents and radionucleotides in the management of gynecologic neoplasms. Am. J. Obstet. Gynecol. **139:** 877–885.
32. MILLER, K. W. & D. M. SMALL. 1983. Trioleincholesteryl oleate-cholesterol-lecithin emulsions: structural models of triglyceride-rich lipoproteins. Biochemistry **22:** 443–451.
33. HALBERT, G. W., J. F. B. STUART & A. T. FLORENCE. 1984. The incorporation of lipid-soluble antineoplastic agents into microemulsions—protein-free and analogues of Low Density Lipoprotein. Int. J. Pharmaceut. **21:** 219–232.
34. DAVIS, S. S. & L. ILLUM. 1986. Colloidal delivery systems. *In* Site Specific Drug Delivery. E. Tomlinson & S. S. Davis, Eds.: 93–110. Wiley. Chichester.
35. ILLUM, L., S. S. DAVIS & P. WEST. 1987. The effect of surface properties on the fate of intravenously administered emulsions.
36. LUBRAN, M. & J. D. PEARSON. 1958. A screening test for steatorrhoea using, ¹³¹I-labelled triolein. J. Clin. Pathol. **11:** 165–169.
37. TONAKI, H., T. M. SABA, L. W. MAYRON & E. KAPLAN. 1976. Phagocytosis of gelatinized "R.E. Test Lipid Emulsion" by Kupffer cells: electronmicroscopic observations. Expl. Mol. Path. **25:** 189–201.
38. ILLUM, L., S. S. DAVIS, R. H. MULLER, E. MAK & P. WEST. 1987. The organ distribution

and circulation time of intravenously injected colloidal carriers sterically stabilised with a block copolymer Poloxamine 908. Life Sci. **40:** 367–374.

39. GUDEWICZ, P. W., J. MOLNAR, M. Z. LAI, D. W. BEEZHOLD, G. E. SIEFRING, R. B. OFEDO & L. LORAND. 1980. Fibronectin-mediated uptake of gelatin-coated latex particles by peritoneal macrophages. J. Cell Biol. **87:** 427–433.

40. VERMESS, M., D. H. M. LAU, M. D. ADAMS, R. M. HOPKINS, G. B. HOEY, G. GRIMES, D. C. CHATTERJI, M. GIRTON & J. L. DOPPMAN. 1982. Biodistribution study of ethiodized oil emulsion 13 for computed tomography of the liver and spleen. J. Comp. Assisted Tomogr. **6:** 1115–1119.

41. JEPPSSON, R. & S. ROSSNER. 1975. The influence of emulsifying agents and of lipid soluble drugs on the fractional removal rate of lipid emulsions from the blood stream of the rabbit. Acta Pharmacol. Toxicol. **37:** 134–144.

42. LOPEZ-BERESTEIN, G., R. L. JULIANO, K. MEHTA, R. MEHTA, T. MCQUEEN & R. L. HOPFER. 1986. Liposomes in antimicrobial therapy. *In* Targeting of Drugs with Synthetic Systems. G. Gregoriadis, J. Senior & G. Poste, Eds.: 221–228. Plenum Press. New York.

43. LOPEZ-BERESTEIN, G., V. FAINSTEIN, R. HOPFER, K. MEHTA, M. P. SULLIVAN, M. KEATING, M. G. ROSENBLUM, R. MEHTA, M. LUNA, E. M. HERSH, J. REUBEN, R. L. JULIANO & G. P. BODEY. 1985. Liposomal amphotericin B for the treatment of systemic fungal infections in patients with cancer. A preliminary study. J. Infect. Dis. **151:** 704–710.

44. WASHINGTON, C. & S. S. DAVIS. 1987. An emulsion formulation of Amphotericin B. UK. Patent application 8714652.

45. MEHTA, R., R. LOPEZ-BERESTEIN, R. HOPFER, K. MILLS & R. JULIANO. 1984. Liposomal amphotericin B is toxic to fungal cells but not to mammalian cells. Biochim. Biophys. Acta **770:** 230–234.

Membrane-to-Membrane Transfer
of Lipophilic Drugs Used against Cancer
or Infectious Disease[a]

R. L. JULIANO,[b,c] SAYED DAOUD,[b,c]
HANS-JURGEN KRAUSE,[b] AND C. W. M. GRANT[d]

[b]Department of Pharmacology
University of Texas Medical School
Houston, Texas 77096
and
[d]Department of Biochemistry
University of Western Ontario
London, Ontario

INTRODUCTION

The plasma membrane, as well as intracellular membranes, are potentially important sites of action for cytotoxic drugs, since membranes play a vital role in cell organization and function. However, there are relatively few clinically utilized drugs that have, as a major feature of their action, disruptive effects on the organization or functional activities of membranes. One reason for this is that such membrane active drugs are likely to be extremely toxic to tissues and organs whose physiological functions rely on ion gradients; this would include, of course, such vital organs systems as the kidney, the cardiovascular system, and the central nervous system. If, however, one could obtund the toxic effects of membrane active drugs on host systems, while maintaining cytotoxic potency to pathogens or to tumor cells, then membrane active agents could provide an exciting new avenue for therapy of infectious or neoplastic disease. This would be of particular importance in the arena of cancer chemotherapy. Most current antineoplastic drugs act on the biosynthesis, replication, or stability of DNA and thus have similar, predictable toxicities usually involving organs with rapidly dividing cell populations. Drugs that act on membranes should offer a different spectrum of toxicities and thus would be able to complement and provide a valuable adjunct to therapeutic regimens using "conventional" anticancer drugs. It was with these concepts in mind that we began, some years ago, to explore the possibility of using drug carrier systems to manipulate the pharmacodynamic behavior of membrane-active drugs.

A phospholipid vesicle–based delivery system (liposomes) seemed an ideal choice as a carrier for membrane-active drugs. Most drugs of this type are highly hydrophobic entities and, as such, can be readily accommodated by intercalation into the phospholipid bilayer membranes of liposomes. Thus, liposomes provide a convenient means for formulation of otherwise insoluble drugs. We also hypothesized that the use of a

[a]Supported by grants from the National Institute of Health (CA 36840) and the Elsa Pardee Foundation (R.L.J.) and by a University of Western Ontario development grant (C.W.M.G.).
[c]Present Address: Department of Pharmacology, University of North Carolina Medical School, Chapel Hill, NC 27514.

phospholipid carrier would have dramatic effects on the kinetics, tissue distribution, and possibly on the toxic/therapeutic ratios (i.e. the therapeutic index) of lipophilic membrane active drugs. One of our first studies[1] simply investigated the effects of lipophilic drugs on liposome stability and physical properties. More recently, our laboratories, as well as collaborating laboratories, have investigated the toxic, therapeutic, and mechanistic consequences of incorporating membrane-active drugs in liposome carriers.

One of the most exciting developments thus far concerns the polyene antibiotic amphotericin B (AMB). This drug is a mainstay in the therapy of serious systemic fungal infections, such as those occurring prevalently in immunocompromised patients suffering from leukemias, lymphomas, or AIDS, or in those intentionally immunosuppressed for organ transplantation.[2] Amphotericin B is a very lipophilic agent that readily partitions into membranes. The drug can then form a complex with membrane sterols leading to the creation of transmembrane channels that allow the egress of ions and critical small metabolites, thereby eventuating death of the cell. Thus, amphotericin B belongs in the category of substances known as channel-forming ionophores.[3] The drug can be used in man because it displays a somewhat higher affinity for ergosterol, the primary fungal sterol, than for cholesterol, the major sterol of mammalian cells.[4,5] Nonetheless, amphotericin B is an extremely toxic substance whose utilization is almost universally accompanied by unpleasant acute side effects and by chronic impairment of renal function.

During the last four years, a series of studies has demonstrated that the incorporation of AMB into liposomes of an appropriate type, permits a marked reduction in the toxicity of the drug to animals, with full retention of therapeutic efficacy in the treatment of systemic fungal infections.[6,7] This has been followed by a preliminary clinical trial of liposome-incorporated AMB, which seemed quite promising.[8] In this report we go on to explore the mechanism of action of liposomal AMB and demonstrate that the enhanced therapeutic index observed *in vivo* can most likely be understood in terms of a fundamental alteration of the ability of the drug to partition into different types of cellular membranes.

Recently, we have also extended the use of liposome carriers for membrane-active drugs to the arena of antitumor therapy. Valinomycin is a cyclic depsipeptide with remarkably selective ionophoric activity for potassium.[9] It has been widely employed as a mobile ionophore in studies of cell membrane function. Valinomycin has been shown to display considerable antitumor activity in murine tumor models; however, it has not been extensively developed as an anticancer drug because of its profound host toxicity.[10,11] Recently, we have shown that the incorporation of valinomycin in an appropriate liposomal carrier can markedly reduce host toxicity with maintenance of substantial antitumor activity, using the murine P388 leukemia as a model system.[12] In this report, we will discuss these observations as well as possible mechanistic bases for the effects seen *in vivo*.

RESULTS AND DISCUSSION

Studies on the Mechanism of Action of Liposomal Amphotericin B

It has previously been shown that the incorporation of amphotericin B (AMB) into multilamellar liposomes composed of dimyristoyl phosphatidyl choline/dimyristoyl phosphatidyl glycerol (7:3 molar ratio) produces a marked reduction in the *in vivo* toxicity of the drug as compared to its current clinical formulation (Fungizone®, a deoxycholate micelle of AMB). An approximately twenty-fold reduction in toxicity is

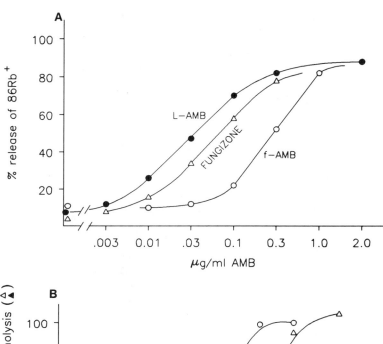

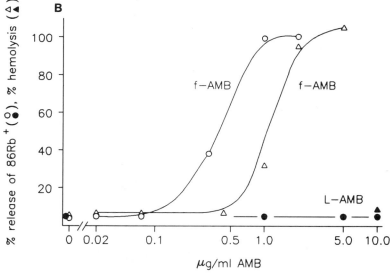

FIGURE 1. AMB effects on ion fluxes in yeast cells and erythrocytes. (A) Candida. The release of $^{86}Rb^+$ during a 90-min interval at 37°C caused by various concentrations of free or liposomal AMB was measured. Points are means of triplicate determinations. Liposomal AMB (●——●), Fungizone (△——△), and Free AMB (○——○). (B) Erythrocytes. The release of $^{86}Rb^+$ and the hemolysis induced by various concentrations of free or liposomal AMB during 60-min incubation at 25°C was determined. Points are means of triplicate determinations. Free AMB with ^{86}Rb release (○——○), free AMB with hemolysis (△——△), L-AMB with ^{86}Rb release (●——●), and L-AMB with hemolysis (▲——▲).

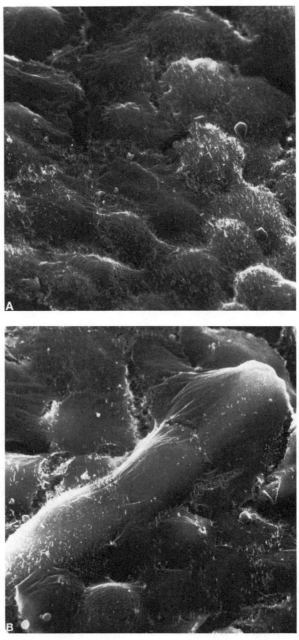

FIGURE 2. Effects of AMB on kidney cell cultures. (A) Control LLCPK₁ culture, (B) Culture treated with free AMB 10 (μg/ml), and (C) Culture treated with liposomal AMB (1000 μg/ml) (legend: 1 cm = 5.5 microns).

observed in mice and a substantial reduction in toxic effects in patients is also manifest.[6,8] Nonetheless, the liposomal formulation of AMB (L-AMB) is at least as potent as Fungizone in therapy of systemic candidiasis in a murine model. Given current understanding of the *in vivo* behavior of liposomes,[13,18] one might postulate several factors capable of contributing to the superior therapeutic index of L-AMB. These might include alterations in drug kinetics, particularly sustained release of drug; altered drug distribution, including enhanced uptake by phagocytic reticuloendothelial cells (which also can take up fungal organisms); and enhanced immunostimulating effects of L-AMB as compared to Fungizone. However, in an important series of preliminary experiments, Mehta *et al.*[14] observed that, while "free" AMB and L-AMB were equally potent in killing candida albicans cells *in vitro*, the only "free" AMB was

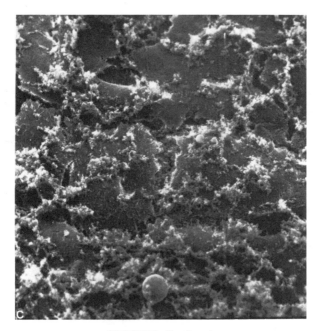

FIGURE 2. Continued

cytolytic to human red cells. In other words, L-AMB displayed an enhanced selective toxicity toward fungal cells in a simple *in vitro* situation. We have recently gone on to perform more extensive mechanistic studies of the actions of AMB and L-AMB on fungal cells and mammalian cells *in vitro*. In these studies we have made use of the fact that cytotoxicity of AMB is related to its actions as a channel-forming ionophore. Thus, we have used ion flux measurements to quantitate AMB actions on fungal and mammalian cell membranes.

The effects of "free" AMB and L-AMB on cation fluxes in yeast cells (candida albicans) and in mammalian erythryocytes are illustrated in FIGURE 1. Thus, "free" AMB and AMB in DMPC/DMPG liposomes are equipotent in inducing ^{86}Rb efflux from yeast cells, with approximately 0.03 μg/ml of either form of drug causing 50%

isotope release in 1 hr. By contrast, while "free" AMB induces ^{86}Rb efflux (and cell lysis at slightly higher doses) in red cells, L-AMB is essentially without effect. This confirms the high degree of selective toxicity of L-AMB for fungal cells as opposed to mammalian cells, a sharp contrast to the relatively non-selective actions of "free" AMB.

The reduced toxicity manifested by L-AMB is not confined to erythrocytes but rather seems to be generally true for a variety of mammalian cells. Thus, we have demonstrated that incorporation of AMB in DMPC/DMPG liposomes reduces the toxicity of the drug to murine macrophages and lymphocytes.[15] Further, the scanning electron micrographs of FIGURE 2 illustrate the relative effects of "free" AMB and L-AMB on LLCPK$_1$ cells (a porcine kidney cell line, which displays many markers characteristic of proximal tubule cells).[16] This is particularly important since the proximal tubule is one of the major sites of AMB toxicity *in vivo*. Thus, FIGURE 2 (A) illustrates the normal morphology of a monolayer of LLCPK$_1$ cells. FIGURE 2(B) shows the effect of 10 μg/ml of "free" AMB; a marked swelling of the cells is observed consistent with disruption of ionic balance. FIGURE 2(C) illustrates cells treated with L-AMB (1000 μg/ml). Despite the fact that large numbers of drug-containing liposomes are adherent to the monolayer, the morphology of the cells is apparently normal. These morphological observations are closely paralleled by functional measurements of protein synthesis and nutrient fluxes in these cells (HJK, unpublished). Thus, in the case of cultured proximal tubule cells, as in the case of erythrocytes, the inclusion of AMB in liposomes confers a remarkable protection against the cytotoxic actions of the drug.

The data of FIGURES 1 and 2 suggest that the membranes of mammalian cells inherently lack susceptibility to the actions of AMB when the drug is presented in liposomal form. We wished to determine if the relative resistance of mammalian cell membranes to L-AMB could be ascribed to the properties of the cell membrane lipids alone, or whether membrane proteins or proteoglycans played a role as well. To pursue this question, we prepared extracts of total red blood cell membrane lipids (RBC lipids), used these lipids to prepare liposomes containing entrapped [86]Rb (RBC liposomes), and then used the radiolabeled liposomes as a "target" to measure the relative actions of free AMB or L-AMB. As seen in FIGURE 3, free AMB caused a 50% release of ^{86}Rb from RBC liposomes, whereas L-AMB failed to cause appreciable isotope release at concentrations up to 160 μg/ml. Thus, liposomes composed solely of RBC lipids, lacking any cellular protein components, are far more sensitive to free AMB than to L-AMB, just as is the case with intact cells. This experiment suggests that it is the physical properties of the membrane lipids that are the prime determinant of the lack of sensitivity of mammalian cells to L-AMB.

We also wished to determine whether the physical properties of the donor liposomes could alter the effects of L-AMB on mammalian cells and on fungal organisms. All of the work described thus far utilized liposomes composed of DMPC/DMPG (7:3), a formulation extensively studied *in vivo*. In FIGURE 4, however, we illustrate some effects of varying the phospholipid composition of the donor liposome on the toxicity of L-AMB to mammalian cells. Thus, AMB liposomes prepared from saturated phosphatidyl cholines (DMPC, DLPC) caused essentially no ^{86}Rb efflux from red cells at concentrations up to 30 μg/ml; by contrast, AMB liposomes prepared from unsaturated phosphatidylcholines (DOPC) were almost as potent as free AMB in causing cation release. Both types of liposomes were equally toxic to candida albicans (data not shown). We have extensively explored the role of liposome composition in the selective toxicity of L-AMB, and have examined the effects of more than 20 distinct compositions.[17] We have varied both the polar head group, substituting the zwitterionic PC head group both with PE (also zwitterionic)

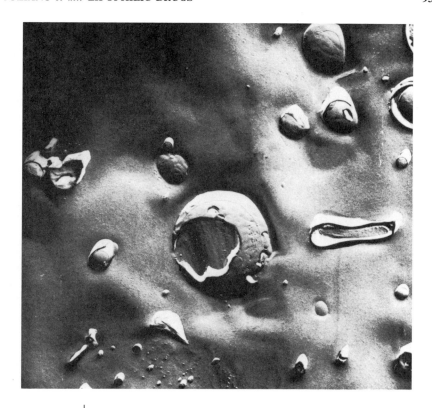

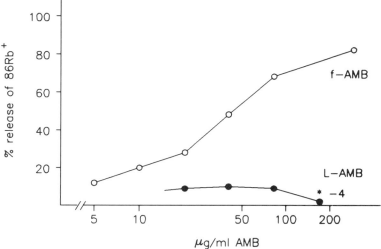

FIGURE 3. AMB effects on ^{86}Rb$^+$ efflux in large unilamellar vesicles prepared from red cell lipids. (A) Freeze-fracture EM of LUVs composed of red cell lipids. (B) Release of ^{86}Rb$^+$ from LUVs composed of red cell lipid was determined. Results are means of triplicate determinations. Free AMB (O—O) and L-AMB (●—●). *The value for this point was less than control.

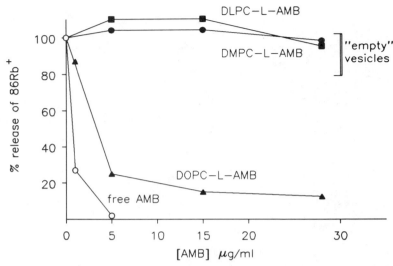

FIGURE 4. Effect of donor lipid composition on AMB-induced $^{86}Rb^+$ release from red cells. The release of $^{86}Rb^+$ from red cells during 60-min incubation at 25°C was determined. Points represent the means of triplicate determinations. The brackets (]]) indicate the range of $^{86}Rb^+$ release caused by various compositions of "empty" liposomes. Free AMB (O—O), AMB in DLPC liposomes (■—■), AMB in DMPC liposomes (●—●), and AMB in DOPC liposomes (▲—▲).

and PG (anionic); we have also examined the effect of varying the acyl chain composition and have studied the effects of including sterols in the formulation. A rough set of rules have emerged from these studies. (1) The prime determinant of toxicity is the acyl chain composition; saturated phosphatidycholine (PC) liposomes (either fluid phase or gel phase) containing AMB are non-toxic to mammalian cells, while unsaturated PC liposomes containing AMB are toxic. (2) Substitution of PE for PC head groups in AMB-containing liposomes has no effect; partial substitution of anionic PG head groups for PC of the same acyl chain composition tends to reduce toxicity to mammalian cells. (3) Cholesterol-containing AMB liposomes remain toxic to fungal cells while displaying low toxicity to mammalian cells; ergosterol-containing liposomes lose potency versus fungal cells and tend to be somewhat toxic to mammalian cells. (4) The toxicities displayed by various formulations of L-AMB are not related to simple physical stability properties. All preparations examined, both those toxic to mammalian cells and those not toxic, bind AMB in a stable fashion and do not release substantial quantities of the drug into free solution.

Since there are such marked differences in the selective toxicity of different formulations of L-AMB, we attempted to ascertain if there were corresponding differences in the physical properties of the liposomes that might explain the pharmacological effects. In particular, we were interested in knowing whether AMB perturbed the bilayer membranes of different liposome types to different degrees. These studies were carried out using freeze-fracture electron microscopy as well as electron spin resonance (ESR) spectroscopy, in order to examine changes in bilayer organization consequent to the intercalation of AMB. As seen in FIGURE 5, the inclusion of a low mol% of AMB in a variety of liposome types produced only minor changes in the observed fracture faces. This suggests that AMB can be incorporated into liposomes without gross perturbation of membrane structure, that the L-AMB preparations are relatively homogeneous and, in particular, that there is no evidence of amorphous structures that might represent AMB aggregates not incorporated into the liposome membranes. The morphological observations are essentially confirmed by the ESR studies illustrated in FIGURE 6. Thus, the phase transition temperatures of several

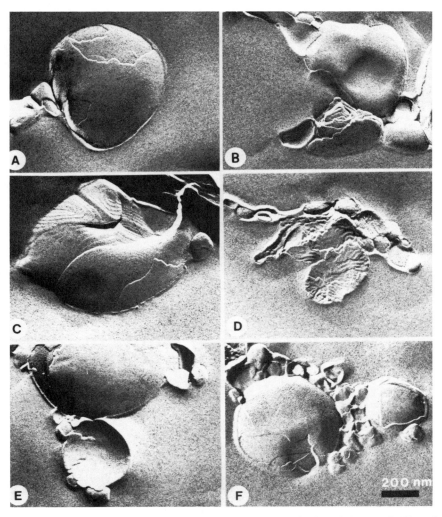

FIGURE 5. Freeze-fracture electron micrographs of liposomes of DOPC (A), DMPC (C), and DSPC (E) formed by hydration of dry films with normal saline. The accompanying micrographs show DOPC with 4.9 mol % AMB (B), DMPC with 3.05 mol % AMB (D), and DSPC with 2.7 mol % AMB (F). Samples were quenched from 20°C. Shadow direction is from bottom to top. Magnification × 71,333.

liposome types including DOPC, DMPC, DSPC, and DMPC/DMPG are only modestly affected (1–2°C shift) by the incorporation of 3–5 mol% of AMB into the bilayer. The first AMB liposome composition (DOPC) is quite toxic to mammalian cells while the remainder are not. Thus, at this time, we have no obvious correlation between the physical properties of L-AMB formulations and their toxicities to mammalian cells.

In summary, the enhanced therapeutic index of L-AMB observed *in vivo* is likely related to the selective toxicity of certain formulations of L-AMB manifested *in vitro*. The prime determinants of this selective toxicity seem to be the lipid composition of the "target" cell membrane and the lipid composition of the "donor" liposomes. In other studies,[17] we have accumulated preliminary evidence that AMB transfers from "donor" liposomes to "target" cells by diffusion of AMB monomers or oligomers through solution, rather than by "collision" of the AMB liposomes with the target cell. Thus, the selective toxicity of L-AMB seems to involve a preferential or selective membrane-to-membrane transfer of the drug, regulated by the physical properties of both "donor" and "target" membranes.

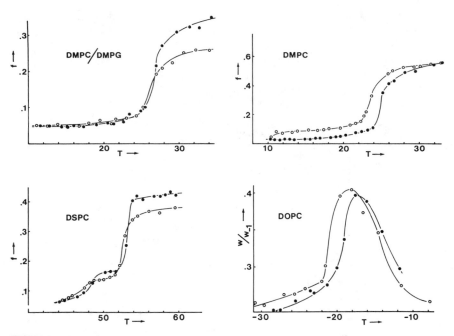

FIGURE 6. Phase Behavior Profiles for liposomes with and without AMB.[17] Curves derived from EPR spectral data displaying the melting characteristics of liposomes used are shown: Filled circles are for lipid alone, open circles denote the presence of AMB. The TEMPO spectral parameter, f, has been plotted for 7:3 DMPC/DMPG (5.0 mol % AMB); DMPC (3.1 mol% AMB); and DSPC (5.0 mol % AMB) as a function of temperature, T, in °C. For DOPC (and its mixture containing 4.9 mol % AMB) the ratio, w/w_{-1}, of midfield to highfield spectral linewidth has been plotted. All samples were in normal saline; the data shown for DMPC/DMPG were derived in the presence of 2 mM Ca^{2+} at pH 7.4. Without Ca^{2+} the curves for DMPC/DMPG and DMPC/DMPG/AMB were virtually identical to those shown, but shifted to lower temperatures by 2.7°C and 2.1°C, respectively.

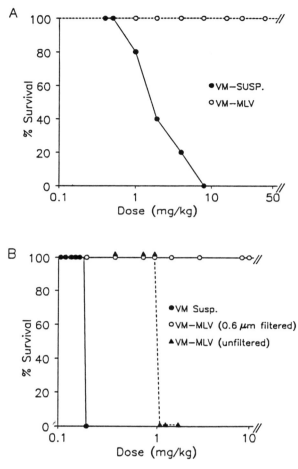

FIGURE 7. Reduction of valinomycin toxicity using liposomes. Groups of 6 B6D2F1, mice each were given injections i.p. (A) or i.v. (B) with free VM or liposomal valinomycin (VM-MLV) and the acute toxicity was monitored for 1 week following the injected dose. The doses of lipid in the VM-MLV preparations ranged from 1–100 mg. In some cases, the VM-MLV preparations were filtered through 0.6 μ Nucleopore filters. Abscissa dose of VM; Liposome composition, DMPC:CH:PS (10:4:1). SUSP, suspension.

STUDIES ON LIPOSOMAL VALINOMYCIN—
A POTENTIAL ANTITUMOR DRUG

Investigations on liposomal AMB, showing that the toxicity of this channel forming ionophore could be markedly reduced via incorporation into liposomes, encouraged us to ascertain whether the toxicity of other membrane active drugs could be reduced in a similar fashion. In these studies we sought to extend the strategy developed with the antifungal drug AMB, to the arena of cancer chemotherapy. We began to work with

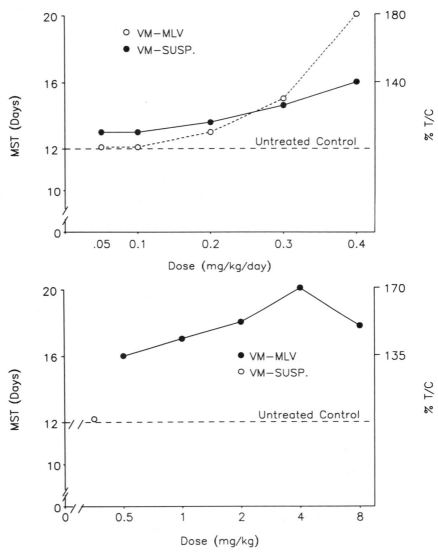

FIGURE 8. (Top) Antitumor activity of free or liposomal valinomycin against P388 leukemia. B6D2F1 mice were inoculated with 1×10^4 P388 leukemic cells i.p. on day 0; i.p. treatment was started on day 1 for 5 days with free VM or liposomal valinomycin. The doses of VM ranged from 0–0.4 mg/kg, which is the MTD for free VM. Liposome composition, DMPC:CH:PS (10:4:1). MST, median survival time and SUSP, suspension. (Bottom) Effect of a single high dose of liposomal valinomycin on P388 mice. B6D2F1 mice were inoculated with 1×10^4 P388 cells i.p. on day 0 and treated i.p. 24 hr later with single variable doses of MLV-VM or free VM. Liposome composition, DMPC:CH:PS (10:4:1). MST, median survival time; SUSP, suspension.

valinomycin, a cyclic peptide with potassium selective ionophoric activity. Although this compound exhibits considerable activity in several animal tumor screens, it has been considered to be too toxic for development as an anti-cancer drug.[11] We incorporated valinomycin, a highly lipophilic substance, into multilamellar liposomes; preliminary investigations suggested that a composition containing DMPC:Chol:PS (10:4:1 molar ratio) could confer some protection against valinomycin toxicity while providing a stable, easily formulated preparation. We then began to investigate, in some detail, the toxicity and antitumor efficacy of this preparation in the P388 murine tumor model.

The data shown in FIGURE 7 illustrate how profoundly the incorporation of valinomycin into liposomes affects the toxicity of the drug. Whereas "free" valinomycin (an ethanolic suspension) displayed an LD_{50} of approximately 1 mg/kg when given i.p. or 0.2 mg/kg given i.v., the respective LD_{50}s for the liposomal form of the drug were >50 mg/kg i.p. and 10 mg/kg i.v. Interestingly, the mean size of the liposomal valinomycin preparation was an important determinant of toxicity when the drug was given intravenously. The decrement in toxicity is achieved without loss of antitumor potency. Thus, when small doses of free or liposomal valinomycin (in a multiple i.p.

TABLE 1. Therapeutic Effect of i.v. Administered Valinomycin on i.v. P.388 Leukemia: Free and Liposomal (DMPC:CH:PS) Valinomycin Were Used at 25% of Their MTDs

Treatment	Valinomycin Total Dose (mg/kg)		Median Survival Time (Days)		% T/C	
	VM Suspension	VM-MLV	VM Suspension	VM-MLV	VM Suspension	VM-MLV
Single	0.045	2.50	9(8)	9(8)	100	100
Daily (1–9)	0.405	22.50	9(8)	13(8)	100	144
Every 12 hr × 3	0.270	15.00	9(8)	12.5(8)	100	138
Untreated control			9(12)			

Relative percentages of median survival of test and control animals. Numbers in parenthesis, number of B6D2F1, mice.

dose format) are compared, the liposomal drug is as potent as the free in terms of increasing the survival of tumor-bearing animals (FIG. 8a). Further, since liposomal valinomycin is so much less toxic then free drug, large single doses of the liposomal drug can be given that produce substantial antitumor effects; single doses of free valinomycin, at the maximal tolerated dose, display no antitumor action (FIG. 8b). Thus, in some circumstances, liposomal valinomycin is actually more efficacious than free drug as well as displaying lower toxicity.

The antitumor actions of liposomal valinomycin are manifested against disseminated leukemia as well as against the intraperitoneal form of the disease. Thus, as shown in TABLE 1, liposomal valinomycin, given intravenously, can produce substantial increases in the survival of animals with disseminated leukemia; by contrast, free valinomycin, is ineffective in this context. Presumably then, the liposomal drug is able to reach and exert its cytotoxic effects on systemically disseminated leukemia cells, not just on cells confined to the peritoneal cavity. It should be noted, however, that therapy of intravenously injected P388 leukemia requires intravenous injection of the liposomal drug; i.p. administration of liposomal valinomycin is ineffective in treatment of disseminated disease (data not shown).

In contrast, to the case of liposomal AMB, we do not presently have a clear picture of the mechanisms underlying the enhanced therapeutic index of liposomal valinomycin. It is possible that valinomycin is selectively toxic to transformed cells, as has been suggested by Kleuser et al.[19] and that the incorporation of valinomycin in liposomes enhances this selectivity. Alternatively, the reduced toxicity we have observed with the liposomal form of the drug may be due to the protection of critical organs caused by changes in pharmacokinetics and/or drug distribution. This may allow expression of sufficient direct toxicity to tumor cells to cause substantial impairment of tumor growth, while avoiding unsupportable toxicity to the host. Finally, we must also consider the possibility that liposomal valinomycin may prove to be a strong immuno-stimulating agent, and that the impairment in tumor growth is consequent to activation of host defense systems, most likely macrophages. These questions are currently under investigation.

SUMMARY

Use of liposomal drug delivery systems can enhance the therapeutic potential of membrane active anti-cancer and anti-infectious drugs. Thus, the therapeutic index of the important antifungal agent amphotericin B is markedly improved via incorporation of the drug into liposomes. The mechanistic basis of this effect seems to be an increase in the selectivity of the drug at the cellular level. Thus, free amphotericin B can readily partition into both fungal and mammalian membranes and can cause toxicity to both types of cells, giving rise to the notorious in vivo toxicity of this drug. By contrast, when amphotericin B is formulated in certain types of liposomes, the drug still readily partitions into fungal membranes but can no longer partition into animal cell membranes, thus markedly reducing its toxicity. Liposomes can also be used to reduce the toxicity of membrane-active antitumor drugs. Thus, the peptide ionophore valinomycin is far less toxic to animals when presented in liposomal form. Nonetheless, the drug retains useful antitumor activity in this form. The underlying basis of the enhanced therapeutic index of liposomal valinomycin is unknown at this time but is being explored. The development of membrane-active anti-tumor drugs, in conjunction with liposomal delivery systems, could be an important new approach in cancer chemotherapy. While no anticancer drug is likely to be free of toxic side effects, the toxicities engendered by membrane-active antitumor drugs are likely to affect a different spectrum of tissues and organs than those caused by "conventional" antitumor drugs. Thus membrane-active drugs could complement existing drugs and provide a valuable adjunct to therapy.

REFERENCES

1. JULIANO, R. L. & D. STAMP. 1979. Interaction of drugs with lipid membranes: Characteristics of liposomes containing polar or non-polar anti-tumor drugs. Biochim. Biophys. Acta **586:** 137–145.
2. MEDOFF, G., J. BRAJTBURG, G. S. KOBAYASHI & J. BOLARD. 1983. Antifungal agents useful in therapy of systemic fungal infections. Annu. Rev. Pharmacol. Toxicol. **23:** 303–330.
3. OUCHINNIKOV, Y. A. 1979. Physico-chemical basis of ion transport through biological membranes: inophores and ion channels. Eur. J. Biochem. **94:** 321–336.
4. KERRIDGE, D. 1979. The polyene macrolide antibiotics. Postgrad. Med. J. **55**(647):653–656.
5. READIO, J. D. & R. BITTMAN. 1982. Equilibrium binding of amphotericin B and its methyl ester and borate complex to sterols. Biochim. Biophys. Acta **685**(2):219–224.

6. LOPEZ-BERESTEIN, G., R. MEHTA, R. L. HOPFER, K. MILLS, L. KASI, K. MEHTA, U. FAINSTEIN, M. LUNA, E. M. HERSH & R. L. JULIANO. 1983. Treatment and prophylaxis of disseminated candida albicans infections in mice with liposome encapsulated amphotericin B. J. Infec. Dis. **147:** 939–945.
7. JULIANO, R. L., G. LOPEZ-BERESTEIN, R. L. HOPFER, R. MEHTA, K. MEHTA & K. MILLS. 1985. Selective toxicity and enhanced therapeutic index of liposomal polyene antibiotics in systemic fungal infections. Ann. N.Y. Acad. Sci. **446:** 390–402.
8. LOPEZ-BERESTEIN, G., V. FAINSTEIN, R. HOPFER, M. SULLIVAN, M. ROSENBLUM, R. MEHTA, M. LUNA, E. HERSH, J. REUBEN, K. MEHTA, R. L. JULIANO & G. BODEY. 1985. A preliminary communication: treatment of systemic fungal infections in cancer patients with liposome encapsulated Amphotericin B. J Infect. Dis. **151:** 704–710.
9. PRESSMAN, B. L. & M. FAHIM. 1982. Pharmacology and toxicology of the monovalent carboxylic ionophores. Annu. Rev. Pharmacol. Toxicol. **22:** 465–490.
10. SUFFNESS, M. & J. DOUROS. 1980. Miscellaneous natural products with antitumor activity. Med. Chem. **16:** 465–487.
11. REPTA, A. J. 1981. Formulation of investigational anticancer drugs. *In* Topics in Pharmaceutical Sciences, D. D. Breimer & P. Speiser, Eds: 131–151. Elsevier/ North-Holland Biomedical Press. Amsterdam.
12. DAOUD, S. & R. L. JULIANO. 1986. Reduced toxicity and enhanced antitumor effects in mice of the ionophoric drug valinomycin when incorporated into liposomes. Cancer Res. **46:** 5518–5523.
13. POZNANSKY, M. & R. L. JULIANO. 1984. Biological approaches to the controlled delivery of drugs: a critical review. Pharmacol. Rev. **36:** 277–336.
14. MEHTA, R., B. LOPEZ-BERESTEIN, R. HOPFER, K. MILLS & R. L. JULIANO. 1984. Liposomal amphotericin B is toxic to fungal cells but not to mammalian cells. Biochim. Biophys. Acta **770:** 230–234.
15. MEHTA, R., K. MEHTA, G. LOPEZ-BERESTEIN & R. L. JULIANO. 1985. Effect of liposomal amphotericin B on murine macrophages and lymphocytes. Infect. Immun. **47:** 429–433.
16. YONEYAMA, Y. & J. E. LEVER. 1984. Induction of microvillar hydrolase activities by cell density and exogenous differentiation inducers in an established kidney epithelial cell line (LLC-PK$_1$). J. Cell. Physiol. **121:** 64–73.
17. JULIANO, R. L., C. W. M. GRANT, C. BARBER & M. A. KALP. 1987. Mechanism of the selective toxicity of amphotericin B incorporated into liposomes. Mol. Pharm. **31:** 1–11.
18. PAPAHADJOPOULOUS, D. 1987. Ann. N.Y. Acad. Sci. (this volume.)
19. KLEUSER, B., H. REITER & C. ADMA. 1985. Selective effects of valinomycin on cytotoxicity and cell cycle arrest of transformed vs. nontransformed rodent fibroblasts *in vitro*. Cancer Res. **45:** 3022–3028.//0A

Magnetic Microspheres for the Targeted Controlled Release of Drugs and Diagnostic Agents[a]

DAVID F. RANNEY AND HOLLY H. HUFFAKER

Laboratory of Targeted Diagnosis and Therapy
Department of Pathology
University of Texas Health Science Center
Dallas, Texas 75235

INTRODUCTION

Pharmaceutical agents with very high toxicities or production costs, short circulation times, and low plasma stabilities may require special methods of delivery in order to limit systemic side effects, deposit acceptable fractions of the injected dose in target tissues, and control local bioavailability in a manner that treats target cells or microorganisms but not bystander cells.[1] Criteria for drug targeting vary, but, the most standard one in the pharmaceutical industry is that the therapeutic index should increase by at least one-half to one order of magnitude. Hence, true targeting causes drug levels in liver, bone marrow, kidney, and other major sites of toxicity to rise by less than one-third to one-tenth of the increment achieved in the selected target organ (tissue). There are two exceptions to this. The first is "site-avoidance targeting," in which drug is allowed to reach therapeutic levels in multiple nontarget as well as target sites, provided it avoids major organ(s) of toxicity. A second exception occurs when the objective is to localize a relatively nontoxic drug for reasons of rapid plasma clearance, biodegradation, high production costs, or limited commercial availability.

The difficulty of targeting drugs *in vivo* using high-molecular-weight and supramolecular carriers (e.g., monoclonal antibodies and drug-receptor conjugates, polymeric drugs, liposomes, and standard microspheres) is that the body contains not one, but three major test tubes: the blood-vascular, extracellular, and intracellular compartments. Except for reticuloendothelial organs, which have highly porous sinusoidal endothelium, the remaining organs exhibit microvascular barriers that severely restrict the extravasation of drug carriers above ca. 3–5 nm in molecular diameter.[2,3] This means that many potential carriers of sufficient molecular size to encode receptor-binding information are excluded from the extravascular compartment of normal target organs other than liver, spleen, bone marrow, and (variably) kidney. Diseased regions of organs (e.g., infarcts, infections, and tumors) exhibit variable breakdown of microvascular barriers. For example, in experimental tumors whose vascular filtration properties have been sized using fluoresceinated dextrans, moderate permeabilities are reported for 150,000-dalton species and lower permeabilities for up to 3,000,000-dalton species.[4] Even with partial breakdown, the largest soluble molecules (e.g., drug-DNA complexes), molecular microaggregates (of 3–100 nm) and the smallest

[a]Studies were supported by National Institutes of Health CA15673; the Departments of Pathology and Radiology, University of Texas Health Science Center, Dallas; and grants from the Upjohn Company, Eli Lilly, and the Dallas Foundation for Health Education and Research.

particles (≥ 50 nm in diameter) experience rates of lesional accumulation that are generally too slow to compete with faster rates of active hepatic clearance. Due primarily to this problem, the peak tissue concentrations of monoclonal antibodies are frequently only 1.5–3 times higher in tumors than surrounding normal tissues,[5] and only one-third to one-tenth as high in tumors as in liver.[5] This highlights the major challenges facing drug targeting *in vivo*, namely, that the initial biodistribution of drug carrier and its transport into the tissue compartment (second test tube) are the primary bioengineering problems that must be solved before the possibilities of cell-receptor binding and cell uptake can be meaningfully addressed.

In developing efficient approaches to targeting, it is instructive to observe how the body localizes its own biopharmaceuticals in diseased tissues. It does this by inducing targeted extravascular migration of drug carriers in the form of white blood cells, which produce controlled tissue release of proteolytic enzymes, potent toxins (e.g., interleukin 2, tumor necrosis factor, and lymphotoxin) and oxygen-free radicals.[6] Normal bystander cells, which lie in the microenvironment of disease, are frequently damaged and occasionally killed, however, these effects are minimized by the controlled manner in which the most potent toxins are released. Long-lived lipid peroxides are formed secondarily. These mediators, together with elevated tissue metabolites and fragments of coagulation proteins[7] induce opening of endothelial-cell junctions. Microvascular filtration is increased nonspecifically for plasma albumin, alpha globulins, antibodies, polymeric drugs, and diagnostic polymers. Because most white-cell toxins are degraded locally, the remainder of the body is relatively protected except in very severe disease. Naturally occurring inflammatory mediators are largely nonspecific in relation to the surface receptors of microorganisms and tumors. In designing drug carriers, immunologically specific targeting may be undesirable because of target heterogeneity, which results from mutation and cell cycle–dependent modulation of surface antigens. Additionally, tumors have the capacity to shed surface antigens and survive when perturbed by drug-receptor conjugates and cytolytic antibodies.[8] In this context, a "magic shotgun pellet" may be preferable to a "magic bullet" from the standpoints of efficacy and general pharmaceutical utility.

Given these biological barriers and responses, the major objectives of drug targeting must be to produce localized, controlled release of broad-spectrum agents within the extracellular compartment of the desired organs or tissues. The most immediate "targets" for circulating carriers are endothelial cells because they reside in the same compartment as the carriers. Efficient transport across microvascular barriers can be achieved by one of three means: (1) magnetic dragging of specialized microparticles directly through endothelium and basement membrane[9–11] (2) facilitated transport of specific ligand-drug conjugates (biochemical targeting),[12,13] or coated microparticles (bioadhesion targeting)[13,14] across endothelium as a result of ligand binding to luminal surface antigens or receptors, and (3) transient, regional opening of endothelial junctions combined with vascular infusion of drug carriers that become sequestered in the extracellular compartment.[13,15] For each approach, it is important to decide if the objective is to traverse (or permeabilize) (1) normal endothelium—the requisite target for delivering physiologic mediators—or (2) structurally altered endothelium—the requisite target for treating tumors and infections that induce biochemical and physical changes in the adjacent endothelium. It is also necessary to protect endothelial cells and normal parenchymal cells from the instantaneous bioavailability of toxic agents.[13,15,16] Hence, carriers with a stabilized entrapment matrix, such as microspheres, may be preferable to free drugs, polymeric drugs, and unstabilized liposomes, all of which make portions of their drug available as they interact with the first cell membranes encountered *in vivo:* red cells, white cells, and vascular endothelium.

TRANSVASCULAR MAGNETIC MICROSPHERES

Magnetic localization is the most efficient method yet developed for targeting agents other than stable hormones. Up to 60% of an injected dose can be deposited and control-released in selected nonreticuloendothelial organs. This efficiency is achieved at significant cost. Magnetic targeting is an expensive, technical approach that requires specialized manufacture and quality control of microspheres and that depends on specialized magnets for targeting, advanced techniques for monitoring, and trained staff to perform the procedures. Multiple body regions can be treated, but this must be accomplished sequentially. Magnets must be used that have relatively constant gradients, in order to avoid focal overdosing with toxic drugs. A portion (ca. 40–60%) of the Fe_3O_4, which is entrapped to magnetize spheres, is deposited permanently in target tissue. The total dose of iron required to treat a 1,000 g tumor is about 7 mg. Whereas extensive epidemiologic evidence in hematite miners indicates that Fe_3O_4 (magnetite) deposition at 100-fold higher levels is nontoxic to lung over occupational lifetimes,[17] magnetic drug targeting is likely to be approved only for very severe diseases that are refractory to other approaches. Such targeting will be limited to specialized centers; and to anti-tumor, anti-fungal, transplantation, and CNS agents that are highly toxic or labile. These include adriamycin, amphotericin B, certain neuropeptides, immunosuppressives, prostaglandins, white-blood-cell chemoattractants (e.g., f-met-leu-phe), interleukin 2, tumor necrosis factor; and potentially in the future, magnetized white blood cells and labile gene vectors for which efficient tissue deposition is required to reconstitute the involved organ(s). Despite these problems, there are three major advantages to magnetic targeting: (1) it achieves therapeutic responses in target organs at only one-tenth of the free drug dose; (2) it affords controlled drug release within target tissues for intervals of 30 minutes to 30 hours, as desired; and (3) it avoids acute drug toxicity directed against endothelium and normal parenchymal cells.

Magnetic microspheres are made by mixing water-soluble drugs (or lipophilic drugs + water-soluble adducting agents) and 10-nm magnetite particles in an aqueous solution of the matrix material (typically albumin), emulsifying this mixture in biodegradable oil, ultrasonifying or shearing to produce submicron particles, stabilizing the matrix by controlled heating or chemical cross-linking, extracting the oil with a volatile organic solvent (typically hexane or ether), and lyophilizing the preparation to dryness. Resulting spheres have a magnetite content of ca. 20% (by weight). They also have a shelf life of greater than one year at 22°C. No "burst" release of drug occurs during storage. An electron micrograph of the original magnetic microspheres (containing adriamycin) is shown in FIGURE 1.

MECHANISMS OF TARGETING

Magnetic microspheres are usually injected either into the arterial supply to the target organ for high-efficiency systemic targeting, or intravenously for high-efficiency pulmonary targeting or medium-efficiency systemic targeting. Because these spheres are considerably smaller than the 4-μm size that distinguishes nonembolizing from embolizing particles, they would normally pass through target capillaries and be cleared by liver, spleen, and bone marrow ($t_{1/2}$ of 20 min). However, because they are subjected to an extracorporeal gradient magnetic field of 0.55–0.8 Tesla, they are captured in small arterioles and capillaries of the magnetic targeting volume. Using high-efficiency vascular routes in two rat models, approximately 55% of injected spheres were localized in the magnetic segment of rat tail tissue (0.8 Tesla field),[9,11] and 40% of the injected spheres were localized in the thoracic viscera (35% in lungs and 5% in heart; 0.55 Tesla field).[13,18] In the second model, microsphere localization occurred within seconds of injection.[18] At linear flow rates below 0.75 cm/sec, magnetic force exceeds microvascular flow force. Spheres are dragged up the magnetic gradient and caused to pass both between and through endothelial cells into the interstitium of adjacent tissues.[9-11,18,19] Intravascular capture is complete within 2–5 minutes.[18] Extravascular migration is complete within 15 minutes, as determined morphometrically.[18] Plasma levels of the entrapped agent reach peak values at about 2 minutes and then fall quickly as spheres captured initially on the luminal surfaces of endothelium are dragged out into the interstitium.[18] By electron microscopy, transen-

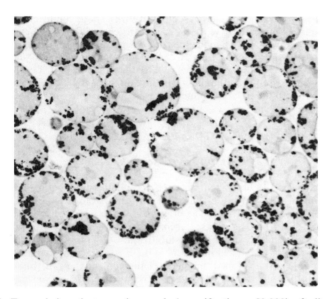

FIGURE 1. Transmission electron micrograph (magnification $\times 50,000$) of albumin microspheres containing entrapped Fe_3O_4 and adriamycin. Spheres range from ca. 0.35 to 1.6 μm in diameter. Small black particles are micoaggregates of 10-nm Fe_3O_4. Albumin matrix appears grey; adriamycin is not visualized by this method. (Adapted from Widder et al.[11,19])

dothelial migration of micron-sized albumin spheres is seen to be nontoxic to endothelium. This is true for both placebo and drug-containing spheres (adriamycin and amphotericin B).[9-11,18,19]

MAGNET DESIGN

Microsphere targeting depends on the force exerted on magnetically susceptible particles by a gradient magnetic field. The relationship of force, field gradient, and the magnetic moment of particles is expressed in the general equation: $F = M \cdot \nabla H$; where F = force on particles, M = magnetic moment of particles after saturation magnetization (see text below), and ∇H = magnetic field gradient.[20] This equation indicates that particles with increased magnetic moments will experience a force sufficient for extravascular migration at reduced field gradients. The earliest targeting studies demonstrated that satisfactory localization of microspheres with 20% Fe_3O_4 (by weight) could be achieved in rat organs using magnets of 0.55–0.8 Tesla, 0.01 Tesla/mm (gradient) and 0.4–0.8-cm (diameter) pole faces positioned next to the target tissue (normal lungs and tail tumors).[9–11,18] In subsequent attempts to treat dog-limb sarcomas using adriamycin microspheres, a larger, 1.8-Tesla electromagnet was used that had a single, chisel-shaped pole piece 10 cm in width.[21] Technical problems were encountered initially due to field inhomogeneity, which caused focal overcapture of microspheres. An optimal solution to this problem lies in using a field whose gradient is nearly constant throughout the targeting volume, and having the microspheres flow initially through a high-field region, which magnetizes them to saturation levels just prior to microvascular capture. These conditions are met by a quadripolar field configuration[13] (FIGURE 2) (P. Antich and D.F. Ranney, unpublished studies). As tested by computer modeling, this design produces a field gradient whose magnitude varies by less than 15% across the targeting volume. A 2-Tesla electromagnet of this configuration will produce the required gradient of 0.01 Tesla per mm over the 40-cm pole gap required for human targeting. Such magnets can be constructed for one-fifth to one-tenth the cost of a magnetic resonance imager.

PROTOTYPE CARRIERS

Anti-Tumor Microspheres

Adriamycin was the first agent selected for magnetic targeting because it was effective against a wide variety of human solid tumors but also caused irreversible, dose-dependent cardiomyopathy.[22] The original albumin microspheres contained 4.5% drug (by weight).[9–11] This was released according to first-order kinetics with $t_{1/2}$'s of 15 min to 8 hr, depending on matrix stabilization.[23] Transarterial targeting was performed using a rat-tail model in which an 0.8 Tesla gradient magnet was oriented perpendicular to a distal, 4-cm ("magnetic") segment of the tail. In representative studies, 215 μg of spheres were localized per gram of tissue (wet weight) in the "magnetic" tail segment, while only 25 μg per gram were cleared by liver—a ratio of 8.6:1 favoring the target tissue.[9–11,19] Drug release was documented histologically by the appearance of diffuse adriamycin fluorescence in tissues surrounding localized spheres.[19] Resulting drug concentrations were monitored by fluorescence measurements of tissue extracts (TABLE 1). In subsequent studies, malignant Yoshida sarcomas, were grown in the tails of Holtzman rats. These tumors underwent complete remission in 75% of animals following a single transarterial magnetic targeting of microsphere adriamycin at 0.5 mg/kg given 6–8 days after tumor inoculation ($N = 12$).[24] By contrast, no remissions were achieved with free drug at 10 times the dose (5 mg/kg i.v.) given either intra-arterially or intravenously on days 1, 5, and 9 ($N = 10$). In a second study performed with Yoshida sarcomas, microsphere-targeted vindesine sulfate produced total remission of tumors in 85% of rats at both 0.5 and 2.5 mg/kg.[25] Free vindesine was ineffective at 0.5 mg/kg and was lethal due to toxicity at 2.5 mg/kg. Spontaneous canine osteogenic sarcomas have been largely refractory to intra-arterially targeted adriamycin spheres (R.C. Richardson, personal communication). Other agents have yet to be tested in the canine model. The LD_{50} dose of 1-micron (diameter) placebo albumin-magnetite spheres in CBA mice is 1,250 mg/kg (D.F. Ranney, unpublished studies). Hence, the ratio of toxic dose of placebo spheres

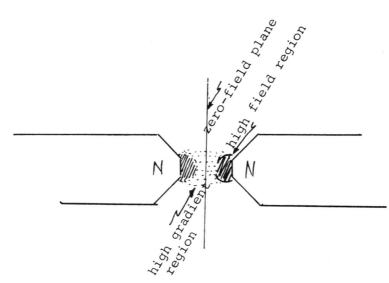

FIGURE 2. Diagram of quadripolar magnetic field for improved homogeneity of microsphere localization. Uniform gradient region is shown as dotted and high-field region as cross-hatched. A zero-field region exists at the midplane between pole pieces. Other arrangements are made possible by introducing additional pole pieces. In order to avoid microsphere aggregation in the infusion syringe, injections are performed near the zero-field region.

to effective dose of adriamycin spheres is 113:1. The use of albumin as a matrix material has also proved safe from the standpoint of allergic reactions. None were observed in 50 patients who received serial injections of large (diagnostic) albumin microspheres over a course of 3 weeks to 12 months.[26] The tendency of albumin to become phagocytized and cleared from target sites within 8 hours of localization may functionally limit the interval of controlled drug release that can be achieved in target tissues.[19,26–28] However, this problem can be overcome by using more inert carrier materials such as polymers of the intermediary metabolites, poly-L-lactic and polyglycolic acids. These remained at their original subcutaneous injection sites for intervals

TABLE 1. Localization of Microsphere-Delivered and Free Adriamycin[a]

Form of Drug	Dose[c] (mg/kg)	Magnet[d]	Tissue Concentrations[b] (μg/g wet weight)	
			Target Tail Skin	Liver
Microsphere	0.05	−	<1	<1
	0.05	+	3.9	<1
Free	0.05	−	<1	<1
	5.00	−	3.3	15.0

[a]Adapted from Widder *et al.*[11,19]
[b]At 30 minutes after infusion; limits of detection 1 μg/g.
[c]Drug and microspheres infused into the ventral caudal artery of tail.
[d]0.8 Tesla field.

of months to years.[13,29] Improved magnets and carriers are under development that could make selected human applications feasible.[13]

Chemoattractant Microspheres

Neutrophil chemoattractant, f-met-leu-phe, was selected as the first biomodulator for magnetic targeting because it was lethal when administered freely in the circulation at concentrations above ca. 2×10^{-7} M, and it required regional localization in order to meet the objective of facilitating local inflammation. In a recently developed rat-lung model, almost all of the intravenously injected microsphere f-met-leu-phe became localized in either lungs (25%) and heart (3%), or liver (49%) and spleen (8%).[18] In order to produce acute effects, the $t_{1/2}$ of peptide release was designed to be 20 minutes. Because of the low total dose (15.7 μg/kg), high efficiency of pulmonary targeting, and rapid reticuloendothelial clearance of untargeted agent, free blood levels remained below 1.9×10^{-8} M (10 times lower than the acute LD_{50} concentration).[18] Within target tissues, controlled release and the hydrophobic nature of f-met-leu-phe facilitated membrane binding and maintained a tissue reservoir of entrapped plus released agent. Total tissue levels stayed nearly constant over a post-targeting interval of 5 to 70 minutes, at 2.9×10^{-6} M and 2.7×10^{-6} M, respectively (150 times the peak free-plasma concentration). Locally released f-met-leu-phe broadcasted an attractant signal to circulating neutrophils that migrated out of adjacent arterioles and capillaries into the interstitium next to microsphere fragments. When the injected dose was selected to produce tissue levels above ca. 3.3×10^{-8} M, extravascular neutrophils were activated to release O_2^- and lysosomal enzymes.[13,18,30] This resulted in local acute tissue injury and edema. If the injected dose was lowered by a factor of 3.3, chemoattraction occurred without significant neutrophil activation (D.F. Ranney, unpublished results). Targeted f-met-leu-phe also attracted alveolar macrophages, which engulfed almost all excess microsphere material that passed across alveolar septa into the small air spaces.[13,18] By this means, excess f-met-leu-phe was detoxified and cleared in the sputum. Targetable f-met-leu-phe could be used in experimental as well as therapeutic applications. For example, in pulmonary medicine, it could be used (1) as a test for new drugs that block lung elastin destruction in smokers; (2) as a method to study relationships between acute alveolar damage and adult-type respiratory distress syndrome (ARDS); and (3) as an adjuvant therapy for patients with deep pulmonary aspergillosis (in whom hyphal forms predominate and are susceptible to extracellular killing by neutrophil products).

Magnetic Neutrophils

In certain clinical states, the indirect approach of targeting chemoattractant may not work due to generation of chemotactic factor inactivators or neutrophil-directed inhibitors of chemotaxis. These disorders include Hodgkin's disease, chronic lymphocytic leukemia, sarcoidosis, alcoholic cirrhosis, hemodialysis, Chron's disease, and severe infections (especially abdominal abscesses with neutrophil anergy). Hence, a method was developed for making the cells ingest Fe_3O_4 particles so that they could be targeted directly by magnetic means (D.F. Ranney and P. Meunier, unpublished studies). Normal human blood was processed to enrich for granulocytes and eliminate erythrocytes.[31] The enriched cells were adhered to specially treated culture plates, which allowed subsequent detachment without cellular damage. Nonadherent cells (mostly lymphocytes) were discarded. Magnetite particles of 10–50 nm were opsonized with human IgG, in order to facilitate ingestion by neutrophils via their Fc receptors. The adherent cells (granulocytes + monocytes) were allowed to ingest opsonized magnetite for 60 minutes. Excess magnetite was removed by washing, cells detached by gentle agitation, and single-cell suspensions made in normal saline. Magnetized granulocytes retained 80% of their functional activity, as assessed by a stimulated chemiluminescence assay for oxygen free-radical generation.[30] Magnetite ingestion was assessed in two ways. (1) It was visualized cytologically using a Prussian blue iron stain and was present intracellularly (ca. 60%) and extracellularly (ca. 40%) in both neutrophils (predominant cell type) and monocytes (minor). (2) The cells were tested by nuclear magnetic resonance (NMR) methods in which the quantity of cell-associated magnetite was approximated by its effect on the apparent T_2 relaxation time (T_2^*) of surrounding water protons. By the latter method, each adherent cell carried an average of 7 to 20 pg of magnetite (= range for three donor preparations). This represented 0.8–2.2% magnetite (by weight). We predicted this would be too low for neutrophil capture *in vivo*, however, significant magnetic localization did occur, as described below.

   In vivo targeting was performed by injecting $0.5–1.0 \times 10^6$ adherent cells i.v. into neutropenic test mice. To achieve lung localization, a 0.55-Tesla magnet was placed perpendicular to the right chest wall during the post-injection interval of 1 to 20 minutes. Mice were sacrificed at 40 minutes, lungs inflated to constant size with intratracheal formalin, and neutrophils quantified morphometrically (TABLE 2). Magnetic targeting increased the numbers of pulmonary neutrophils by a multiple of 2.6 compared to the nonmagnetic controls. The magnetic neutrophils were also capable of responding *in vivo* to f-met-leu-phe administered intratracheally. Why did targeting work at the low cellular magnetite contents measured above? Gamma-camera[32] and histologic images (D.F. Ranney and P. Meunier, unpublished studies) of lungs at 2, 20, and 40 minutes post-injection have revealed that *in vitro* processing of donor granulocytes causes them to bioadhere transiently to arteriolar and capillary endothelium of the recipient lung. This occurs for all categories of cells (with or without magnetite ingestion) and lasts for less than 20 minutes. Hence, the neutrophils that remained in lung at 40 minutes were actually targeted by the combined processes of cellular bioadhesion and magnetic retention. These results show that the biodistribution of functional white cells can be altered by extracorporeal magnetic guidance. They have also prompted new studies that suggest it is possible to target inert microspheres by bioadhesion alone.[13]

Amphotericin B Microspheres

   Invasive pulmonary aspergillosis is a life-threatening condition in neutropenic and immunocompromised patients. Amphotericin B remains the treatment of choice, however, it produces frequent, serious side effects.[33] The major one, nephrotoxicity, occasionally requires interruption of systemic therapy. Since alternative drugs are less effective, the result is compromised patient survival. Because of these problems, we have entrapped amphotericin B in magnetically responsive albumin microspheres for targeting to the lungs (or brain) and reticuloendothelial organs (D.F. Ranney, H. Huffaker, W. Welch, and P. Southern, unpublished studies). This was accomplished by adducting amphotericin B (AMB) to water-soluble γ-cyclodextrin (CD), entrapping the adduct in a fatty-acid–free albumin matrix, and heating the microspheres briefly at 135°C to produce controlled drug release. *In vitro* testing was carried out by suspending microspheres at 10 mg/ml in phosphate-buffered saline and washing once (with magnetic separation) to remove the minor fraction of rapidly released (surface)

TABLE 2. Neutrophils Localized in Target Lung at 40 Minutes

Magnetite in Cells	Magnet Over Target Lung[a]	Cells/cm²[b]
No	No	33.4 ± 2.3
Yes	No	32.0 ± 6.4
Yes	Yes	84.0 ± 7.2

[a]0.55 Tesla field; 0.01 Tesla/mm gradient over target lung.

[b]Sections = 5 μm thick; cells stained histochemically for neutrophil esterase + magnetite iron, as described; $N = 5$.[18]

drug. The washed spheres were resuspended in fresh buffered saline and either tested immediately or incubated in buffer, sedimented by centrifugation, and resuspended to test how much AMB remained in spheres after various intervals of release. Drug was bioassayed in the wells of bacteriological plates streaked with an amphotericin-sensitive strain of *Candida albicans*, which gave reliable quantification of growth inhibition at 24 hours (FIGURE 3). Note that microspheres are restricted to the well chambers, however, both of the wells which contain experimental spheres are surrounded by large zones of growth inhibition. This indicates that AMB-CD adducts

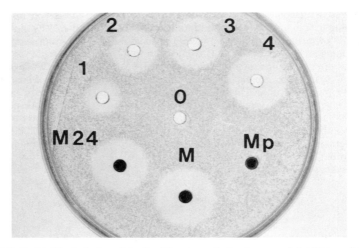

FIGURE 3. Bacteriological plate (Mueller-Hinton agar) showing growth inhibition of *Candida albicans* by microsphere amphotericin B. Plates incubated for 24 hours at 37°C. Samples 1–4, standards of 1:1 γ-cyclodextrin-amphotericin B, added as follows (μg/well): 1.3×10^{-2}, 3.5×10^{-2}, 7×10^{-2}, 1.4×10^{-1}. Sample 0, cyclodextrin alone at the same concentration as in the top cyclodextrin-amphotericin standard. M, Fe_3O_4 fatty acid–free human albumin microspheres containing 1:1 γ-cyclodextrin-amphotericin B, plated immediately after rapid washing and magnetic recovery of the controlled-release fraction. M24, same as M, except the washed spheres were incubated in phosphate-buffered saline for 24 hours at 37°C and recovered by centrifugation at $1750 \times g$ for 15 min, prior to plating at the same concentration as M. Mp, placebo microspheres (formulated as for M, except without amphotericin B). Drug values for M and M24 were read from a standard curve (not shown) of areas generated by standards 1–4. The ratio of M24/M = $(1.2 \times 10^{-1} \mu$g $/ 1.8 \times 10^{-1} \mu$g$) = 0.67$. Hence, the $t_{1/2}$ of amphotericin release in physiologic saline is greater than 24 hours.

(or AMB-CD-albumin complexes) are released in a form that diffuses through the agar gel for distances of greater than 5 mm. This has important implications for therapy of aspergillosis because it suggests that AMB, which would be released from microspheres at the periphery of characteristic lesional microthrombi, should also be capable of diffusing into an adjacent protein coagulum. Hence, microsphere-AMB-CD can probably gain access to sequestered *Aspergillus* hyphae. Results of delayed microsphere plating (FIGURE 3) indicate that the $t_{1/2}$ of AMB release in physiologic solutions is greater than 24 hours. Data (not shown) indicate that AMB is detectable in microspheres for up to 5 days of incubation in buffer. Hence, controlled bioavailability is compatible with maintenance of anti-fungal activity.

Preliminary experiments were carried out *in vivo* to test the acute pulmonary toxicity of AMB-CD microspheres. They were injected i.v. into CBA mice and magnetically targeted to lung (0.55-Tesla gradient field) in numbers calculated to

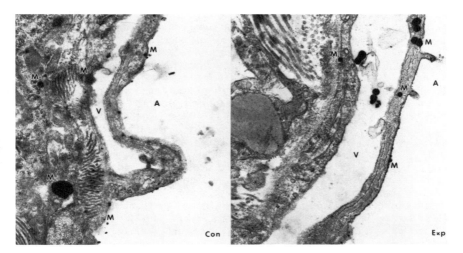

FIGURE 4. Electron micrograph (magnification $\times 15,000$) of CBA mouse lung 70 minutes after magnetic i.v. targeting of amphotericin microspheres. Exp, targeted Fe_3O_4 fatty acid–free human albumin microspheres containing 1:1 γ-cyclodextrin-amphotericin B (see text for injected dose). Con, targeted placebo microspheres formulated as for Exp, except without amphotericin. M, microspheres; V, vascular space; A, airspace.

deliver a supratherapeutic dose of AMB (lung dose equal to that delivered by 5 mg/kg of free AMB-desoxycholate). Based on the time required for induction of acute endothelial toxicity by f-met-leu-phe,[18] the present mice were sacrificed at 70 minutes. Light microscopic sections (not shown) revealed homogeneous microsphere localization and gave no evidence of septal edema, inflammatory cells, or hemorrhage. At 70 minutes, the majority of spheres had already migrated through endothelium into the interstitium. However, in isolated foci, clusters of spheres remained in or near capillary walls. Representative electron micrographs of these foci are shown in FIGURE 4. The endothelium that contained microspheres revealed no evidence of vesiculation, membrane redundancy, or vacuolation characteristic of acute toxicity. These results provide compelling evidence for an absence of endothelial toxicity during transcapillary migration of AMB-CD spheres. Controlled bioavailability also appeared to protect adjacent interstitium and epithelium from acute toxic effects of AMB. Efficacy studies are pending in immunosuppressed mice with experimentally induced pulmonary aspergillosis.

Interleukin 2 Microspheres

Interleukin 2 (IL-2) is a 15,000 MW glycoprotein made by activated T lymphocytes, that increases host cellular immune responses and augments resistance to certain tumors and infections.[34] Multiple cellular activities are boosted *in vivo,* including T helper cells, cytotoxic T cells, natural killer (NK) cells, and possibly also macrophages.[34,35] IL-2 is an ideal biopharmaceutical for experimentation because it is available as a cloned gene product and the recombinant human molecule is also active in mice. High doses of IL-2 have been reported to mediate regression of established pulmonary and hepatic metastases from selected murine tumors[36] and disseminated human tumors (particularly melanomas and renal cell carcinomas) that were unresponsive to conventional therapy.[34] A marked lymphocytic infiltrate of Leu 4+, Leu 2+, and Dr(+) cells is documented to have been induced by IL-2 in one regressing human melanoma.[34] Despite these promising findings, tumor treatment is fraught with difficulties. IL-2 is cleared rapidly from the plasma ($t_{1/2}$ = 3–6 minutes).[37] Consequently, it must be administered in extremely high doses (e.g., up to 3 million units/kg) over a 2–3 week interval in order to induce tumor regression.[34] High-dose treatment costs between \$30,000 and \$100,000 per round of therapy and entails severe toxicity, including: anemia (requiring multiple transfusions), severe thrombocytopenia, fever, marked hypotension, gastritis, azotemia, jaundice, skin eruptions, malaise, and confusion.[38] IL-2 also induces a capillary leak syndrome (increased capillary permeability) that can lead to severe (occasionally fatal) pulmonary edema and ascites that require aggressive management with diuretics and intubation in an intensive-care environment.[34,38]

Because of these almost unacceptable limitations on classical administration of IL-2, we are developing a controlled-release, microsphere form of agent that is adaptable to selected organ targeting by either magnetic or passive (embolic) localization (H. Huffaker and D.F. Ranney, unpublished studies). Bioassays of drug release have been carried out by adding serial dilutions of microsphere supernatants to an IL-2-responsive, CTLL-2 cell line, culturing for 16 hours, quantifying the pulsed incorporation of [³H]thymidine, and reading the experimental IL-2 units from a standard curve produced by free agent. By chemically cross-linking the carrier matrix, we have achieved controlled release with $t_{1/2}$'s of up to 42 minutes, and longer times are anticipated. Availability of a targetable, controlled-release form of IL-2 would allow localization in regions of residual tumor and infection in much the same way as occurs naturally when lymphocytes themselves localize and release IL-2.[39] Targeted delivery may also overcome the prohibitive costs associated with systemic administration. It has been suggested that IL-2's property of increasing capillary permeability could be used to increase tissue access of monoclonal antibodies.[34] In order for this to work in practice, permeability changes would need to be induced selectively in the regions around tumor rather than systemically, as occurs with free IL-2 (D.F. Ranney and P. Antich, work in progress). This is because lesional access of secondarily administered antibody occurs by a largely nonspecific process of ultrafiltration, which takes place wherever there is increased microvascular permeability. If this occurs in large organs, such as lungs and liver (established sites of IL-2-induced capillary leak), then antibody is depleted from the circulation and tumor uptake is compromised. Hence, the desired method of IL-2 delivery is one that targets it to tumor per se. Studies are underway to test the *in vitro* boosting of NK cells and the anti-tumor effects of targeted IL-2 *in vivo* (D.F. Ranney, H. Huffaker, M. Tutt, V. Kumar, and M. Bennett, work in progress).

MONITORING

Carrier Localization

In order to avoid normal tissue injury, washed, sized microspheres should be infused at a moderate rate, and appropriate methods should be used for monitoring blood flow and perfusion in target tissue. Magnetic shielding may be necessary to minimize microsphere capture in adjacent body parts (e.g., head vis-a-vis upper arm). It is also important to monitor the mass of microspheres that becomes localized in a given mass of tissue. Knowing this ratio and the *in vitro* release kinetics, one can estimate free tissue levels of drug at various times after targeting. This estimate is

TABLE 3. Effect of Albumin Microspheres[a] on NMR Proton Spin-spin (T_2^*) Relaxation[b] in Rat Target Organs

Organ	Fe_3O_4 in Spheres[c]	Tissue Fe_3O_4[d] ($\mu g/g$ wet wt)	Line Width at $\frac{1}{2}$ Peak Height ($1/\pi \cdot T_2$) (Hz)
Lung	−	0.0	454
	+	54.8	1395
Liver	−	0.0	120
	+	17.6	330

[a]Dose of spheres = 2 mg/kg.
[b]300 MHz NMR spectrometer.
[c]Fe_3O_4 content = 20% (w/w).
[d]Tissue iron measured by acidic oxidation of tissues and graphite-furnace photometry; Fe_3O_4 calculated from lattice formula for the mixed oxide.

crude because tissue enzymes may accelerate drug release and backdiffusion of drug into microvessels may accelerate drug clearance. Carrier dosing can be assessed by standard gamma dosimetry and imaging methods at a resolution of about 0.5–1 cm.[21,40] Alternatively, one can use NMR to evaluate carrier targeting, potentially at submilli-meter resolution. This is based on the capacity of ferromagnetic materials to decrease the apparent T_2 relaxation time (T_2^*) of water protons adjacent to localized spheres. The effect results from micro-inhomogeneities of the externally applied magnetic field, which are introduced by tiny magnetic dipoles of the ferromagnetic particles. It acts across distances of at least 1–3 microns. TABLE 3 shows the NMR spectral effects of targeting Fe_3O_4 microspheres to the right lung of a rat and allowing the escaping spheres to be cleared by liver (D.F. Ranney and R. Nunnally, unpublished studies). Although these early studies were performed on freshly excised organs, recent reports indicate that a related change (image darkening) occurs in standard proton magnetic resonance images.[41] This should make it possible to determine noninvasively at high resolution if microspheres have distributed evenly or unevenly by anatomic subre-gion.[21]

Drug Release and Tissue Effects

Because magnetic drug targeting reduces free blood levels of drug by a factor of 150, it is difficult to monitor circulating levels and extrapolate to corresponding tissue levels. Hence, drug monitoring must be carried out noninvasively on target tissue per se. This can be approached by performing positron emission tomography with labeled metabolic precursors and modeling the initial reaction kinetics of label within the major cellular compartment of the tissue. Alternatively, monitoring can be performed by NMR imaging and spectroscopy. For example, the rate of drug release from spheres might be monitored by attaching a paramagnetic label to the drug or to a substance

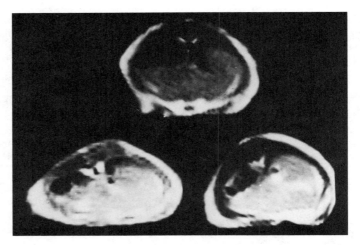

FIGURE 5. Magnetic resonance images at mid-liver of prone Sprague-Dawley rats, performed to demonstrate hydration and release of gadolinium chelate (Gd-DTPA) from dextran microspheres. Images are oriented transaxially and acquired at 5-mm thickness using a spin-echo pulse sequence (TR, 0.5 sec; TE, 26 msec). Experimental rats (lower panels) were imaged at post-injection times optimized for their respective agents. Upper image, uninjected control; lower left image, 15 min after i.v. injection of soluble Gd-DTPA (0.3 mmol Gd/kg); lower right image, 40 min after i.v. injection of Gd-DTPA-dextran microspheres (0.06 mmol Gd/kg). Both Gd rats had prominent liver brightening due to paramagnetic T_1 relaxation of water protons by hydrated (released) Gd chelate. As assessed by image-intensity analyses, microsphere-Gd was 11 times more potent than soluble DTPA-Gd, indicating selective uptake of microspheres by liver. Also, image enhancement by soluble Gd-DTPA had faded almost completely by 40 min, indicating Gd washout. (Adapted from Ranney et al.[42])

that is released at the same rate as drug. Paramagnetic substances (e.g., the metal ion, gadolinium, Gd^{+3}) are ones that become oriented in an external magnetic field but lose their orientation when the field is removed. In contrast to ferromagnetic materials (e.g., Fe_3O_4 above), paramagnetic ions and ion chelates have the following properties. They (1) act on susceptible nuclei (e.g., water protons) at distances of angstroms rather than microns; (2) produce preferential T_1-type rather than T_2-type relaxation at the low doses used *in vivo;* and hence, (3) induce brightening rather than darkening of magnetic resonance images. A paramagnetically tagged drug must be fully dissolved before adjacent water protons can move to within the short distances required for accelerating their magnetic relaxation. Consequently, only the fraction of drug that has been fully hydrated and released from microspheres should be detectable in target tissue. As an initial test of this hypothesis, we prepared heat-stabilized dextran microspheres to which had been chelated Gd^{+3}.[42] These spheres were designed to remain intact long enough for spontaneous particulate clearance by the livers of recipient rats, however, they were also designed to dissolve within 30 minutes of rehydration, so that all Gd^{+3} chelate would be rapidly released. The effect of injecting these spheres i.v. is shown in FIGURE 5.[42] Substantial image brightening of liver occurred at therapeutically relevant doses of microspheres. By contrast, microspheres that contained the same quantity of GD^{+3} chelate entrapped in a slowly releasing albumin matrix ($t_{1/2}$ = 8 hours) gave no enhancement at 30 minutes (data not shown). From these results, we conclude that, for microspheres with rapid and intermediate release kinetics, it should be possible to approximate the quantities of free tissue drug by paramagnetic methods (provided that tissue Gd^{+3} concentrations remain below levels at which T_2 effects predominate). For water-soluble drugs, this method may also allow the noninvasive measurement of capillary backdiffusion. It should be noted, that Gd-dextran microspheres were nontoxic, and there was almost complete clearance of Gd^{+3} chelate from test rats within 2 weeks of injection (as assessed by radioisotopic ^{153}Gd; P. Kulkarni and D.F. Ranney, unpublished studies). Hence, these new spheres may be a valuable diagnostic agent in their own right.

Targeting of Diagnostic Agents

The preceding microspheres contained no ferromagnetic material, and hence were incapable of extracorporeal guidance. However, in special experimental and clinical situations, it may be necessary to guide diagnostic agents selectively to nonreticuloendothelial organs. These include cases in which (1) systemic toxicity is high (e.g., fluorodeoxyglucose), (2) dose requirement is high (e.g., magnetic resonance image enhancement), and (3) tissue access is low (e.g., transport of circulating neuropeptides into brain). Ferromagnetic microspheres can provide the highly selective targeting required in these instances.

CONCLUSION

Magnetic drug targeting is a technologically involved but highly efficient means of delivering a select group of pharmaceuticals to single or multiple regional targets. For several new biopharmaceuticals, it is the only way at present to avoid toxic blood levels, distribute drugs homogeneously in target tissues, achieve adequate tissue levels, control bioavailability within tissues, and produce local effects with recombinant protein and peptide mediators.

ACKNOWLEDGMENTS

We thank Dr. Peter Antich for assistance with the section on magnet design, and Mrs. Carla Peacock for preparing the manuscript.

REFERENCES

1. VARGA, J. M. & N. ASATO. 1983. *In* Polymers in Biology and Medicine. E. P. Goldberg, Ed. **2:** 73–88. John Wiley and Sons, New York.
2. MAJNO, G. 1965. *In* Handbook of Physiology. Philip Dow, Ed. **3:** 2293–2375. American Physiological Society. Washington, D.C.
3. SIMIONESCU, M., N. SIMIONESCU & G. E. PALADE. 1975. J. Cell Biol. **67:** 863-885.
4. JAIN, R. K. 1985. Biotechnol. Progr. **1:** 81–94.
5. PIMM, M. V. & R. W. BALDWIN. 1984. Eur. J. Clin. Oncol. **20:** 515–524.
6. HATCH, G. E., D. E. GARDNER & D. B. MENZEL. 1978. J. Exp. Med. **147:** 182–195.
7. DANG, C. V., W. R. BELL, D. KAISER & A. WONG. 1985. Science **227:** 1487–1490.
8. OLD, L. J., E. STOCKERT, E. A. BOYSE & J. H. KIM. 1968. J. Exp. Med. **127:** 523–539.
9. WIDDER, K. J., A. E. SENYEI, S. D. REICH & D. F. RANNEY. 1978. Proc. Am. Cancer Res. **19:** 17.
10. SENYEI, A. E., K. J. WIDDER, S. D. REICH & D. F. RANNEY. 1978. Fed. Proc. Fed. Am. Soc. Exp. Biol. **37:** 316.
11. WIDDER, K. J., A. E. SENYEI & D. G. SCARPELLI. 1978. Proc. Soc. Exp. Biol. Med. **158:** 141–146.
12. GILLIS, C. N. & J. D. CATRAVAS. 1982. Ann. N.Y. Acad. Sci. **384:** 458–474.
13. RANNEY, D. F. 1986. Biochem. Pharmacol. **35:** 1063–1069.
14. LOPES, J. D., M. DOS REIS & R. R. BRETANI. 1985. Science **229:** 275–277.
15. NEUWELT, E. L., P. A. BARNETT, M. GLASBERG & E. P. FRENKEL. 1983. Cancer Res. **43:** 5278–5285.
16. ADAMSON, I. Y. R. 1984. Environ. Health Perspect. **55:** 25–36.
17. STOCKINGER, H. E. 1984. Am. Ind. Hyg. Assn. J. **45:** 127–133.
18. RANNEY, D. F. 1985. Science **227:** 182–184.
19. WIDDER, K. J., A. E. SENYEI & D. F. RANNEY. 1979. Adv. Pharmacol. Chemotherapy **16:** 213–271.
20. PURCELL, E. M. 1965. Berkeley Physics Course. **2:** 369. McGraw-Hill. New York.
21. BARTLETT, J. M., R. C. RICHARDSON, G. S. ELLIOTT, W. E. BLEVINS, W. JANAS, J. R. HALE & R. L. SILVER. 1984. *In* Microspheres and Drug Therapy: Pharmaceutical, Immunological and Medical Aspects. S. S. Davis, L. Illium, J. G. McVie & E. Tomlinson, Eds.: 413–426. Elsevier Science Publishers. Amsterdam.
22. ALEXANDER, J., N. DAINIAK, H. J. BERGER, L. GOLDMAN, D. JOHNSTONE, L. REDUTO, T. DUFFY, P. SCHWARTZ, A. GOTTSCHALK & B. L. ZARET. 1979. N. Eng. J. Med. **300:** 278–283.
23. WIDDER, K. J., A. E. SENYEI & D. F. RANNEY. 1980. Cancer Res. **40:**3512–3517.
24. WIDDER, K. J., R. M. MORRIS, G. POORE, D. P. HOWARD, JR. & A. E. SENYEI. 1981. Proc. Natl. Acad. Sci. USA **78:** 579–581.
25. MORRIS, R. M., G. A. POORE, D. P. HOWARD & J. A. SEFRANKA. 1984. *In* Microspheres and Drug Therapy: Pharmaceutical, Immunological and Medical Aspects. S. S. Davis, L. Illum, J. G. McVie & E. Tomlinson, Eds.: 439. Elsevier Science Publishers. Amsterdam.
26. RHODES, B. A., I. ZOLLE, J. W. BUCHANAN & H. N. WAGNER, JR. 1969. Radiology **92:** 1453–1460.
27. ZOLLE, I., B. A. RHODES & H. N. WAGNER, JR. 1970. Intl. J. Appl. Radiat. Isot. **21:** 155–167.
28. PETRIEV, V. M., T. R. BOCHKOVA, D. G. KHACHIROV & S. V. SERYI. 1976. Med. Radiol. **21:** 39–44.
29. HIGASHI, S., Y. YAMAMURO, Y. KATUTANI, Y. IKADA, S-H. HYON & K. JAMSHIDI. 1985. *In* Advances in Drug Delivery Systems. A. M. Anderson & S. W. Kim, Eds.: 167. Elsevier-North Holland. Amsterdam.
30. HATCH, G. E., D. E. GARDNER & D. B. MENZEL. 1978. J. Exp. Med. **147:** 182–195.
31. LOHR, K. M. & R. SYNDERMAN. 1982. J. Immunol. **129:** 1594–1599.
32. WORTHEN, G. S., C. HASLETT, L. A. SMEDLY, A. J. REES, R. S. GUMBAY, J. E. HENSON & P. M. HENSON. 1986. Fed. Proc. Fed. Exp. Biol. Med. **45:** 7–12.
33. STAMM, A. M. & W. E. DISMUKES. 1983. Chest **83:** 911–917.

34. LOTZE, M. T., A. E. CHANG, C. A. SEIPP, C. SIMPSON, J. T. VETTO & S. A. ROSENBERG. 1986. J. Am. Med. Assoc. **256:** 3117–3124.
35. HERBERMAN, R. B. 1985. Cancer Treat. Rep. **69:** 1161–1164.
36. ROSENBERG, S. A., J. J. MULE, P. J. SPIESS, C. M. REICHERT & S. L. SCHWARZ. 1985. J. Exp. Med. **161:** 1169–1188.
37. DONOHUE, J. H. & S. A. ROSENBERG. 1983. J. Immunol. **130:** 2203–2208.
38. MOERTEL, C. G. 1986. J. Am. Med. Assoc. **256:** 3141.
39. HARRIS, G. 1979. *In* Drug Carriers in Biology and Medicine. G. Gregoriadis, Ed.: 167–190. Academic Press. New York.
40. SCHLAFKE-STELSON, A. T. & E. E. WATSON, Eds. 1986. Proc. Fourth Intl. Radiopharm. Dosimetry Symp.: 1–700. Oak Ridge Associated Universities. Oak Ridge, TN.
41. STARK, D. D. & J. T. FERRUCCI, JR. 1985. Diagnostic Imaging **7:** 118–127.
42. RANNEY, D. F., J. C. WEINREB, J. M. COHEN, S. SRIKANTHAN, L. KING-BREEDING, P. KULKARNI & P. ANTICH. 1986. *In* Contrast Agents in Magnetic Resonance Imaging. V. M. Runge, C. Claussen, R. Felix & A. E. James, Jr., Eds.: 81–87. Excerpta Medica, Princeton, NJ.

Biopharmaceutics of Microparticulate Drug Carriers

J. E. O'MULLANE, P. ARTURSSON, AND E. TOMLINSON[a]

Advanced Drug Delivery Research
Ciba-Geigy Pharmaceuticals
Horsham
West Sussex RH12 4AB
United Kingdom

INTRODUCTION

The concept of site-specific drug delivery is an old one, but it is only recently that full consideration has been given to the ways in which this might be achieved in practice, due largely to the advent of the new biosciences.[1] Clearly, a drug's therapeutic index, as measured by its pharmacological response and safety, relies on the access and specific interaction of the drug with its candidate receptor, whilst minimizing its interactions with non-target tissues. Peptide drugs illustrate the case where failure in the clinic may not be due to a poor intrinsic activity, but rather to transport factors including widespread disposition, rapid catabolism and excretion, variable or inefficient extravasation, and the subsequent high dosing levels required to obtain a therapeutic effect.[2]

Site-specific drug delivery may be achieved by using carrier systems, where reliance is placed on exploiting both the innate pathway(s) that these carriers have, and the protection that they can afford to drugs during transit through the body. The use of a carrier opens up a range of opportunities for adjusting both drug access to its site of action and its pharmacological response that are not necessarily available by simple chemical modification of the drug alone.

Such carriers can be broadly categorized as soluble (macro)molecular drug conjugates and drug-bearing particulates. In this present paper, we shall consider some of the key pharmaceutical and biopharmaceutical aspects of microparticulate carriers ranging in size from 20 nm to 20 μm diameter. Such particles can be monolithic or capsular in construction; they have been proposed as drug carriers largely due to the features given in TABLE 1. These properties will be examined in some detail later, although we note here that carriers differ widely in these features. For example, small, unilamellar vesicles have a low drug-bearing capacity in relation to the composite mass of the carrier, whereas it is theoretically possible to synthesize a monolithic particulate carrier from bioactive peptides such that the carrier is composed entirely of this material.

We have argued that the strategy for site-specific drug delivery should be based on consideration of the *d*isease and drug *a*ccess, *r*etention, and *t*iming in its interaction with the target (DART).[3] Thus, in the treatment of a disease with a carrier system we need to have a clear understanding of the inherent anatomical and (patho)physiological opportunities (and constraints) for site-specific drug delivery, the intravascular or extravascular location of the target, the chronopharmacology of the drug, and the

[a]To whom correspondence should be addressed.

120

target site response, in addition to the potential side-effects and the clinical utility of the therapeutic system.

The ability to leave the blood pool (extravasate) in a reproducible, efficient, and (perhaps) specific manner is often central to drug action mediated by the use of carriers. Since the potential for particulate extravasation is limited, it is argued that the use of these carriers will probably be restricted to targets within discrete anatomical compartments, to intravascular targets, or to extravascular targets at highly specialized areas of endothelia, or where the pathology at the site permits particle extravasation. We shall discuss each of these in turn.

DISCRETE ANATOMICAL COMPARTMENTS

Several anatomical compartments exist where the placement of particulates will lead to their retention due to either the physical properties of the environment or the biophysical interactions of particles with the cellular components of the target tissue. This approach is best applied where a persistent and sustained presentation of drug is required at the target site. Compartments of relevance here include the eye, joints, and respiratory tract although we also detail the nasal passage and the gastrointestinal tract.

TABLE 1. Perceived Advantages of Microparticulate Drug Carriers

Relatively high payload of drug
Protection of drug and non-target tissues from each other
Controlled and sustained release of drug
Novel biological pathways of carrier followed by drug

The *eye,* and the cornea in particular, are easily accessible targets though dilution by lacrimal fluid, but washout effects[4] present difficulties in being able to retain microparticulate drug carriers at the cornea for more than a few hours. In recent years emulsions, liposomes, and latex preparations have been developed,[5,6] though with limited success. Gurny has described a novel approach using the ability of a nanoparticle suspension (having an adsorbed drug) to gel in the neutral pH environment of the cul-de-sac of the eye.[7] The rapid change in the viscoelastic properties of the particle suspension from fluid to gel ensures ocular retention of the dosage form and results in an improved therapeutic profile of the drug compared to a solution of the free drug applied topically.

The *intraarticular* injection of liposomes and monolithic particles has been examined in the treatment of both cancer and chronic inflammation. The persistence of such materials within the joint is related to their size, with larger particles (7 to 15 μm in diameter) being retained for longer periods.[8] There is also evidence that particles may be phagocytosed by the fixed macrophages within the synovium.[9] The intraarticular administration of liposomes containing the sterol cortisol palmitate has been successfully used to treat experimental arthritis in the knee joints of rabbits at relatively low doses of the drug,[10,11] although other issues, such as the host compatability of the carrier and the cost and suitability of alternative colloidal systems, have reduced the potential use of this novel mode of treatment.

Upon their inhalation, the access and retention of microparticulates within the *lung* depends on a number of factors, including the dynamics of air flow within the lung, the limiting diameter of the bronchioles, the ability of particles to translocate to the tracheobronchial lymph nodes, and the avoidance of the mucociliary escalator. Recent work has shown that instilled microspheres larger than 7 μm are effectively lodged in the pulmonary region. Particles of 3 μm to 7 μm in diameter, instilled into the lungs of beagle dogs can translocate to the tracheobroncheal lymph nodes[12] and appear to be extracellularly accumulated.[13] Small liposomes of 50 nm are retained for many hours, though those depositing in the tracheal bronchial regions are physically cleared within 6 hours by the mucociliary escalator.[14] Liposomes have, however, been used effectively to provide a sustained input to the lung tissue leading to an increase in drug efficacy and a decrease in drug toxicity.[15]

The *intranasal* route has been explored as a non-invasive alternative for the sustained input of peptides and proteins into the blood. Indeed, the serum levels of drugs after intranasal administration compare favorably with intravenous administration in certain cases.[16] Conventional nasal formulations are rapidly cleared from the nose, which has prompted the development of bioadhesive gels in order to prolong the residence time of, for example, insulin and calcitonin.[17] Bioadhesive microparticulates have recently been proposed as an alternative to the gel formulations.[18] Such particles would have pharmaceutical advantages to gels in offering greater control over the surface properties and drug release. Studies on the retention, side-effects (such as irritability), and elimination of intranasally administered particles will show whether these carriers hold promise as alternatives to current intranasal preparations.

The introduction of carriers into the systemic circulation via the *oral* route has largely been an unrealized ambition. Carriers have to survive mechanical disruption, drastic fluctuations in pH, resist the attack by digestive enzymes and surfactants, must have a significant residence time within the gastrointestinal tract at the site of absorption, and also enter and penetrate the epithelial barrier. The small intestine is the segment of the gastrointestinal tract with the highest absorption capacity and is made up of an anatomically continuous barrier of cells that permits the passage of low molecular weight materials by simple diffusion and other higher molecular weight materials either by specific (nutrient) processes or by cellular vesicular processes. Particles can pass in a specialized case where the epithelial barrier is immature (as demonstrated by the passage of spheres of 20 nm in suckling mice.[19] Interestingly, in the fully competent gastrointestinal tract, specialized cells lining the intestine can absorb indigenous bacteria and transport these through into the Peyers' patches of the gut-associated lymphoid tissue.[19] There are also other examples of M cell-mediated transport of viruses[21] and carbon particles.[22]

A key question is whether the M cell provides a suitable means of uptake of particulate carriers from the gastointestinal tract. Present evidence suggests that the capacity of these absorptive cells and the translocation of materials onwards from the uptake site are limiting factors in being able to utilize the system in a general way. However, since mucosal immune responses are initiated within Peyer's patches it can be postulated that a drug-carrier system sample through the M cells could be used in oral immunization to bring an appropriate immunomudulator to the attention of the mucosal immune system.

Claims have frequently been made that drugs given orally within liposomes have an enhanced intestinal absorption. Evidence suggests that if so, this is due to a protection of the drug or an enhanced drug availability at the mucosal surface rather than a transfer of intact liposomes.[23] Other microparticulate systems, such as albumin microspheres[24] and polymethylmethacrylate particles,[25] have been examined for peroral absorption. In the latter case, it was concluded that intact particles are not absorbed across the gastrointestinal tract. Although evidence for the transcellular passage of 200 nm diameter polystyrene latex particles was provided over 25 years ago, we are not aware that this has been examined subsequently.[26]

In conclusion, current evidence suggests that the transport of intact carriers across the gastrointestinal tract is restricted to exceptional and unusual circumstances.

INTRAVASCULAR TARGETS

The introduction of microparticulate carriers into the vasculature opens up a range of opportunities to targets either within the vasculature or to extravascular targets accessible via the capillary endothelium. In the discussion that follows, consideration will be given to the size and surface chemistry of microparticulates, and the extent to which these features dominate the processes of access and retention.

3.1 Capillary Filtration

The access afforded to microparticulate carriers will be governed primarily by the limiting diameter of the capillary bed that it will encounter upon parenteral administration.[27] Particles larger than the narrowest capillary bed will become filtered by virtue of their size. Thus, such particles injected intravenously (apart from the portal vein) will become entrapped in the capillaries of the lung.[28] This phenomenon has been exploited in the diagnostic use of radiolabeled human serum albumin microspheres (HAM) for the scintigraphic examination of tumor masses within the lung.[29] As a consequence, it has been proposed that large drug-loaded microspheres (larger than 7 μm in diameter) could be used in the treatment of lung diseases, such as emphysema. Martodam *et al.*[30] have demonstrated the feasibility of covalently attaching a peptide-linked inhibitor of human leukocyte elastase to the surface of HAM and the passive targeting of such a system to the lungs. Microspheres were found to be entrapped in the lungs and to have an extended half-life as compared to underivatized microspheres. Although it was shown that *in vitro* activity of the inhibitor was retained after coupling, *in vivo* activity of the construct was not demonstrated.

Capillary filtration by the lungs by large particles can be avoided by intra-arterial administration, and has its use in both diagnostic and therapeutic applications. For example, Torchilin has used microspheres of Sephadex to which thrombolytic enzymes including fibrinolysin, streptokinase, and urokinase were bound. Approximately 10–80 mg enzyme can be bound to one gram of carrier, and was found to be highly effective in the treatment of thrombi accessible via catheterization. A successful lysis of an experimental thrombus in a dog femoral artery was obtained by administration of a dose of immobilized fibrinolysin 100 times lower than was required by intravenous injection of the free enzyme.[31] There are serious doubts on the potential applications of the Sephadex carrier as there are difficulties in chemically linking drugs to the carrier matrix and the carrier is degraded only very slowly. In contrast, biodegradable starch microspheres can contain large amounts of entrapped enzymes and are rapidly degraded *in vivo*.[32]

Intra-arterial delivery of drugs using microparticulate systems to cancer masses typically uses one of the two approaches. In the first case the drug is incorporated into the particle matrix;[33] the access of the carrier and its retention are controlled by the pathophysiology of the tissue and the release of the drug is controlled by the system variables of the microsphere preparation. For example, the intraarterial administration of a bolus of particles of a diameter greater than 15 μm in rabbits bearing V2 carcinomas was found to result in a distribution of the particles to tumor capillaries, in preference to the surrounding (normal) capillaries by a factor of four.[34] This effect would appear to be due to a quantitative greater capillary supply to the tumor compared with the supply to the normal tissue.[35] In the second case, the co-administration of particles and drug in solution is postulated to increase the dwell time of the drug within the local vasculature, thus increasing the probability for extravasation.[36]

The working hypothesis, in both of these cases, is that at the point of blockage, there will be a high concentration of drug for an extended period of time. It is assumed that this leads to an increased concentration of the drug at its pharmacological receptor. This hypothesis is largely unproven. In the case of emphysema, for example, it is accepted clinically that the target site is the interstitium of the lung.[37] It is yet to be demonstrated that there is a benefit in using drugs coupled to microspheres as opposed to using free drug in being able to access the interstitium of the lung from the blood pool. It has also been shown that the access of the carrier and its retention are controlled by hemodynamic considerations.[38] The trapping of a microsphere at the trunk level of the arterial tree will restrict the blood supply to the branches, creating areas of ischemia. The erosion of the particle would be expected to proceed most rapidly on the side of the microsphere in contact with the flowing blood. A disadvantage in this process would be that the released drug would be carried in the efferent blood rather than be restricted to the target site. As the microsphere diameter is reduced by surface erosion, it passes up to the narrower branches where it will become

TABLE 2. Cells of the MPS[40]

Kupffer cells (stellate cells lining the walls of the hepatic sinusoids)
Blood-borne macrophages
Tissue macrophages (histiocytes)
Reticulum cells (of the reticular connective tissue)
Hotega cells (microglia of the central nervous system)

trapped again. The process of erosion continues until the particle has reached a size at which it escapes the narrowest capillary and may then be sequestered by cells of a mononuclear phagocytic system.

3.2 Mononuclear Phagocytic System

Particles small enough to avoid capillary filtration are generally cleared from the circulation by cells of the mononuclear phagocytic system (MPS). This system is a connective tissue of cells mesenchymal in origin (TABLE 2). Other cells, primarily the endothelial cells of the liver, take part in the clearance of small particles by the liver by non-phagocytic endocytosis. The main functions of the MPS include the clearance of a large variety of potentially harmful substances from the plasma, catabolism of macromolecules, participation in the immune response, and the synthesis and secretion of various effector molecules.

Normally, when colloidal particles are injected intravenously, about 90% are removed from the circulation by the Kupffer cells, 5% by the spleen, and the few remaining percent by the bone marrow.[39] The circuitry of the blood is such that the spleen and liver are in series and the bone marrow in parallel;[40] the dominance of the liver as the site for clearance reflects the accessibility and capacity of uptake of these macrophages rather than reflecting a paucity of macrophages at other sites. There is, however, considerable species variation, with the rabbit (in particular) exhibiting a greater bone marrow uptake than other observed species.[41] It is becoming clear that the extent of particle clearance by the MPS is determined primarily by the physicochemical nature of the surface, although other factors, such as the nature of the particle matrix, particle stability, and physiological state of the species can be important.[42]

The phagocytosis of particulates by the MPS and phagocytic cells in culture is understood to be mediated by the adsorption of plasma proteins by a process known as opsonization.[43] The opsonized particle adheres to the phagocytic cell membrane and is subsequently engulfed by the phagocytosing cell. The surface of macrophages bears over thirty receptors, including those to the Fc portion of immunoglobulins and the C3b component of complement.[44] Opsonins mediate the onset of phagocytosis by their ability to bind to the particle surface and to the target receptors on phagocytes. Since the Fc region is common to all immunoglobulins, regardless of antigenic specificity, IgG can act as a bridge between the macrophage and the foreign material that is to be engulfed.

The phagocytosis of foreign particulates depends on opsonic selectivity and specificity for surface structures.[45] In addition to the well-described involvement of IgG and complement C3 in the phagocytosis of natural particles,[46] there is also firm evidence for the involvement of other proteins, such as fibronectin,[47] in the opsonization and phagocytosis of synthetic particulate carriers. (For a review of the interaction of liposomes with serum proteins see Bonte & Juliano.[48])

Surface manipulations can result in qualitative and quantitative alterations in opsonization and thence macrophage uptake. Such effects are clearly demonstrated by the chemical modification of the erythrocyte.[49] For example, mild chemical treatment of erythrocytes *in vitro* with N-ethylmalemide results in splenic extraction after reinjection. More severe treatment of erythrocytes with glutaraldehyde leads to Fc-mediated clearance by the liver. Differences can also be seen in selectivity to cell populations within the liver. The removal of sialic acid from red cells exposes the terminal galactosyl residues, resulting in hepatocyte uptake—whereas the sequential removal of galactose residues causes N-acetylglucosamine or mannose to be revealed, leading to the uptake of erythrocytes by the Kupffer cells.

The processes of opsonization and phagocytosis of synthetic microparticulate carriers are not as clearly defined as they are for carriers of biological origin. It has been shown, for example, that phagocytosis of polystyrene latex particles *in vitro* can occur in the absence of plasma proteins.[50] It is generally accepted, however, that proteins are prime mediators in the interaction of colloidal particles with phagocytic cells. Wilkins and Meyers found that colloids incubated in plasma, regardless of initial surface charge, acquired the same final charge due to the adsorption of plasma proteins.[51] It was suggested, at that time, that the effect was due to adsorption of albumin (as this is the most abundant protein in plasma). Subsequent studies have shown that interfacial adsorption of proteins on to colloids rarely proceeds in accordance with the relative concentration of proteins in the mixture. Fibrinogen, for example, is found to adsorb preferentially on to polystyrene latex from mixed solutions of albumin, fibrinogen, and IgG.[52] Although there is an extensive literature on the adsorption of proteins on to planar surfaces,[53–55] there is no definitive correlation between the adsorption of proteins on to colloids and the effects that this has on the uptake of the colloid by cells of the MPS *in vivo*. The effects of particle surface modification to reduce protein adsorption will be returned to in the section on the avoidance of MPS.

Targeting to the Cells of the MPS

The MPS can be regarded as either a constraint to site-specific delivery or an opportunity for targeting. Many parasitic, viral, and enzyme storage diseases are associated with cells of the MPS, making them an attractive target using phagocytosed particulate drug carriers. Several life-threatening infectious diseases, such as Leishmania, and systemic fungal infections have been successfully treated using this approach in both experimental animals and in man.[56,57] The use of liposome-encapsulated drugs in the treatment of various disease states of the MPS has been reviewed elsewhere.[58]

It is clear that macrophages can react dramatically to soluble (macro)molecular and particulate stimuli by releasing some of one hundred or so substances that exhibit the full range of activities from the induction of cell growth to the promotion of cell death.[59] Targeting of gamma-interferon, or other immunomodulators, to macrophages transforms these cells into more competent host defense cells with the capacity to kill tumor cells.[60] Carrier-mediated macrophage activation has been successfully exploited to inhibit metastatic spread in experimental animals,[61] and could be useful clinically in cases where there is a low burden of tumor cells.

Avoidance of MPS

We can conclude from the foregoing discussion that the interaction of particles with the MPS is a limitation to the use of particulate carriers in terms of their access to intravascular and extravascular sites. How then may the MPS be avoided? Some suggested approaches are listed in TABLE 3.

MPS blockade. The rationale governing the principle of MPS blockade is that, if the MPS system can be preloaded with a saturating dose of material, successive doses of the same (or different) material stand a better chance of accessing other target tissues. Dextran sulfate,[39] aggregated albumin, colloidal gold stabilized with gelatin,[62] latex beads,[49] and liposomes[63] have all been used to explore this phenomenon. It is understood that macromolecules such as dextran sulfate aggregate plasma proteins to generate a complex that is avidly sequestered by the MPS. It has been argued[64] that MPS blockade can be viewed as a depletion of opsonic serum factors, although other studies have shown that liposomes incubated in serum failed to reverse a blockade induced by a dose of untreated liposomes.[65] Dosing regimens and materials used to effect the blockade may be responsible for the differences observed. In terms of a mechanism of clearance, it has been suggested that the reduction in phagocytosis after loading of macrophages with particles is due to a loss in surface adhesion sites rather than to a limitation in phagocytic capacity or particle loading of macrophages.[50]

The success of MPS blockade in permitting access of carriers to other tissue sites is variable. For example, it has been demonstrated that blockade with dextran sulfate produces a redistribution of sheep erythrocytes to the spleen and bone marrow.[39] Blockade with latex particles has shown to lead to an increase in lung uptake of a test dose of the same particles in rat[63] and rabbit.[66] Illum found that when the MPS system of the rabbit was blocked with dextran sulfate instead of latex, a similar increase in lung uptake could be observed, but in this case there was a redistribution of latex particles over an eight-day period from the lungs to the liver.[66] It is plausible in this case that the particles intially trapped in the lungs were microaggregates that were subsequently removed.

The approach of MPS blockade for site-specific drug delivery does not appear to be clinically viable at the present time due to unpredictable and inefficient uptake of particles at other sites. Moreover, saturation of macrophages must be considered to be unattractive due to an inactivation of these important host-defense cells.

Hopkins has discussed another blockading approach that uses monoclonal antibodies to the low affinity Fc receptors of macrophages.[67] Some encouraging results have been obtained in the chimpanzee with the half-life of immune complex-coated red cells being increased from 50 min to 23.5 hr.

Altering surface properties of particulates. The biophysical behavior of particles in biological fluids has recently been considered by Norde.[68] His analysis suggests that two steps, i.e. the adsorption of proteins to the particle surface and the adhesion of the modified particle to the target (or non-target) cell membrane, are most important in determining the fate of the carrier in the biological environment. A third event, namely particle-particle interactions resulting from ionic interactions or macromolecular (protein) adsorption, also needed to be considered.

In ideal (non-biological) systems, colloidal suspensions may be stabilized against aggregation by a combination of electrostatic, dispersion, hydration, and steric forces. Colloidal particles will repel one another through long-range (Coulombic) forces and attract each other through short-range (van der Waals) interactions. Particles carrying a net charge may be stabilized by electrostatic repulsive interactions. If the ionic composition is altered such that the charges are negated, aggregation of the dispersion may occur.

TABLE 3. Approaches for Avoiding Uptake of Particulate Carriers by the Mononuclear Phagocytic System

Approach	Example
Blockade of MPS	
by saturation	Dextrans, empty liposomes
by competitive receptor occupancy	Anti-receptor antibodies
Alteration of surface	
charge	Charged liposomes
hydrophilicity	Nanoparticles
hydrophobic + steric stabilization	Poloxamer copolymers adsorbed to poly-strene-latex
Mimics of cells	Erythrocyte ghosts

In biological fluids, repulsive forces can be overcome by both physiological salt concentrations and the cross-bridging of proteins to adjacent particles. For example, fibronectin has been shown to adsorb to liposomes causing their aggregation.[69]

Surface charge is also an important factor influencing the interaction of particulates with macrophages. Evidence has been provided that shows that the incorporation of sterylamine (a positively charged lipid) into liposomes enhances the uptake of these particles by peritoneal macrophages *in vitro*.[70] In contrast with this is the observation that neutral and negatively charged liposomes are cleared more rapidly from the circulation than positively charged liposomes.[71] It is clear that the interactions of particles with proteins and lipoproteins can affect the surface properties of the particle and influence the pattern of distribution *in vivo*.

Steric stabilization. It has been postulated that phagocytosis will be reduced or abolished if the surface of the particle is modified in such a way as to diminish protein adsorption and/or cell adhesion events.[69] One way of reducing protein adsorption and cell adhesion is to introduce a hydrated (i.e. hydrophilic) polymer at the surface of the particle.[72] A high potential energy barrier is then created that can effectively negate short-range attractive forces. The hydration effect is enthalpic in origin and the stabilization effect is manifested by osmotic and mixing components, which are entropic in origin.[73] The effectiveness of the steric barrier is determined by the physicochemical features of the stabilizing polymer, the thickness of the adsorbed coat, and the density of surface coverage.[72]

A priori it is expected that the best stabilizing effect will be produced where the polymer is covalently grafted to the particle surface, such that desorption (in biological fluids) is prevented. An alternative approach of Illum and Davis has been to adsorb block copolymers of poloxamer[74] or poloxamine types[75] onto hydrophobic polystyrene latex, in order to examine the effect this has on the clearance of the particles by the MPS.

Poloxamers are A-B-A copolymers, where A is poly(oxyethylene) (POE) and B is

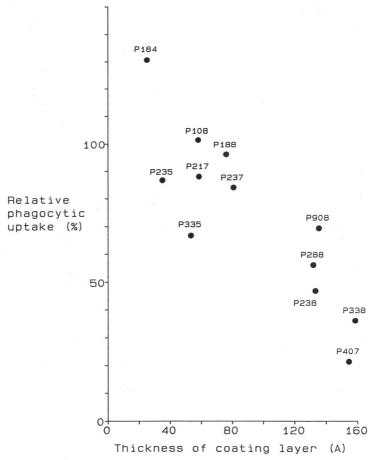

FIGURE 1. The relationship between thickness of the coating layer of poloxamers and poloxamines on polystyrene particles and their relative phagocytic uptake by mouse peritoneal macrophages. (From Illum *et al.*[76] With permission from *Biomaterials*.)

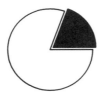

                    Poloxamer 237   Poloxamer 338

FIGURE 2. Adsorption of [^{125}I]Fibrinogen onto polystyrene latex with and without adsorbed coats of block copolymers. (■) Relative fibrinogen adsorption.

poly(oxypropylene) (POP). The block copolymer is understood to orientate at the surface such that the hydrophobic POP moiety anchors the copolymer to the surface and the POE acts as the stabilizing chain. The most effective copolymers in causing the particles to avoid clearance by the MPS are those that have a large hydrophobic block and large hydophilic block within the same molecule. The reasons for this are two fold. First, the hydrophobic block anchors the polymer to the hydrophobic particle surface (preventing its desorption by plasma components). Second, a large hydrophilic block produces an effective adsorbed coat thickness that would be predicted to minimize protein adsorption and particle-particle/particle-cell interactions. In a recent study on the phagocytosis of particles coated with poloxamers and poloxamines, it was demonstrated that a decrease in uptake was indeed correlated with an increased thickness of the adsorbed coat[76] (an adsorbed layer thickness of around 15 nm was most effective, see FIGURE 1). In addition, the chemical properties of the stabilizing chains and the density of surface coverage are important factors in determining the extent of stabilization.

In an attempt to examine the mechanism of uptake in more detail, we have measured the adsorption of fibrinogen onto uncoated and poloxamer-coated particles (having a mean diameter of 330 nm),[77] their aggregation behavior, and the distribution of these particles *in vivo*. Poloxamer 237–coated particles had an adsorbed layer thickness of 12.8 nm compared to 18.5 nm for Poloxamer 338–coated particles (as measured by photon correlation spectroscopy (PCS)).

FIGURE 2 gives data for the maximum isothermal adsorption of fibrinogen (at 310 K) onto Poloxamer 237–coated and Poloxamer 338–coated latex in relation to uncoated latex. The uncoated particles were found to strongly adsorb fibrinogen *in vitro* (causing aggregation of the particles). The Poloxamer coats reduced protein adsorption *in vitro* (Poloxamer 338 being more effective than Poloxamer 237), although a limited aggregation of Poloxamer 237-coated particles was noted. FIGURE 3 gives the distribution of particles ten minutes after an i.v. bolus dose in mice. Uncoated particles were found primarily in the liver and lungs. These results are higher than lung values found by other workers but are consistent with our own *in vitro* data, suggesting that lung accumulation is due to an aggregation of particles upon injection, followed by mechanical filtration of the formed aggregates. Poloxamer 237–coated particles were cleared predominantly by the liver, whereas Poloxamer 338-coated particles remained in the blood pool. The results suggest that particle-cell interactions are reduced by the steric coat of poloxamer 338 but not with poloxamer 237.

The adsorption of a steric coat of Poloxamer 338 has also been used to obtain a reduction in the phagocytosis of parenteral lipid emulsions.[78]

Beukers[79] describes a similar approach using natural materials, such as albumin, to obtain a negatively charged hydrophilic coat of protein on polystyrene latex. Uncoated

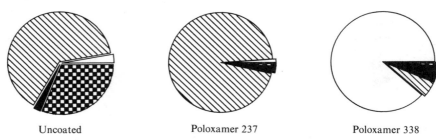

FIGURE 3. Distribution of intravenously injected bolus dose of polystyrene latex after 10 min (in mice). (□) blood, (◨) liver, (■) spleen, and (◪) lung.

particles were phagocytosed to a far greater extent than particles with an adsorbed coat of albumin.

Mimics of Blood Cells

It is possible that steric stabilization is akin to the mechanisms whereby natural particles, such as erythrocytes, escape detection by cells of the MPS. For example, the surface of erythrocytes is covered with a dense packing of carbohydrate chains producing a hydophilic coat of approximately 16 nm thick.[80] It can be postulated that the packing of the chains is such that protein-cell and cell-cell interactions are minimized.

Some groups have attempted to exploit the properties of erythrocytes in order to increase the circulating times of synthetic particles. Utsumi *et al.*[81] have demonstrated that the incorporation of the sialoglycoprotein from erythrocytes into liposomes resulted in a marked suppression in their liver clearance. In another study,[82] modified liposomes were prepared by covalently attaching a sialoglycopeptide to phosphatidylethanolamine. Small unilamellar liposomes were found to be cleared less rapidly than two types of similarly modified multilamellar liposomes; the blood halftime was increased from 0.8 hr to 1.4 hr. However, it must be observed that the results are not very dramatic in terms of being able to obtain a system with a comparable lifetime of circulation to the erythrocyte (circa 90–100 days).

Other Intravascular Targets

Blood cells may be considered as intravascular targets that may be recognized by ligands including antibodies, hormones, and simple sugars. It is possible that microparticles can be targeted to leukemic lymphocytes *in vitro*.[33] In addition, the covalent attachment of anti-rat erythrocyte F(ab')2 antibody to liposomes has been shown both to enhance their binding to erythrocytes *in vivo* and to reduce their uptake by the liver.[84]

A recent review of the interaction of liposomes with blood cells *in vivo* concludes that efforts to alter the passive (natural) accumulation of these particles in the liver and spleen has been unsuccessful.[85] Since peripheral blood-borne monocytes are easily accessible and have the ability to extravasate the circulation and to differentiate into tissue macrophages, a pathway exists, in theory, for accessing a large variety of tissues.

The vascular endothelium can be regarded as a tissue containing organ-specific and disease-related antigenic determinants.[86] There are a number of cardiovascular diseases where the exposure of subendothelial structures leads to localized thrombogenesis. Arteries can be experimentally denuded to expose the underlying basement membrane connective tissues in order to model this effect. It has been shown that liposomes with incorporated anti-collagen or anti-human fibronectin antibodies are selectively bound to endothelial free zones of these arterial segments.[87] Such liposomes could, by their presence, prevent platelet adhesion and thrombus formation, as well as being carriers for anti-thrombogenic drugs.

EXTRAVASCULAR TARGETS

Both anatomical and physiological features of the capillary endothelium determine the opportunities for extravasation of particulate carriers (TABLE 4).

Extravasation of macromolecular and particulate materials in normal endothelia is possible via specialized endothelial gaps, by vesicular processes of a fluid-phase, and/or a constitutive and/or non-constitutive receptor-mediated type, or when carried within extravasating cells.

Continuous Endothelium

Capillaries with continuous endothelia and an uninterrupted basement membrane are the most widely distributed. Although low molecular weight solutes freely diffuse through this barrier, macromolecules with a Stokes-Einstein radius larger than serum albumin extravasate slowly if at all.[88]

Endothelial cells exhibit vesicular endocytosis of both the fluid phase and the constitutive and the non-constitutive receptor-mediated types.[67] Since such vesicles are considered to be between 20 to 100 nm in diameter, limits are set that determine the extent to which particles can utilize these pathways. For example, it has been shown that liposome particles of 30–80 nm diameter are not able to pass through the alveolar membrane.[89] In a recent electron microscopy study of albumin-coated gold particles (5 nm in diameter), evidence has been presented for binding and transcytosis in lung, heart, and diaphragm endothelium *in vitro*.[90] Although no binding could be demon-

TABLE 4. Anatomical Features of Endothelial Barriers

Type/Characteristics	Tissue
Continuous	
Tight junctions, vesicular transport, continuous basement membrane	Skeletal, smooth and cardiac muscles, connective tissue, central nervous system, pancreas, gonads, lung
Discontinuous	
Fenestrated	
Interruptions 20–80 nm, thin membrane 4–6 nm, continuous basement membrane	Exo- and endocrine glands, gastrointestinal tract, renal glomeruli, peritubular capillaries
Sinusoidal	
Gaps of 150 nm, basement membrane absent in liver, interrupted in spleen and bone marrow	Liver, spleen, bone marrow

strated *in vivo* (when the complex was in competition with native serum albumin) it has been suggested that albumin receptors may provide a specific mechanism for the transport of albumin and hence for albumin-coated particles.

Endothelial hyperpermeability at sites of inflammation is well established, although protein extravasation may vary considerably between different pathological conditions. Thus, the leakage of serum proteins is larger in rheumatoid arthritis than in osteoarthritis.[91] Endothelial extravasation has also been probed in the granuloma pouch assay using liposomes with entrapped albumin. No extravasation of liposomes could be observed under conditions that allowed leakage of the albumin.[92] Corresponding differences in the retention of serum proteins can be expected in different inflammatory conditions.

The opportunities for extravasation of particulates may also vary with the etiology of the disease. Thus the intravenous injection of small particles can be used to image joints of patients with active rheumatoid disease,[93] though not when the disease is in remission. It has been suggested that the accumulation is due to phagocytic activity within the synovium. This mechanism could perhaps be exploited as a means of obtaining a sustained release of drugs within the inflamed synovium.

Discontinuous Endothelium

From the features listed in TABLE 4, it can be seen that under normal conditions discontinuous endothelium provides the best opportunity for the extravasation of particulates. An early demonstration of extravasation from sinusoidal capillaries was made with liposomes containing ligands for the galactose receptor of liver parenchymal cells (hepatocytes).[94] Low density lipoprotein (LDL) has been used to explore the surface features of carriers in relation to targeting to liver cell populations in more detail. LDL are natural monolithic particles of mean diameter 22 nm, composed of a neutral lipid core with a surface film of polar lipids and apolipoproteins, which are able to pass through the liver sinusoids, enter the space of Disse and interact with the hepatocytes. The specificity of the interaction is between the apolipoprotein ligand on the surface of LDL and receptors on the hepatocyte surface. The acetylation of the apolipoprotein causes it to be taken up by an endocytic pathway by liver endothelial cells rather than by the hepatocytes.[95] Galactose-LDL are preferentially sequestered by the Kupffer cells of the liver. Many other studies show that the modification of surface ligands can cause a redistribution of particles within the liver as well as to other organs, such as the spleen.[96] The redistribution of particles often reflects the diverse carbohydrate recognition systems in the liver and the spleen and illustrates the principle that the surface of the particles, of the correct size, may be altered to enable them to be taken up not only by specific organs but by specific cell types within that organ.

PHARMACEUTICS

Biological molecules, such as albumin and phospholipids, have gained wide acceptance as matrix materials in the preparation of monolithic and capsular particles. It is generally assumed that such molecules have an inherent biocompatability, although, as the manufacture of, for example, albumin microspheres involves the physical or chemical denaturation of the protein, this property cannot be assumed. Some of the pharmaceutical considerations that arise with the use of monolithic carrier systems are given in TABLE 5 and will be used here to draw comparisons between these and lipid vesicles.

Submicron macroaggregates of albumin can be produced by simple crosslinking of aqueous solutions of albumin with bifunctional reagents, such as glutaraldehyde.[97] These preparations are irregular in shape and have a broad range of size. Spherical micron-sized microspheres can be prepared by the crosslinking of a water-in-oil emulsion followed by recovery and washing to remove the contaminating oil phase. Such microspheres can be mechanically fractionated by passage through sieves of defined mesh size.

The simple dispersion, by shaking, of amphipathic lipids (such as phospholipids) in aqueous buffers, at low molar ratios of lipid to water, results in the formation of multilamellar vesicles (MLV) consisting of concentric shells of lipid and water. These vesicles typically have a broad range of size (between 300–3,500 nm), which can be improved by simple filtration procedures. When an MLV preparation is subjected to ultrasonic irradiation, small unilamellar vesicles (SUV) can be produced (20–50 nm diameter) that can be fractionated by size exclusion chromatography. The preparation of liposomes has been extensively reviewed elsewhere.[98]

TABLE 5. Pharmaceutical Considerations in the Development of Monolithic Particulate Carriers[27]

(1)	Core materials
(2)	Route of preparation with respect to (3–8)
(3)	Size
(4)	Drug incorporation
(5)	Type and amount of drug
(6)	Drug release (*in vitro* and *in vivo*)
(7)	Drug stability during (2) and (9)
(8)	Microsphere stability (*in vitro* and *in vivo*)
(9)	Storage
(10)	Surface properties
(11)	Presentation (e.g. free flowing, freeze-dried etc.)

Low molecular weight, water-soluble drugs can be incorporated into monolithic carriers during manufacture by dissolving the drug in the solution, which constitutes the disperse phase of the emulsion. FIGURE 4 gives the incorporation of a number of water-soluble compounds into microspheres and demonstrates the effectiveness of this approach in terms of loading. We have also incorporated a high molecular weight bioactive peptide into microspheres during manufacture, as well as being able to produce spheres composed entirely of this material. The stability of the drug during manufacture is an important consideration in the preparation of monolithic drug-carriers. It has been found, for example, that the use of glutaraldehyde as a crosslinking agent for the carrier causes a breakdown of the cytostatic methotrexate.[99]

Water-soluble drugs can be incorporated into the aqueous compartment of the liposome during manufacture to an extent that is determined by the aqueous solubility of the drug and the aqueous phase volume of the liposome type. Some typical figures for encapsulation efficiencies are SUV (1%) and MLV (15%).[100] Lipophilic drugs can be incorporated into the hydrophobic membrane if the intercalation does not induce a disruption of the structure of the membrane.

Many factors influence the release of drug from a monolithic drug carrier such as

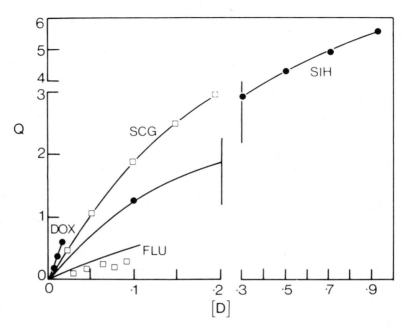

FIGURE 4. Incorporation of water-soluble compound into 10–20 μm HSA microspheres showing the relationship between the amount (mg) of compound incorporated per 10 mg of formed sphere (Q) and the original disperse-phase compound concentration ([D]). SIH, SCG, DOX, and FLU refer to sodium iodohippurate, sodium chromoglycate, doxorubicin, and 5-fluorouracil, respectively. Drawn lines represent 100% incorporation. (From Tomlinson et al.[118] With permission from Elsevier.)

(1) the position of the drug in the microsphere, (2) size and density of the sphere, (3) the extent and nature of the crosslinking, (4) the physicochemical type and molecular weight of the drug, and (5) the nature of interactions between the drug and the microsphere.[27] Low molecular weight water-soluble drugs are typically released from the carrier in a biexponential fashion, i.e. a fast release phase (burst-effect), followed by a much slower first-order release phase. FIGURE 5 illustrates this effect and shows the influence of the degree of crosslinking on the rate of release of the drug from a proteinaceous matrix. It is clear that the burst effect poses a problem in obtaining a controlled release of drug from the microsphere. With peptide-entrapped drugs, we have shown that the release of the drug is dependent on the degradation of the carrier material.

Control of drug release from liposomes can be achieved by manipulating the composition of the constituent lipids such that the vesicle membrane is leaky at high pH[85] or fluid at temperatures just above physiological.[101]

Monolithic carriers can be freeze dried and stored for up to six months with no apparent loss of drug.[57] Small microparticles can be sterile filtered to remove contaminating microorganisms, though other methods of sterilization must be considered for larger particles. Autoclaving may induce drug leakage but can be applied when the drug can be absorbed into the carrier system after manufacture. Drug-containing particles can be sterilized by irradiation given that the radiation dose does not induce the degradation of the drug or carrier matrix.

Poor *in vitro* stability of liposomes has led to various attempts being made to produce stable liposome preparations, such as the formulation of stable polymerized vesicles,[102] proliposomes,[102] and a renewed interest in new freeze-drying techniques as means of preserving liposomes.[104] Another disadvantage is that pure starting materials are relatively expensive and as a result various artificial vehicles prepared from less expensive materials such as non-ionic surfactants have been considered.[105] Many of the available oils and emulsifiers, however, are regarded to be of low biocompatability.[106]

TOXICITY

The use of particulate carriers can be considered in terms of both altered dispersion of the drug as well as possible protection of the body from any unwanted side-effects that the drug may have. However, attention needs to be given to the nature of the carrier materials themselves in terms of the potential toxicities that may arise from the matrix materials and/or the influence that the formed carrier itself can have.

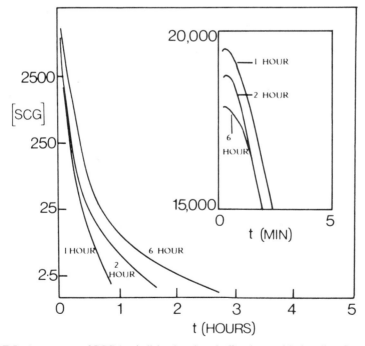

FIGURE 5. Appearance of SCG (ng/ml) in phosphate buffer eluent with time (in a flow through system), showing the influence of crosslinking with 1% glutaraldehyde (given next to the curves) on release. The detail shows release over the first five minutes. (From Tomlinson *et al.*[118] With permission from Elsevier.)

A common approach in the search to avoid carrier toxicity has been to choose materials that are of endogenous origin (e.g., albumin and phospholipids). Alternatively, materials that have been used as implants have been chosen (e.g. poly(lactic acid) and poly(alkylcyanoacrylate)). However, a recent study by Smith and Hunneyball shows that poly(lactic acid) microspheres were toxic to macrophages although the same material showed an excellent biocompatibility as an implant,[107] revealing the importance of the presentation of the material to the biological environment.

If the carrier is installed in the circulation, it will eventually be phagocytosed by macrophages, a process that is well known to cause the release of a variety of inflammatory mediators.[59] Although inflammatory substances are released upon phagocytosis of natural particles, such as erythrocytes and microorganisms, it could be argued that an increased, dose-related, loading of macrophages, with a subsequent increased release of inflammatory products, will accompany the injection of a bolus dose of microparticles. Thus, microparticle-loaded macrophages are likely to have a reduced phagocytic capacity resulting in an increased risk of infections.[108] Impaired macrophage function may also affect the normal catabolism of serum amyloid A, a protein that can cause failure of vital organ functions.[109] Microparticle-loaded liver macrophages also have a reduced capacity to perform cytochrome-P450 mediated drug metabolism.[110] However, microparticles that stimulate macrophages to a limited degree—thereby increasing host defense functions without the introduction of severe inflammatory reactions—may be used as adjuvant drug carriers in the treatment of inflammatory and neoplastic diseases.

The immunological responses induced by carriers are ubiquitous and can be initiated by the matrix material itself and/or the drug. Antibodies against phospholipids can be initiated by immunization with liposomes and it is thought that antibody-liposome interactions can destabilize liposomes.[111] Naturally occurring antibodies against polysaccharides, such as dextran or chemically modified starch, have caused severe type III anaphylactic reaction in humans.[112] Other carrier matrices, such as albumin, have been used extensively for radioimaging purposes without immunological side effects coming to light.[27] A more worrisome consideration is the induction of toxic responses by covalently coupling drugs to carrier matrices.[113] Penicillin, for example, when covalently linked to a soluble carrier is treated as a hapten by the immune system with the consequent development of drug-carrier specific antibodies. The same drug, encapsulated within a liposome, produced no such immune response.[114] However, when haptens are covalently linked to liposomal phospholipids, significant levels of antibodies are produced, demonstrating the immunopotentiating effects of firm attachment of the drug to the carrier matrix.[111] The immune response against a covalently linked drug is likely to be dependent on the type of carrier and the drug. Anti-drug antibody formation is less likely if the carrier is of endogenous origin or if the drug is immunosuppressive. The hapten-carrier concept also applies when various targeting moieties, such as sugar residues, are attached to the microparticles. Glycosylation of proteins, for example, may render them immunogenic.[115] Introduction of a targeting moiety may also result in an altered acute toxicity. Although galactosamine enhances the delivery of P(HPMA) to the liver,[116] it has been demonstrated that galactosamine produces a profound liver toxicity.[117]

CONCLUDING REMARKS

It is clear from this brief summary that there are severe limitations on the ability of particulate, site-specific drug carriers to reach extravascular sites in the body. Although much of the early work on particulates was with liposomes used for accessing cancers, it is now apparent that the use of particulate carriers in the treatment of extravascular tumor masses can only be regarded as sensible in two special cases: as part of a strategy that involves targeting immunomodulatory agents to monocytes and where it is possible to alter the availability of drug to a healthy though drug-sensitive tissue (i.e. so-called negative targeting or site avoidance).

The advantages of particulate systems have always been addressed in terms of unique biological pathways (that drugs can follow), protection of the drug and the body from one another and the amount of drug that may be carried. In addition, there are many variations in structure and type of particulates that render their abilities to cause drug to become available either through an active or a passive process.

The disadvantages are quite clear. Although access and retention within discrete anatomical compartments and to targets within the cardiovasculature and the lymphatic system are readily accessible, the large majority of targets outside these regions, in particular extracellular and intracellular extravascular targets, are probably not accessible, and other modalities will need to be used to reach such regions.

REFERENCES

1. TOMLINSON, E. 1986. *In* Site-Specific Drug Delivery: Cell Biology, Medical and Pharmaceutical Aspects. E. Tomlinson, & S. S. Davis, Eds.: 1–26. John Wiley. Chichester, UK.
2. TOMLINSON, E., S. S. DAVIS & L. ILLUM. 1986. *In* Delivery Systems for Peptide Drugs. S. S. Davis, L. Illum & E. Tomlinson, Eds.: 351–355. Plenum Press. New York.
3. TOMLINSON, E. 1987. Adv. Drug Delivery Rev. Vol. 1 (In press.)
4. CHRAI, S. S., T. F. PATTON, A. MEHTA & J. R. ROBINSON. 1973. J. Pharm. Sci. **62:** 1112–1121.
5. HARA, S., S. ISHIGURO & K. MIZUNO. 1985. Ophthalmol. Visual Sci. **26:** 1631–1634.
6. ALGERVE, P. & B. MARTINI. 1985. Acta Ophthalmalogica 63 (Supp 173): 107–110.
7. GURNY, R., T. BOYE & H. IBRAHIM. 1985. J. Controlled Released **2:** 353–361.
8. NOBLE, J., A. G. JONES, M. A. DAVIS, C. B. SLEDGE, R. I. KRAMER & E. LEVINI. 1983. J. Bone Joint Surg. **65A:** 381–389.
9. RATCLIFFE, J. H., I. M. HUNNEYBALL, C. G. WILSON, A. SMITH & S. S. DAVIS. 1984. *In* Microspheres and Drug Therapy. Pharmaceutical, Immunological and Medical Aspects. S.S. Davis, L. Illum, J. G. McVie & E. Tomlinson, Eds.: 345–346. Elsevier. Amsterdam.
10. DINGLE, J. T., J. C. GORDON, B. L. HAZELMAN, C. G. KNIGHT, D. P. P. THOMAS, N. C. PHILLIPS, I. H. SHAW, F. J. T. FILDES, J. E. OLIVER, G. JONES, E. A. TURNER & J. S. LOWE. 1978. Nature **271:** 372–373.
11. FEHR, K., M. VELVART, K. ROOS & H. G. WEDER. 1985. Therapiewoche 2986–2998.
12. SNIPES, M. B., G. T. CHAVEZ & B. A. MUGGENBURG. 1984. Environ. Res. **33:** 333–342.
13. LEHNERT, B. E., Y. E. VALDEZ & C. C. STEWART. 1968., Exp. Lung Res. **10:** 245–266.
14. JULIANO, R. L. & H. N. McCULLOUGH. 1980. J. Pharmacol. Exp. Ther. **214:** 381–387.
15. MUFSON, D. & F. C. SZOKA. 1985. Pharm Technol. **1:** 16–21.
16. SU, S. E., K. M. CAMPANATE, L. G. MENDELSOHN, G. A. KERCHNER & C. L. GRIES. *In* Delivery Systems for Peptide Drugs. S. S. Davis, L. Illum & E. Tomlinson, Eds.: 221–232. Plenum Press. New York.
17. MORIMOTO, K., K. MORISUKA & A. KAMADA. 1985. J. Pharm. Pharmacol. **37:** 134–136.
18. ILLUM, L. 1987. *In* Delivery Systems for Peptide Drugs. S. S. Davis, L. Illum & E. Tomlinson, Eds.: 205–210. Plenum Press. New York.
19. MATSUNO, K., T. SCAFFNER, H. A. GERBER, C. RUCHTI, M. W. HESS & H. COTTIER. 1983. J. Reticuloendothelial Soc. **33:** 263–273.
20. OWEN, R. L., N. F. PIERCE, R. T. APPLE & W. C. CRAY. 1986. J. Infect. Dis. **153:** 1108–1118.
21. WOOLF, J. L., D. H. RUBIN, R. FINBERG, R. S. KAUFFMAN, A. H. SHARPE, J. S. TRIER & B. N. FIELDA. 1981. Science **212:** 471–472.

22. JOEL, D. D., J. D. LAISSUE & M. E. LeFEVRE. 1978. J. Reticuloedothelial Soc. 72: 440–451.
23. CHANG, C.-M. & N. WEINER. 1987. Int. J. Pharmaceutics 37: 75–87.
24. KLIPSTEIN, F. A., R. F. ENGERT & W. T. SHERMAN. 1983. Infect. Immun. 39: 1000–1003.
25. NEFZEGER, M., J. KREUTER, R. VOGES, E. LIEHL & R. J. CZOK. 1984. J. Pharm. Sci. 73: 1309–1312.
26. SANDERS, E. & C. J. ASHWORTH. 1961. Exp. Cell Res. 22: 137–145.
27. TOMLINSON, E. 1983. Int. J. Pharm. Tech. Prod. Mfr. 4: 49–56.
28. AL-JANABI, M. A. A., A. Y. HEYAM & A. M. AL-SALEM. 1984. Int. J. Appl. Radiat. Isot. 35: 209–214.
29. WIDDER, K. J., P. A. MARINO, R. M. MORRISS, D. P. HOWARD, G. A. POOR & A. E. SENYEI. 1983. Eur. J. Cancer Clin. Oncol. 19: 141–147.
30. MARTODAM, R. R., D. Y. TWUMASI, I. E. LIENER, J. C. POWERS, N. NISHINO & G. KREJCAREK. 1979. Proc. Natl. Acad. Sci. USA 76: 2128–2132.
31. TORCHILIN, V. P. 1983. In Targeted Drugs. E. P. Goldberg, Ed.: 127–152. John Wiley. New York.
32. ARTURSSON, P., P. EDMAN, T. LAASKO & I. SJOHOLM. 1984. J. Pharm. Sci. 73: 1507–1513.
33. BURGER, J. J., E. TOMLINSON, E. M. A. MULDER & J. G. McVIE. 1985. Int. J. Pharmaceutics 23: 333–345.
34. BLANCHARD, R. J. W., I. GROTENHUIS, J. W. LE FAVRE & J. F. PERRY. 1965. Proc. Soc. Exp. Biol. Med. 118: 465–468.
35. LINDELL, B., K. F. ARONSEN, U. ROTHMAN & H. O. SJÖGREN. 1977. Res. Exp. Med. 171: 63–70.
36. LINDBERG, B., K. LOTE & H. TEDER. 1984. In Microspheres and Drug Therapy. Pharmaceutical, Immunological and Medical Aspects. S.S. Davis, L. Illum, J. G. McVie & E. Tomlinson, Eds.: 153–189. Elsevier. Amsterdam.
37. SNIDER, G. L., J. KLEINERMAN, W. M. THURLBECK & Z. H. BENGALI. 1985. Am. Rev. Resp. Dis. 132: 182–185.
38. TUMA, R. F. 1984. In Microspheres and Drug Therapy. Pharmaceutical, Immunological and Medical Aspects. S. S. Davis, L. Illum, J. G. McVie & E. Tomlinson, Eds.: 189–203. Elsevier. Amsterdam.
39. BRADFIELD, J. W. B. 1980. Br. J. Exp. Path. 61: 617–623.
40. BRADFIELD, J. W. B. 1984. In Microspheres and Drug Therapy. Pharmaceutical, Immunological and Medical Aspects. S. S. Davis, L. Illum, J. G. McVie & E. Tomlinson, Eds.: 25–36. Elsevier. Amsterdam.
41. DOBSON, E. L. 1957. In Physiopathology of the Reticuloendothelial System. B. N. Halpern, B. Benacerraf & J. F. Delafresnaye, Eds.: pp 97. Blackwell. Oxford.
42. GREGORIADIS, G., J. SENIOR, B. WOLFF & C. KIRBY. 1985. Ann. N.Y. Acad. Sci. 446: 319–340.
43. WRIGHT, A. E. & S. R. DOUGLAS. 1903. Proc. R. Soc. London 72: 357–370.
44. SHARMA, S. D. 1986. Clinics Immunol. Allergy 6: 1–28.
45. CHUDWIN, D. S., S. G. ARTRIP, A. KORENBLIT, G. SCHIFFMAN & S. RAO. 1985. Infect. Immunol. 50: 213–217.
46. SHAW, D. R. & F. M. GRIFFIN. 1981. Nature 289: 409–411.
47. VAN DE WATER, L., S. SCHROEDER, B. CRENSHAW & R. O. HYNES. 1981. J. Cell Biol. 90: 32–39.
48. BONTE, F. & R. L. JULIANO. 1986. Chem. Phys. Lipids. 40: 359–372.
49. WAGNER, H. N., M. A. RAZZAK, R. A. GAERTNER, N. P. CAINE & O. T. FEAGIN. 1962. Arch. Int. Med. 110: 90–135.
50. LEHNERT, B. E. & C. TECH. 1985. J. Immunol. Meth. 78: 337–344.
51. WILKINS, D. T. & P. A. MEYERS. 1966. Br. J. Exp. Path. 47: 569–576.
52. LENSEN, H. G. W., D. BARGEMAN, P. BERGVELD, C. A. SMOLDERS & J. FEIJEN. 1984. J. Clin. Sci. 99: 1–8.
53. LEE, R. G., C. ADAMSON & S. WAN KIM. 1974. Thromb. Res. 4: 485–490.
54. BAIER, R. E. & R. C. DUTTON. J. Biomed. Mater. Res. 3: 191–206.
55. MORRISSEY, B. W. 1977. Ann. N.Y. Acad. Sci. 283: 50–64.

56. LOPEZ-BERENSTEIN, G., R. MEHTA, R. L. HOPFER, K. MILLS, L. KASI, K. MEHTA, V. FAINSTEIN, M. LUNA, E. M. HERSH & R. L. JULIANO. 1983. Br. J. Infect. Dis. **5:** 939–945.
57. ALVING, C. R. 1986. *In* International Encyclopedia of Pharmacology and Therapeutics. G. M. Ihler, Ed.: 281–330. Pergamon Press. New York.
58. SCHROIT, E. J., I. R. HART, J. MADSEN & I. J. FIDLER. 1983. J. Biol. Response Modifiers **2:** 97–100.
59. NATHAN, C. F. 1987. J. Clin. Invest. **79:** 319–326.
60. BUGELSKY, P., R. KIRSCH, J. M. SOWINSKI & G. POSTE. 1985. Am. J. Pathol. **118:** 419–424.
61. FIDLER, I. J. 1980. Science. **208:** 1469–1471.
62. WAGNER, H. N. & M. IIO. 1964. **43.** 1525.
63. DAVE, J. & H. M. PATEL. 1986. Biochim. Biophys. Acta **888:** 184–190.
64. SABA, T. M. & N. R. DI LUZIO. 1969. Am. J. Physiol. **216:** 197–205.
65. KAO, Y. K. & R. L. JULIANO. 1981. Biochim. Biophys. Acta **677:** 453–461.
66. ILLUM, L., N. W. THOMAS & S. S. DAVIS. 1986. J. Pharm. Sci. **75:** 16–22.
67. HOPKINS, C. R. 1986. *In* Site-Specific Drug Delivery: Cell Biology, Medical and Pharmaceutical Aspects. E. Thomlinson & S. S. Davis, Eds.: 27–48. Wiley. Chichester, UK.
68. NORDE, W. 1984. *In* Microspheres and Drug Therapy. Pharmaceutical, Immunological and Medical Aspects. S. S. Davis, L. Illum, J. G. McVie & E. Tomlinson Eds.: 39–59. Elsevier. Amsterdam.
69. HSU, M. J. & R. L. JULIANO. 1982. Biochim. Biophys. Acta **720:** 411–419.
70. SCHWENDENER, R. A., P. A. LAGOCKI & Y. E. RAHMAN. 1984. Biochim. Biophys. Acta **772:** 93–101.
71. SENIOR, J. H. 1987. Crit. Rev. Ther. Drug. Carrier Syst. 1987. **3:** 123–193.
72. NAPPER, D. H. 1983. *In* Polymeric Stabilisation of Colloidal Dispersions. pp 197–215. Academic Press. London.
73. OTTEWILL, R. H. 1977. J. Colloid. Interface Sci. **58:** 357–373.
74. ILLUM, L. & S. S. DAVIS. 1984. FEBS Lett. **167:** 79–82.
75. ILLUM, L., S. S. DAVIS, R. H. MULLER, E. MAK & P. WEST. 1987. Life Sci. **40:** 367–374.
76. ILLUM, L., L. O. JACOBSEN, R. H. MULLER, E. MAK & S. S. DAVIS. 1987. Biomaterials **8:** 113–117.
77. O'MULLANE, J. E., C. J. DAVISON, K. PETRAK & E. TOMLINSON. 1987. Biomaterials. (Submitted for publication.)
78. DAVIS, S. S. & P. HANSRANI. 1985. Int. J. Pharmaceutics **23:** 69–77.
79. BEUKERS, H., F. A. DEIERKAUF, C. P. BLOM, M. DEIERKAUF & J. C. RIEMERSMA. 1978. J. Cell Physiol. **97:** 29–36.
80. VIITALA, J. & J. JARNEFELT. 1985. Trend in Biochem. Sci. Oct.: 392–395.
81. UTSUMI, S., H. SHINOMIYA, J. MINAMI & S. SONODA. 1983. Immunol. **49:** 113–120.
82. HAGA, M., F. KATO, M. YOSHIDA, F. KOHARA & Y. KATO. 1986. Chem. Pharm. Bull. **36:** 2979–2988.
83. VIDAL, M., J. SAINTE-MARIE, J. R. PHILIPPOT & A. BIENVENUE. 1985. EMBO J. **4:** 2461–2468.
84. SINGHAL, A. & C. M. GUPTA. 1986. FEBS. Lett. **201:** 321–326.
85. SCHROIT, A. J., J. MADSEN & R. NAYAR. 1986. Chem. Phys. Lipids **40:** 373–393.
86. AUERBACH, R., L. ALBBY, L. W. MORRISEY, M. TU & J. JOSEPH. 1985. Microvasc. Res. **29:** 401–411.
87. SMIRNOV, V. N., S. P. DOMOGATSKY, V. V. DOLGOV, V. B. HVATOV, A. L. KLIBANOV, V. E. KOTELIANSKY, V. R. MUZYKANTOV, V. S. REPIN, B. V. SAMOKHIN, B. V. SHEKHONIN, M. D. SMIRNOV, D. D. SVIRIDOV, V. P. TORCHILIN & E. I. CHAZOV. 1986. Proc. Natl. Acad. Sci. USA **83:** 6603–6607.
88. TAYLOR, A. E. & D. N. GRANGER. 1984. Handb. Physiol. **6:** 467–520.
89. POSTE, G., C. BUCANA, A. RAZ, P. BUZELSKI, R. KIRSH & I. J. FIDLER. 1982. Cancer Res. **42:** 1412–1422.
90. GHITESCKU, L., A. FIXMAN, M. SIMIONESCU & N. SIMIONESCU. 1986. J. Cell Biol. **102:** 1304–1311.
91. WALLIS, W. J., P. A. SIMKIN & W. B. NELP. 1987. Arthritis Rheum. **30:** 57–63.

 92. POSTE, G. 1983. Biol. Cell. **47:** 19–38.
 93. WILLIAMS, B. D., M. M. O'SULLIVAN, G. S. SAGGU, K. E. WILLIAMS, L. A. WILLIAMS &
      J. R. MORGAN. 1986. Brit. Med J. **293:** 1143–1144.
 94. GHOSH, P., P. K. DAS & B. K. BACHAWAT. 1982. Arch. Biochem. Biophys. **213:** 266–
      270.
 95. VAN BERKEL, T. J. C., J. KARKRUIJT, L. HARKES, J. F. NAGELKERKE, H. SPANJER &
      H.-J. M. KEMPEN. 1986. *In* Site-Specific Drug Delivery: Cell Biology, Medical and
      Pharmaceutical Aspects. E. Tomlinson & S. S. Davis, Eds.: 49–68. Wiley. Chichester,
      UK.
 96. KIWADA, H., H. NIMURA & Y. KATO. 1985. Chem. Pharm. Bull. **33:** 2465–2482.
 97. SOKOLOSKI, T. D. & G. P. ROYER. 1984. *In* Microspheres and Drug Therapy. Pharmaceu-
      tical, Immunological and Medical Aspects. S. S. Davis, L. Illum, J. G. McVie & E.
      Tomlinson, Eds. 295–307. Elsevier.Amsterdam.
 98. SZOKA, F. & D. PAPAHADJOPOULOS. 1980. Ann. Rev. Biophys. Bioeng. **9:** 467–508.
 99. OPPENHEIM, R. C. 1981. Int. J. Pharmaceutics 1981. **8:** 217–234.
100. POZNANSKY, M. J. & R. L. JULIANO. 1984. Pharmacol. Revs. **36:** 277–336.
101. SULLIVAN, S. M. & L. HUANG. 1986. Proc. Natl. Acad. Sci. USA **83:** 6117–6121.
102. MEHTA, R., M. J. HSU, R. L. JULIANO, H. J. KRAUSE & S. L. REGEN. 1986. J. Pharm Sci.
      75: 579–581.
103. PAYNE, N. I., P. TIMMINS, C. V. AMBROSE, M. D. WARD & F. RIDGWAY. 1986. J. Pharm.
      Sci. **75:** 325–329.
104. CROWE, J. H., B. J. SPARGO & L. M. CROWE. 1987. Proc. Natl. Acad. Sci. USA
      15: 1537–1540.
105. BAILLIE, A. J., A. T. FLORENCE, L. R. HUME, G. T. MUIRHEAD & A. ROGERSOM. 1985. J.
      Pharm. Pharmacol. **37:** 863–868.
106. DAVIS, S. S., J. HARDGRAFT & K. J. PALIN. 1983. *In* Encyclopedia of Emulsion
      Technology. P. Becher, Ed. **2:** 159–160. Marcel Dekker. New York.
107. SMITH, A. & I. M. HUNNEYBALL. 1986. Int. J. Pharmaceutics **30:** 215–220.
108. NUGENT, K. M. 1984. J. Leu. Biol. **36:** 123–132.
109. FUKS, A. & D. J. ZUCKER-FRANKLIN. 1985. J. Exp. Med. **161:** 1013–1028.
110. PETERSON, T. C. & K. W. RENTON. 1984. J. Pharmacol. Exp. Ther. **229:** 299–304.
111. ALVING, C. R. 1986. Chem. Phys. Lipids **40:** 303–314.
112. RICTER, A. W. & H. I. HEDIN. 1982. Immunol. Today **3:** 132–138.
113. RIHOVA, B. & I. RIHA. 1985. CRC Crit. Rev. Therap. Drug Carrier Systems **1:** 311–374.
114. DE HAAN, P., E. CLAASSEN & N. VAN ROOIJEN. 1986. Int. Arch. Allergy Appl. Immunol.
      81: 186–188.
115. WITZUM, J. L., U. P. STEINBRECHER, M. FISHER & A. KESANIEMI. 1983. Proc. Natl.
      Acad. Sci. USA **80:** 2757–2761.
116. DUNCAN, R., L. C. W. SEYMOUR, L. SCARLETT, J. B. LLOYD, P. REJMANOVA & J.
      KOPECEK. 1986. Biochim. Biophys. Acta **880:** 62–71.
117. CHOJKIER, M. & J. FIERER. 1985. Gastroenterology **88:** 115–121.
118. TOMLINSON, E., J. J. BURGER, E. M. A. SCHOONDERWOERD & J. G. McVIE. 1984. *In*
      Microspheres and Drug Therapy. Pharmaceutical, Immunological and Medical
      Aspects. S. S. Davis, L. Illum, J. G. McVie & E. Tomlinson, Eds: 75–89. Elsevier.
      Amsterdam.

Drug Delivery to Macrophages for the Therapy of Cancer and Infectious Diseases

RICHARD KIRSH, PETER J. BUGELSKI,
AND GEORGE POSTE

Smith Kline and French Laboratories
Philadelphia, Pennsylvania 19101

INTRODUCTION

The role of cells of the mononuclear phagocyte system (MPS), which includes the Kupffer cells in the liver; alveolar, splenic, lymph node, and bone marrow macrophages; tissue histiocytes; and circulating blood monocytes, in host defense against neoplastic and infectious disease has attracted increasing attention over the past ten years.[1-4,58] This interest stems from three principal aspects of the functional behavior of mononuclear phagocytes. First, when activated,[a] mononuclear phagocytes display significant cytotoxicity towards neoplastic cells and invading microorganisms while leaving "normal" host cells completely unharmed. Second, mononuclear phagocytes will infiltrate sites of infection and neoplastic lesions thus circumventing the need to target therapeutic agents to such sites. Third, agents that activate the tumoricidal and microbiocidal properties of mononuclear phagocytes augment host defense against tumors and infectious disease. Collectively, these observations, coupled with the disappointing results obtained in both clinical and experimental trials with immunologically specific therapeutic modalities mediated by T- and B-lymphocytes, have led to renewed interest in the functions of macrophages in host defense and renewed interest in the therapeutic value of augmenting the immunologically non-specific tumoricidal and microbiocidal properties of mononuclear phagocytes in the therapy of cancer and infectious diseases.

The ability to selectively target drugs to specific cells within the body has been one of the most coveted goals in experimental and clinical therapeutics. To this end, a wide variety of macromolecular, particulate, and cellular matrices have been proposed for use as drug carrier systems. These include antibodies, dextrans, plasma proteins, polynucleotides, red blood cells, polymorphonuclear leukocytes, gelatin or albumin microspheres, synthetic polymeric nanoparticles, multiphase microemulsions, and liposomes. Many of these systems have failed to fulfill their initial promise but interest in targetable drug delivery systems remains high.[10,56]

Current information on the application of liposomes to drug delivery *in vivo*, with particular emphasis on their use for the selective delivery of antibiotics and biological response modifiers (BRM) to mononuclear phagocytes will be reviewed. Although liposomes have received considerable attention in experimental therapeutics, surprisingly little emphasis has been given to evaluation of the issues of toxicity and pharmaceutical formulation required for successful commercialization of these car-

---

[a]The term "activated macrophage" will refer to macrophages that display tumoricidal and/or microbiocidal activity.

riers to fulfill their widespread clinical use. The importance of these issues cannot be overstated and will be addressed in this article.

Liposome Targeting to the Mononuclear Phagocyte System

Targeting of liposomes to any specific cell type *in vivo* requires the completion of several independent steps[9,10] including: access to the appropriate target cell, selective interaction with the target cell, and uptake by the target cell with little or no uptake by non-target cells. Furthermore, the drug must remain associated with the liposomes until it is delivered to the target cell and the liposome-drug complex must not induce unacceptable levels of toxicity.

Numerous studies have shown that the majority of liposomes injected i.v. localize primarily in the liver, spleen, and bone marrow irrespective of size, charge, or structural class.[9,10] Tissue fractionation and ultrastructural studies have established that liposome retention in these organs is due primarily to their uptake by mononuclear phagocytes lining the vascular sinusoids in these organs.[11] In addition to uptake by the fixed phagocytic cells in these organs, liposomes can also be phagocytosed by circulating blood monocytes within the vascular system.[11]

Although clearance by Kupffer cells lining hepatic sinusoids represent the major fate for liposomes administered intravenously, liposomes can also interact with the liver parenchymal cells (hepatocytes). Small sonicated unilamellar (SUV) liposomes can be taken up by hepatocytes as intact particles.[11,12] In contrast, uptake of intact liposomes of larger size, such as large multilamellar vesicles (MLV) by hepatocytes, if it occurs, is limited.[11,12] This is presumed to be due to the inability of the larger particles to penetrate the gaps in the endothelial lining of the hepatic sinusoids. Exchange of phospholipids between large MLV liposomes and hepatocytes has been described.[12] This can occur either via direct phospholipid exchange or via indirect transfer of liposomal lipids to high density lipoproteins (HDL), which in turn transfer lipid to hepatocytes. Scherphof and his colleagues have obtained evidence that suggests that lipids from liposomes taken up by phagocytic Kupffer cells in the liver can be transferred subsequently to hepatocytes.[12] However, the more important observation from the standpoint of designing therapeutic strategies is that liposomes of diverse size and composition can be delivered as intact particles, together with any associated therapeutic or diagnostic agent, to Kupffer cells.

The other major sites of liposome retention after i.v. injection are in the mononuclear phagocytes of the spleen and the bone marrow. Liposome accumulation in the spleen is enhanced under conditions where hepatic uptake of liposomes is eliminated. Splenic retention thus represents "spillover" of liposomes from the liver. Saturation of the ability of splenic macrophages to remove liposomes results, in turn, in "spillover" of liposomes to bone marrow macrophages. Multiple injections of liposomes can eventually "exhaust" the capabilities of macrophages in the liver, spleen, and bone marrow to clear liposomes and other particles with resulting toxicity due to impaired reticuloendothelial function.[9,10]

Apart from the reports of uptake of intact small sonicated SUV liposomes by hepatocytes,[12] there is no evidence of uptake of i.v. administered liposomes as intact structures by cells other than mononuclear phagocytes of the RES and circulating blood monocytes.

The clearance of liposomes from the circulation and their tissue disposition is analogous to the behavior of other inert particulate materials injected i.v., including colloidal carbon, erythrocytes, immune complexes, and various artificial particulate drug carriers (such as latex particles, nanoparticles, and microspheres).[9,10]

The localization of liposomes injected i.v. in cells of the mononuclear phagocyte system, though frustrating to investigators who wish to direct liposomes to other cells, offers a potentially powerful method for targeting therapeutic agents to these cells. This type of targeting will be referred to as "passive targeting" since it simply exploits the natural fate of liposomes and other particles to be taken up by mononuclear phagocytes following i.v. injection.

STRATEGIES FOR MACROPHAGE ACTIVATION IN EXPERIMENTAL THERAPEUTICS

The Activated Macrophage

As mentioned previously, the central role of the mononuclear phagocyte system (MPS) in host defense is well documented.[13,14] In addition to its classical role as a scavenging system for the clearance of foreign materials, immune complexes, dead or effete cells, and cell debris from the circulation, the MPS is now known to be important in determining the outcome of various forms of shock, tissue ischemia, and drug therapy.[13] Considerable attention has also been devoted to the role of activated macrophages in host defense against invading bacteria, parasites, and tumor cells.[14] The term "activated macrophage" is an operational definition and is used differently by various authors to describe acquisition of a variety of functions that are not exhibited by resident tissue macrophages. Diverse examples of the use of the term activation can be found: referring to activated macrophages as cells that show oxidative metabolism, but lack microbiocidal or tumoricidal activity; in other instances to macrophages that exhibit microbiocidal but not tumoricidal activity; while yet other authors, including ourselves, limit the use of the term to macrophages that exhibit both microbiocidal and tumoricidal properties. In this chapter, the term will be used solely to describe macrophages that exhibit microbiocidal and tumoricidal activities. Acquisition of tumoricidal properties is usually accompanied by other phenotypic alterations including: increased phagocytosis, secretion of neutral proteases and acid hydrolases, synthesis and release of arachidonic acid metabolites, expression of an altered ectoenzyme profile, the ability to suppress natural killer-cell activation, and an enhanced ability to kill intracellular microorganisms.[15–17] In this review, macrophages that display a biochemical and/or physiological profile different from resident tissue macrophages, but which do not express tumoricidal activity, will be referred to as stimulated macrophages.

Pathways of Macrophage Activation

Macrophages can be rendered tumoricidal by a wide variety of naturally occurring and synthetic agents either by agents that act directly or by agents that induce other cells to release mediators that evoke macrophage activation.[2] Currently there are two major classes of macrophage-activating agents that merit consideration as potential therapeutic candidates: (1) microbial cell wall components and structural analogs related to these agents and (2) various lymphokines.[58]

The direct activation of macrophages is induced by interaction with agents such as bacterial endotoxin (lipopolysaccharide, LPS), lentinin, glucan, and with diverse bacteria such as *Mycobacteria, Propionibacteria, Nocardia*, or subunits isolated from the cell walls of these microorganisms.[17–29]

Most of the microbial cell wall–derived materials are unsuitable for clinical use due to significant toxicities. In addition, detailed structural characterization of many of the components responsible for macrophage activation by these materials has yet to be accomplished. One notable exception is the water-soluble, low molecular weight synthetic dipeptide, N-acetyl-muramyl-L-alanyl-D-isoglutamine, referred to as muramyl dipeptide (MDP). MDP is the smallest structural unit (M_r 459), capable of inducing all of the adjuvant activities of mycobacteria in a water-in-oil emulsion (complete Freund's adjuvant).[21,22] MDP has been shown to stimulate a wide variety of macrophage functions *in vitro* including secretion of prostaglandins and collagenase, generation of superoxide anion, release of interleukin-1, and to augment macrophage-mediated bacteriocidal and tumoricidal activities.[21,22] *In vivo,* MDP has been shown to protect experimental animals against lethal infection by a range of bacteria,[23–31] parasites,[30] fungi,[24–27] and viruses.[32,33] However, MDP although far less toxic than intact mycobacteria, is also far less effective than intact bacteria in activating macrophages *in vivo* because its efficacy *in vivo* is limited by its extremely rapid clearance (90% of MDP injected intravenously i.v. can be detected in the urine within 2 hr).[34]

Indirect macrophage activation can be achieved by lymphokines released by antigen- or mitogen-stimulated lymphocytes and which interact with specific receptors on the macrophage surface.[35] This activity is referred to by the predictable designation, macrophage-activating factor (MAF), but the exact identity of the mediator(s) involved and whether different subpopulations of macrophages are activated by different mediators in lymphokine preparations is still unknown.[62–64]

Current limitations in lymphokine purification and the production of standardized and pharmaceutically stable lymphokine preparations dictate that the lymphokine preparations containing MAF activity vary markedly in their biological activities. In particular, the crucial question of whether there is a single, specific lymphokine that can be classified as MAF or whether such activity is in fact caused solely by other lymphokines such as gamma-interferon (IFN-γ), is currently an area of intense investigation. MAF activity and IFN-γ share many physicochemical and biological characteristics including co-purification by a variety of chromatographic procedures, similar chemical stabilities and abilities to induce an oxidative burst and expression of microbiocidal and tumoricidal properties.[65–72] Conversely, several groups have demonstrated MAF activity in culture supernatants from T-cell lines that contain no detectable IFN-γ activity in association with materials whose physicochemical and immunological properties are distinct from IFN-γ.[73–76] The biological effects of this group of MAFs have some overlap with the effects IFN-γ with respect to shared induction of macrophage-mediated cytotoxicity. However, several significant differences can be cited. First, interferon-induced, macrophage-mediated cytotoxicity requires the presence of a second signal, supplied by bacterial endotoxin, for induction of the tumoricidal phenotype,[46] whereas MAF-induced tumoricidal activity is independent of a second signal.[49] Second, the non-interferon MAF does not induce the expression of Fc receptors or Class I or II histocompatibility antigens and does not have direct antiviral activity whereas interferon elicits these effects.[51] However, formal proof of the existence of a specific lymphokine with macrophage activation activity that is distinct from gamma-interferon must await cloning of the gene and rigorous chemical analysis of the gene product(s).

Effective cancer therapy with macrophage-activating agents will not only require compounds that are non-toxic and non-immunogenic, but that are also capable of activating those macrophages that are refractory to lymphokine-mediated activation either as a result of an active suppression phenomenon imposed by other immune cell subsets or to the passive decay in the responsiveness of macrophages to activation by lymphokines that accompanies their migration from the blood stream into the tissues.[52]

LIPOSOME-MEDIATED ACTIVATION OF MACROPHAGES *IN VIVO*

Antineoplastic Therapy

Liposomes and other particulates offer an efficient system for the delivery of materials to mononuclear phagocytes *in vivo*. Studies on the disposition of intravenously injected liposomes have demonstrated that in common with other particulate materials, liposomes localize selectively in organs with high levels of mononuclear phagocyte activity such as the liver, spleen, and bone marrow, as well as circulating to blood monocytes.[9,11,53] This passive localization of liposomes within macrophages and monocytes facilitates selective delivery of liposome-associated materials to these cells *in vivo*. In addition to the delivery of materials to mononuclear phagocytes, entrapment of materials in liposomes serves several other useful functions. Encapsulation of biologically labile materials within liposomes will protect them from premature inactivation or degradation within the circulation. Furthermore, compounds such as MDP, which show rapid clearance kinetics when administered as a "free" compound, may show extended retention *in vivo* when administered within liposomes.

Passive localization of i.v. administered liposomes within the macrophages of the MPS can be exploited to deliver BRM agents selectively to these cells to enhance their tumoricidal and/or microbiocidal activity. The systemic administration of liposomes containing either lymphokines or synthetic MDP has been shown to activate macrophage-mediated tumoricidal activity *in vitro* and *in vivo*.[1,58,59]

Liposomes containing MAF, MDP, or human C-reactive protein (CRP) injected i.v. result in significant destruction of established metastases produced by murine tumors of diverse histologic origins.[59-63] In these systems, spontaneous pulmonary and lymph node metastases arising from tumors implanted in the foot pad were established at the start of liposome therapy. Multiple metastatic lesions containing several thousand tumor cells were present at the onset of therapy, which in the absence of therapy, progress rapidly to form large colonies exceeding 2–3 mm in diameter at the time of death. However, when a three-week protocol of therapy was initiated with liposome-encapsulated macrophage activating agents 3–4 days after removal of the "primary" lesion in the foot pad, the majority (about 70%) of treated animals were free of macroscopic or microscopic tumors. Furthermore, in the few animals in the treatment groups that still exhibited residual metastatic disease, the median number of metastatic colonies was still significantly reduced compared with both the untreated control group and animals treated with unencapsulated "free" activating agents.[58,60,61]

The therapeutic efficacy of liposome-encapsulated BRM in rendering pulmonary macrophages tumoricidal in these experimental tumor models is encouraging since the lung is a major site of metastatic disease. Similarly, findings showing that the residual metastatic lesions from experimental animals treated with liposome-encapsulated BRM were populated by tumor cells that remained susceptible to killing by activated macrophages are also encouraging.[58,59,63] The *in vivo* observations are consistent with the lack of success in selecting tumor cell clones with increased resistance to macrophage-mediated killing *in vitro*[58] and reinforces the suggestion that the most important potential factor limiting the clinical use of this approach will not be due to the emergence of resistant tumor cell subpopulations but the extent of tumor burden at the outset of therapy.[58]

The optimal conditions for therapy with liposome-encapsulated macrophage-activating agents and the efficacy of this modality for treatment of metastatic burdens or infections of increasing severity still have to be defined. In addition to the use of clinically relevant models with predictive value, evaluation and development of immunotherapeutic BRM agents will require re-appraisal and modification of existing test protocols. In contrast to conventional cytotoxic chemotherapeutic agents, which are routinely evaluated at the maximum tolerated dose (MTD), BRM agents may exhibit complex response curves, often with biphasic or multiphasic responses. Agents with this profile may often be more effective at lower doses than high dose levels.[66,67] In most instances to date, however, optimum dose response relationships for clinical studies have not been quantified in detail and clinical trials with BRM agents are apparently conducted all too frequently using doses selected in a seemingly arbitrary fashion, other than with the obvious prerequisite of avoidance of extreme toxicity. The superior efficacy of low doses of BRM agents (compared to those BRM agents administered at their MTD) has recently been demonstrated in three experimental rodent tumor models using recombinant interleukin-2, the interferon inducer poly ICLC, and a low molecular weight semisynthetic microbial cell wall fragment FK565.[66,67] Similarly, dosing frequency and the duration of treatment can have profound influences on the therapeutic efficacy of BRM agents.[67] Critical evaluation of the optimal dose-response relationships for BRM agents in the optimization of immunotherapeutic protocols will require a thorough evaluation of the complex pharmacodynamic properties of the BRM agents with respect to the effects of dose, dosing frequency, and duration of treatment on the acquisition and maintenance of the activated phenotype in macrophages *in vivo.*

In addition to the essential prerequisite of successful enhancement of macrophage-mediated cytotoxic activity *in vivo,* a further critical issue in the design of BRM agent-mediated antineoplastic therapies concerns the number and physiological status of macrophages within neoplastic lesions. At this point, it seems highly unlikely that liposome-encapsulated activating agents could serve as a single modality in treating advanced disease. For example, in mice, even allowing for maximal macrophage recruitment into the lung, there are insufficient numbers of pulmonary macrophages to eradicate more than 10^8 tumor cells/lung.[58] As tumor burdens of this size are easily attained, the potential application of macrophage activation is almost certainly not in the elimination of large tumor masses, but in the eradication of the residual tumor following the use of other cytoreductive therapies. Thus, in common with many other antineoplastic regimens, optimal application will involve use in conjunction with other antitumor modalities.[58,77]

Anti-infectives Therapy

Lymphokines encapsulated within liposomes activate macrophages to selectively destroy *Herpes simplex* virus type 2 (HSV-2) infected cells while leaving non-infected cells unharmed.[54,55] In these studies, liposome-encapsulated lymphokines were shown to be at least one thousand times more efficient than "free" unencapsulated lymphokines in rendering macrophages cytolytic towards HSV-2 infected target cells. Moreover, a lipophilic MDP analog (MTP-PE) encapsulated in liposomes is significantly more effective than free MTP-PE in protecting experimental animals against systemic lethal HSV-2 infections.[64] These studies have recently been extended to include therapy of pulmonary viral infections due to HSV-1 and influenza virus.[65] In these studies, liposome encapsulated MTP-PE and liposome-encapsulated ribavirin were more effective than either agent alone in reducing the level of viremia and in increasing the survival time of infected animals.[65] Although free lymphokines or MDP can activate macrophages to lyse virus-infected cells *in vitro,* the efficacy of free BRM agents *in vivo* is limited by their short biological half-life. By encapsulating lymphokines within liposomes, these agents are protected from inactivation and/or degradation within the circulation and can be targeted, albeit passively, to macrophages within the reticuloendothelial system, including circulating blood monocytes. Macrophages can therefore be activated by liposome-encapsulated lymphokines or MDP *in vivo* to destroy virus-infected cells and this approach may provide a powerful strategy for treatment of viral infections.

Liposomes as Carriers for Improved Antibiotic Therapy

As mentioned above, mononuclear phagocytes play an important role in the clearance and destruction of pathogenic microorganisms. However, a number of bacteria, fungi, viruses, and pathogenic protozoa can also replicate intracellularly within macrophages. Intracellular infections caused by these microorganisms are difficult to manage clinically and are often refractory to conventional chemotherapeutic treatment protocols because of poor drug penetration into cells.

Administration of antimicrobial agents in association with liposomes offers a potential solution to this problem. Assuming that infected macrophages retain their phagocytic capacity, the systemic administration of liposomes containing a drug active against the intracellular pathogen provides an efficient method for drug delivery directly to the sites of infection. Such site-specific drug targeting may permit the utilization of lower drug doses relative to the amount of free drug used in traditional therapy and thus reduce the potential for toxic side reactions. The merits of this approach for the chemotherapy of intracellular infections of the MPS caused by bacteria,[68,69] parasites,[70,71] fungi,[72–74] and viruses[64,65,79,80] have been demonstrated over the last few years.

Opportunistic fungal infections caused by *Candida albicans, Aspergillus fumigatus,* and *Rhizopus spp.* are a major problem in immunologically compromised patients, particularly in patients with neoplastic diseases, such as leukemia and lymphomas and, more recently, with AIDS. The prospect of improved therapy of systemic mycoses using liposome-encapsulated drugs is clinically very important. The demonstration that liposome-encapsulated amphotericin B shows reduced toxicity with no loss of efficacy in the treatment of candidosis, histoplasmosis, and cryptococcosis is a major therapeutic achievement.[72–76] If these findings prove to be a general feature of liposome-associated antifungal drugs it may be possible to develop therapeutic protocols with other compounds that display potent antifungal activity but were dropped from further development due to excessive host toxicity.

Liposome-encapsulated antifungal drugs might reasonably be expected to be of limited success in the treatment of infections with the more common opportunistic fungi, where the organisms grow extracellularly. However, selective delivery of antifungal agents to macrophages may still be therapeutically useful. Phagocytic uptake of fungi by macrophages that contain drugs would be expected to enhance intracellular destruction of the phagocytosed organisms. In addition, macrophages that had phagocytosed liposomes-containing drug could conceivably act as a mobile slow-release depot. For example, macrophages that endocytosed liposomes containing antifungal drugs while in the circulation may migrate to the site of infection and release compound locally over a prolonged period.

COMMERCIAL DEVELOPMENT OF LIPOSOME-ASSOCIATED DRUGS

Safety

The safety of a drug carrier system must be evaluated from two standpoints: the toxicity of the carrier itself and the risk of novel, drug-induced toxicities arising from differences in the disposition, pharmacokinetics, and metabolism of carrier-associated drug compared with conventional drug formulations. These criteria must be evaluated under test conditions that mimic, as closely as possible, the dose, frequency, and route of administration envisaged for clinical use.[56]

Single doses of biodegradable particles such as liposomes and albumin microspheres are tolerated well by many animal species.[5–8,10] However, repeated dosing with particulate carriers can impair RES clearance functions. The onset, extent, and duration of RES failure is affected by particle size, dose, number, and frequency of doses. For liposomes, phospholipid composition is also relevant. Impairment of RES function results from sequential saturation and exhaustion of particle clearance capacities in the liver, spleen, and bone marrow.[9] Histologic evidence of bone marrow hypoplasia and alterations in hematopoiesis have been observed in extended i.v. dosing with liposomes.[77] It is therefore necessary to assess the toxic liabilities associated with each proposed dosing schedule and also to evaluate the possibility of novel toxicities associated with each individual phospholipid mixture and activation mediator.

The disposition, pharmacokinetics, and metabolic fate of drugs administered in association with a carrier may differ substantially from conventional formulations of the same agents, and the risk of novel toxicities must therefore be considered. Perhaps the most obvious example concerns the use of liposomes and other particulate carriers to deliver anticancer drugs. By delivering high concentrations of cytotoxic drugs to mononuclear phagocytes in the blood and the RES, this approach may induce toxic ablation of a vital element of host defense. Inhibitors of DNA synthesis might be expected to have little toxic effect on non-dividing macrophage populations, but drugs that impair RNA and protein synthesis may be toxic to such cells. Recent studies have shown that this fear is justified.[9,10] Systemic administration of several anti-tumor drugs encapsulated within liposomes enhanced the metastatic spread of mouse tumors.[9] This effect was not induced by liposomes injected s.c. or i.m. and it was reversed by injecting syngeneic macrophages 12 hours after each treatment cycle, indicating that the iatrogenic enhancement of metastases was probably caused by toxic destruction of mononuclear phagocytes.[10] The case for using liposomes or other particulate carriers for drug delivery in cancer treatment may be seriously flawed if the drug in question destroys host macrophages.

The ability of certain cytotoxic anti-tumor drugs to destroy the RES when administered in association with liposomes was perhaps predictable in light of existing data that identified the RES as the major site of liposome localization *in vivo*. This phenomenon is not unique to liposomes. Impairment of RES function has been reported in mice injected i.v. with erythrocyte ghosts containing encapsulated bleomycin.[78]

In our opinion, the potential risk posed by drug carriers that show appreciable localization in the RES is of sufficient magnitude to preclude their clinical use as carriers for cytotoxic anti-neoplastic drugs until extensive toxicology studies show that ablation of the RES is not induced by the specific drug(s) to be used in clinical studies. Multiple dosing with particulate carriers for long periods also presents the additional risk of RES toxicity induced by the carrier itself.

Commercialization of Liposome-Based Drug Carriers

Widespread application of liposomes or any other particulate drug carriers in clinical therapeutics will obviously require successful commercialization. As with all potential pharmaceutical products, the decision to embark on the high risk, lengthy and expensive development process necessitates not only a clear definition of the scientific and technical merits of the proposed drug design, but a careful examination of both the medical need for alternative approaches and the economic demands of product development.

The potential therapeutic advantages of a liposome-based drug delivery system for activating macrophages *in vivo* have been the subject of numerous scientific reports and need not be discussed further. However, the technological and economic feasibility of commercial development of liposomes for use as drug carriers is far from certain. In order to be successful within the foreseeable future, liposome production must be adapted to convenient, cost-effective, large-scale preparative methods that will not require extensive process development or a substantial capital investment in ultraspecialized instrumentation. Furthermore, the manufacturing process must be carried out under conditions acceptable to the regulatory agencies. The final product must be homogeneous, amenable to large scale production, have at least a 12–18 month shelf life, and offer maximum convenience to the medical community.

Additional uncertainties arise when one considers that the response of the regulatory agencies that govern the manufacturing and marketing of pharmaceutical products to liposomes or other particulate carrier vehicles has largely gone untested. Although there are no clear precedents, the response of the Food and Drug Administration (FDA) in the U.S. to both pro-drugs and implantable controlled-release polymeric matrices suggests that liposome-associated drugs will be treated as new chemical entities (NCE) and be required to undergo the full range of toxicologic, metabolic, and pharmaceutic evaluations required for approval of any new drug administered to patients.

Economic considerations such as these clearly suggest that other particulate microcarrier systems, such as multiphase emulsions, that share many of the advantageous properties of liposomes deserve careful evaluation. Prevailing commercial factors currently favor these alternative drug carriers because they can be produced as pharmaceutically acceptable formulations at far less cost than liposomes. In this regard, one emulsion-based drug delivery system containing diazepam is currently available commercially for parenteral use.

SUMMARY

The mechanisms by which mononuclear phagocytes discriminate between self and nonself, recognize foreign materials, senescent, damaged, old, or effete cells, and tumor cells are unknown. However, regardless of the mechanism(s) involved, once activated by the appropriate signal(s), macrophages are able to selectively recognize and destroy neoplastic cells *in vitro* and *in vivo*.

Liposomes injected intravenously, in common with other particulate or polymeric matrices, localize preferentially in organs with high mononuclear phagocyte activity and in circulating blood monocytes. This behavior allows microparticulates to serve as a convenient system for the selective delivery of encapsulated drugs to cells of the mononuclear phagocyte series *in vivo*. Liposomes are a particularly attractive experimental system because of their capacity to incorporate a wide variety of water-soluble and lipid-soluble drugs. At this time, however, there is no reason to assume that a liposome-based drug delivery system will offer any significant therapeutic advantage compared to other microparticulate drug delivery systems. As in commercial development of any pharmaceutical preparation, considerations of cost-of-goods, shelf life, and acceptance of the formulation and dosing regimen by both physicians and patients will be of major importance in determining success and widespread clinical use.

Liposomes containing macrophage-activating agents are highly effective at augmenting macrophage-mediated tumoricidal activity *in vitro* eradicating tumor metastasis *in vivo,* as well as protecting animals from a wide variety of microbial and viral infections.

Although the demands of solving the scientific and technical problems associated with liposome development are substantial, the rapid rate of progress in biology and in pharmaceutical sciences enhances the prospect of success for at least several aspects of liposome-mediated drug delivery. The next few years will be crucial in determining whether the commercial development of liposomes is feasible or whether they will join the ranks of other drug carrier designs that have failed to fulfill their initial promise.

REFERENCES

1. FIDLER, I. J. & A. RAZ 1981. The induction of tumoricidal capacities in mouse and rat macrophages by lymphokines. *In* Lymphokines. E. Pick, Ed.: 345–64. Academic Press. New York.
2. CHIRIGOS, M. A., M. MITCHELL, M. J. MASTRANGELO & M. KRIM, Eds. 1981. Modulation of Cellular Immunity in Cancer by Immune Modifiers. Raven Press. New York.
3. KLEINERMAN, E. S. & I. J. FIDLER. 1984. Macrophage activation by lymphokines: Usefulness as antineoplastic agents. *In* Novel Approaches to Cancer Chemotherapy. P. S. Sunkara, Ed.: 232–250. Academic Press. Orlando, FL.
4. ADAMS, D. O. & C. F. NATHAN. 1983. Molecular mechanisms operative in cytolysis of tumor cells by activated macrophages. Immunol. Today **4:** 166–167.
5. BRUCK, S. D., Ed. 1982. Controlled Drug Delivery. CRC Press. Boca Raton, FL.
6. CHIEN, Y. W., Ed. 1982. Novel drug delivery systems. Dekker. New York.
7. COUNSELL, R. E. & R. C. PONLAND. 1982. Lipoproteins as potential site-specific delivery systems for diagnostic and therapeutic agents. J. Med. Chem. **25:** 1115–1120.
8. LEVY, R. & R. A. MILLER. 1983. Tumor therapy with monoclonal antibodies. Fed. Proc. Fed. Am. Soc. Exp. Biol. **42:**2650–2656.
9. POSTE, G. 1983. Liposome targeting in vivo: problems and opportunities. Biol. Cell. **47:** 19–30.
10. POSTE, G., R. KIRSH & T. KOESTLER. 1983. The challenge of liposome targeting in vivo. *In* Liposome Technology. G. Gregoriadis, Ed: 1–28. CRC Press. Boca Raton, FL.
11. POSTE, G., R. KIRSH, W. E. FOGLER & I. J. FIDLER. 1982. Analysis of the fate of systemically administered liposomes and implications for their use in drug delivery. Cancer Res. **42:** 1412–1422.
12. SCHERPHOF, G. L. 1982. Interaction of liposomes with biological fluids and fate of liposomes in vivo. *In* Liposome Methodology. L. D. Lesterman & J. Barbet, Eds.: 79–92. INSERM. Paris.
13. ALTURA, B. M. 1980. Reticuloendothelial cells and host defense. Adv. Microcirc. **9:** 252–294.
14. ROSE, N. & B. V. SIEGEL, Eds. 1983. The reticuloendothelial system: a comprehensive treatise. Vol. 4. Immunopathology. Plenum Press. New York.
15. NORTH, R. J. 1978. The concept of activated macrophages. J. Immunol. **121:** 806–809.
16. COHN, Z. A. 1978. The activation of mononuclear phagocytes: fact, fancy and future. J. Immunol. **121:** 813–816.
17. ALEXANDER, P. & R. EVANS. 1971 Endotoxin and double stranded RNA render macrophages cytotoxic. Nature **232:** 76–78.

18. FENICHEL, R. & M. A. CHIRIGOS, Eds. 1985. Immune modulating agents and their mechanisms. Vol. 25. Marcel Dekker. New York.
19. HERSH, E., M. A. CHIRIGOS & MASTRANGELO, Eds. 1981 Augmenting agents in cancer therapy. Progr Cancer Res. Therapy **16.**
20. MIHICH, E., Ed. 1982. Immunological Approaches to Cancer Therapeutics. John Wiley and Sons, New York.
21. LEDERER, E. 1980. Synthetic immunostimulants derived from the bacterial cell wall. J. Med. Chem. **23:** 819–825.
22. CHEDID, L. & F. AUDIBERT. 1985. New approaches for control of infections using synthetic or semi-synthetic constructs containing MDP. Springer Semin. Immunopathol. **8:** 401–412.
23. CHEDID, L., M. PARANT, F. PARANT, P. LEFRANCIER, J. CHOAY & E. LEDERER. 1977. Enhancement of nonspecific immunity to Klebsiella pneumoniae infection by a synthetic immunoadjuvant (N-acetyl-muramyl-L-alanyl-D-isoglutamine) and several analogs. Proc. Natl. Acad. Sci. USA **74:** 2089–2093.
24. DIETRICH, F. M., W. SACKMANN, O. ZAK & P. DUKOR. 1980. Synthetic muramyl dipeptide immunostimulants: Protective effects and increased efficacy antibiotics in experimental bacterial and fungal infections in mice. *In* Current Chemotherapy and Infectious Disease. J. D. Nelson & C. Grass, Eds. **2:** 1730 Am. Soc. Microbiol., Washington, D.C.
25. FRASER-SMITH, E. B. & T. R. MATTHEWS. 1981. Protective effects of muramyl dipeptide analogs against infections of Pseudomonas aeruginosa or Candida albicans in mice. Infect. Immun **34:** 676–683.
26. HUMPHRIES, R. C., P. R. HENIKI, R. W. FERRARESI & J. L. KRAHENBUHL. 1980. Effects of treatment with muramyl dipeptide and certain of its analogs on resistance to Listeria monocytogens in mice. Infect. Immun. **30:** 462–466.
27. MATTHEWS, T. R. & E. B. FRASER-SMITH. 1980. Protective effect of muramyl dipeptide and analogs against Pseudomonas aeruginosa and Candida albicans infections in mice. *In* Current Chemotherapy of Infectious Disease. **2:** 1734. Am. Soc. Microbiol. Washington, D.C.
28. ONOZUKA, K., T. SAITO-TAKI & M. NAKANO. 1984. Effect of muramyl dipeptide analog on Salmonella enteritidis infection in beige mice with Chedial-Higashi syndrome. Microbiol. Immunol **28:** 1211–1221.
29. PARANT, M., F. PARANT & L. CHEDID. 1978. Enhancement of the neonate's nonspecific immunity to Klebsiella infection by muramyl dipeptide, a synthetic immunoadjuvant. Proc. Natl. Acad. Sci. USA **75:** 3395–3399.
30. KIERSZENBAUM, F. & R. W. FERRARESI, 1979. Enhancement of host resistance against Trypanosoma cruzi infection by the immunoregulatory agent muramyl dipeptide. Infect. Immun. **25:** 273–278.
31. KRAHENBUHL, J. L. & R. C. HUMPHRES. 1983. Effects of treatment with muramyl dipeptide on resistance to Mycobacterium leprae and Mycobacterium marinum infection in mice. Immunopharmacology **5:** 329–339.
32. DIETRICH, F. M., B. LUKAS & K. H. SCHMIDT-RUPIN. 1983. MTP-PE (synthetic muramyl peptide): Prophylactic and therapeutic effects in experimental viral infections. Presented at 13th Int. Congr. Chemotherapy, Vienna, Aug. 28–Sept. 2.
33. KOFF, W. C., I. J. FIDLER, S. D. SHOWALTER, M. K. CHAKRABARTY, B. HAMPAR, L. M. CECCORULLI & E. S. KLEINERMAN. 1984. Human monocytes activated by immunomodulators in liposomes lyse herpesvirus-infected but not normal cells. Science **224:** 1007–1009.
34. PARANT, M., F. PARANT, L. CHEDID, A. YAPO, J. F. PETIT & L. LEDERER. 1979. Fate of the synthetic immunoadjuvant, muramyl dipeptide (¹⁴C-labelled) in the mouse. Int. J. Immunopharmacol. **1:** 35–41.
35. POSTE, G., R. KIRSH & I. J. FIDLER 1979. Cell surface receptors for lymphokines. Cell Immunol. **44:** 71–88.
36. ANDREESEN, R., K. J. BROSS, J. OSTERHOLZ & F. EMMRICH. 1986. Human macrophage maturation and heterogeneity: Analysis with a newly generated set of monoclonal antibodies to differentiation antigens. Blood **67:** 1257–1264.
37. SHEN, H. H., M. A. TALLE, G. GOLDSTEIN & L. CHESS. 1983. Functional subsets of human monocytes defined by monoclonal antibodies. A distinct subset of monocytes contains the

cells capable of inducing the autologous mixed lymphocytes cultures. J. Immunol. **130:** 698–705.

38. ZEMBALA, M., W. URACZ, I. RUGGIERO, B. MYTAR & J. PRYJMA. 1984. Isolation and functional characterization of FcR$^+$ and FcR$^-$ human monocyte subsets. J. Immunol. **133:** 1293–1299.

39. SCHREIBER, R. D., J. L. PACE, S. W. RUSSELL, A. ALTMAN & D. H. KATZ. 1983. Macrophage-activating factor produced by a T cell hybridoma: physiochemical and biosynthetic resemblance of γ-interferon. J. Immunol. **131:** 826–832.

40. LE, J., W. PRENSKY, Y. K. YIP, Z. CHANG, T. HOFFMAN, H. C. STEVENSON, I. BALAZS, J. R. SADLIK & J. VILCEK. 1984. Activation of human monocyte cytotoxicity by natural and recombinate immune interferon. J. Immunol. **131:** 2821–2826.

41. SCHULTZ, R. M. 1980. Macrophage activating by interferons. *In* Lymphokine Reports. E. Pick, Ed. **1:** 63–92. Academic Press, Inc. New York.

42. PACE, J. L., S. W. RUSSELL, R. D. SCHREIBER, A. ALTMAN & D. H. KATZ. 1983. Macrophage activation: priming activity from a T-cell hybridoma is attributable to interferon-γ. Proc. Natl. Acad. Sci. USA **80:** 3782.

43. SCHREIBER, R. D., J. L. PACE, S. W. RUSSELL, A. ALTMAN & D. H. KATZ. 1983. Macrophage activating factor produced a T cell hybridoma: physiochemical and biosynthetic resemblance to γ-interferon. J. Immunol. **131:** 826–832.

44. ROBERTS, W. K. & A. VASIL. 1982 Evidence for the identity of murine gamma interferon and macrophage activating factor. J. Interferon Res. **2:** 519–532.

45. KLEINSCHMIDT, W. J. & R. M. SCHULTZ. 1982. Similarities of murine gamma interferon and the lymphokine that renders macrophages cytotoxic. J. Interferon Res. **2:** 291–299.

46. KLEINERMAN, E. S., R. ZICHT, P. S. SARIN, R. C. GALLO & J. FIDLER. 1984. Constitutive production and release of a lymphokine with macrophage activating factor activity distinct from γ-interferon by a human T cell leukemia virus-positive cell line. Cancer Res. **44:** 4470–4475.

47. MELTZER, M. S., M. GILBREATH, C. A. NACY & R. D. SCHREIBER. 1985. Macrophage activation factor from EL-4 cells distinct from murine gamma interferon (IFN). Fed. Proc. **44:** 1697 (Abstr.).

48. CRAWFORD, R., D. HOOVER, D. FINBLOOM, M. GILBREATH, C. NACY, & M. MELTZER. 1985. Physicochemical properties of a human lymphokine (LK) distinct from gamma interferon (IFN) that activates monocytes to kill Leishmania donovani. Fed. Proc. **44:** 1697 (Abstr.).

49. LEE, J. C., L. REBAR, P. YOUNG, R. W. RUSCETTI, N. HANNA & G. POSTE. 1986. Identification and characterization of a human T cell line-derived lymphokine with MAF-like activity distinct from interferon-γ. J. Immunol. **136:** 1322–1328.

50. PACE, J. L., S. W. RUSSELL, B. A. TORRES, H. M. JOHNSON & P. W. GRAY. 1983. Recombinant mouse interferon induces the priming step in macrophage activation for tumor cell killing. J. Immunol. **130:** 2011–13.

51. LEE, J. C., A. M. BADGER, W. J. JOHNSON, C. P. SUNG & P. HORAN. 1986. Human non-gamma interferon macrophage activating actor (MT-2/MAF) elicits multiple and cross-species effects on macrophage activations. Abstract. 6th Intl. Congress Immunol.

52. POSTE, G. & R. KIRSH, 1979. Rapid decay of tumoricidal activity and loss of responsiveness to lymphokines in inflammatory macrophages. Cancer Res **39:** 2582–2590.

53. GREGORIADIS, G., J. SENIOR & A. TROUET, Eds. 1982. Targeting of Drug NATO Advanced Studies Institute Series. Vol. A47. Plenum Press. New York.

54. KOFF, W. C., S. D. SHOWALTER, D. A. SENIFF & B. HAMPAR. 1983. Lysis of herpesvirus-infected cells by macrophages activated with free or liposome-encapsulated lymphokine produced by a murine T cell hybridoma, Infection Immunity **42:** 1067–1072.

55. KOFF, W. C., I. J. FIDLER, S. D. SHOWALTER, M. K. CHAKRABARTY, B. HAMPAR, L. M. CECCORULLI & E. S. KLEINERMAN. 1984. Human monocytes activated by immunomodulators in liposomes lyse herpesvirus-infected but not normal cells. Science **224:** 1007–1009.

56. POSTE, G. & R. KIRSH. 1983. Site-specific (targeted) drug delivery in cancer therapy. Biotechnology **1:** 869–878.

57. FIDLER, I. J., A. RAZ, W. E. FOGLER, P. BUGELSKI, R. KIRSH & G. POSTE. 1980. Design of

liposomes to improve delivery of macrophage-augmenting agents to alveolar macrophages. Cancer Res. **40:** 4460–4466.

58. FIDLER, I. J. & G. POSTE. 1982. Macrophage-mediated destruction of malignant tumor cells and new strategies for the therapy of metastastic disease. Springer Semin. Immunopathol. **5:** 161–174.

59. SCHROIT, A. J. & I. J. FIDLER. 1986. The design of liposomes for delivery of immunomodulators to host defense cells. *In* Medical Applications of Liposomes. K. Yagi, Ed.: 141–150. Japan Scientific Societies Press. Tokyo.

60. FIDLER, I. J., I. R. HART, A. RAZ, W. E. FOGLER, R. KIRSH & G. POSTE. 1980. Activation of tumoricidal properties in macrophages by liposome-encapsulated lymphokines: in vivo studies. *In* Liposomes and Immunobiology. B. H. Tom & H. Six, Ed.: 109–18. Elsevier. New York.

61. DEODHAR, S. D., B. P. BARNA, M. EDINGER & T. CHIANG. 1982. Inhibition of lung metastases by liposomal immunotherapy in a murine fibrosarcoma model. J. Biol. Resp. Modifiers **1:** 27–34.

62. KLEINERMAN, E. S., A. J. SCHROIT, W. E. FOGLER & I. J. FIDLER. 1983. Tumoricidal activity of human monocytes activated in vitro by free and liposome-encapsulated human lymphokines. J. Clin. Invest. **72:** 304–315.

63. FIDLER, I. J. 1986. Optimization and limitations of systemic treatment of murine melanoma metastases with liposomes containing muramyl tripeptide phosphatidylethanolamine. Cancer Immunol. Immunother. **21:**169–173.

64. KOFF, W. C., S. D. SHOWALTER, B. HAMPAR & I. J. FIDLER. 1985. Protection of mice against fatal herpes simplex type 2 infection by liposomes containing muramyl tripeptide. Science **228:** 495–497.

65. GANGEMI, J. D., M. NACHTIGAL, D. BARNHART, L. KRECH & P. JANI. 1987. Therapeutic efficacy of liposome-encapsulated ribavirin and muramyl tripeptide in experimental infection with influenza or herpes simplex virus. J. Infect. Dis. **155:** 510–516.

66. TALMADGE, J. E., J. ADAMS, H. PHILLIPS, M. COLLINS, B. LENZ, M. SCHNEDIER & M. CHIRIGOS. 1985. Immunotherapeutic potential of poly ICLC in murine tumor models. Cancer Res. **45:** 1066–1072.

67. TALMADGE, J. E. & M. A. CHIRIGOS. 1985. Comparison of immunomodulatory and immunotherapeutic properties of biologic response modifiers. Springer Semin. Immunopathol. **8:** 429–443.

68. DESIDERIO, J. V. & S. G. CAMPBELL. 1983. Liposome-encapsulated cephalothin in the treatment of experimental murine salmonellosis, RES: J. Reticuloendothelial Soc. **34:** 279–287.

69. FOUNTAIN, M. W., C. DEES & R. D. SCHULTZ. 1981. Enhanced intracellular killing of Staphylococcus aureus by canine monocytes treated with liposome containing amikacin, gentamicin, kanamycin, and tobramycin. Curr. Microbiol. **6:** 373–376.

70. ALVING, C. R. & E. A. STECK. 1979. The use of liposome-encapsulated drugs in leishmaniasis. Trends Biochem. Sci. **4:** N175–177.

71. NEW, R. R. C., M. L. CHANCE & S. HEATH. 1981. The treatment of experimental cutaneous leishmaniasis with liposome-entrapped Pentostam. Parasitol. **83:** 519–527.

72. TAYLOR, R. L., D. M. WILLIAMS, P. C. CRAVEN, J. R. GRAYBILL, D. J. DRUTZ & W. E. MAGEE. 1982. Amphotericin B in liposomes: a novel therapy for histoplasmosis. Am. Rev. Respir. Dis. **125:** 610–611.

73. LOPEZ-BERESTEIN, G., R. MEHTA, R. L. HOPFER, K. MILLS, L. KASI, K. MEHTA, V. FAINSTEIN, M. LUNA, E. M. HERSH & R. JULIANO. 1983. Treatment and prophylaxis of disseminated infection due to Candida albicans in mice with liposome-encapsulated amphotericin B. J. Infec. Dis. **5:** 939–945.

74. GRAYBILL, J. E., P. C. CRAVEN, R. L. TAYLOR, D. M. WILLIAMS & W. E. MAGEE. 1982. Treatment of murine cryptococcosis with liposome associated amphotericin B. J. Infect. Dis. **145:** 748–751.

75. LOPEZ-BERESTEIN, G., V. FAINSTEIN, R. HOPFER, K. MEHTA, M. P. SULLIVAN, M. J. KEATING, M. G. ROSENBLUM, R. MEHTA, M. LUNA, E. M. HERSH, J. REUBEN, R. L. JULIANO & G. P. BODEY. 1985. Liposome amphotericin B for the treatment of systemic fungal infections in patients with cancer: A preliminary study. J. Infect. Dis. **151** (4): 704–710.

76. SZOKA, F. C., D. MULHOLLAND & M. BARZA. 1987. Effect of lipid composition and liposome size on toxicity and in vitro fungicidal activity of liposome-intercalated amphotericin B. Antimicrob. Agents Chemother. **31:** 421–429.

77. POSTE, G., R. KIRSH & P. BUGELSKI. 1984. Liposomes as a drug delivery system in cancer therapy. *In* Novel Approaches to Cancer Chemotherapy. P. Sunkara, Ed.: 166–231. Academic Press. Orlando, FL.

78. LYNCH, W. E., G. P. SARTIANO & A. GHAFFAR. 1980. Erythrocytes as carriers of chemotherapeutic agents for targeting to the reticuloendothelial system. Am. J. Hematol. **9:** 249–259.

79. KENDE, M., C. R. ALVING, W. L. RILL, G. M. SWATZ, JR. & P. G. CANONICO 1985. Enhanced efficacy of liposome-encapsulated ribavirin against Rift Valley fever virus infection in mice. Antimicrob Agents Chemother. **27:** 903–907.

80. SMOLIN, G., M. OKUMOTO, S. FEILER & D. CONDON. 1981. Idoxuridine-liposome therapy for herpes simplex keratitis. Am. J. Ophthalmol. **91:** 220–225.

Immunotoxins for *in Vivo* Therapy: Where Are We?

DAVID M. NEVILLE, JR.

Laboratory of Molecular Biology
National Institute of Mental Health
Bethesda, Maryland 20894

INTRODUCTION

Immunotoxins are toxins with altered receptor specificity. The alteration is achieved by coupling a monoclonal antibody to the toxin or to a toxin fragment.[1] Immunotoxins (ITs) are designed specifically to kill targeted cells in a mixed cell population. Several immunotoxins have been constructed that have achieved this goal in *in vitro* situations. An example is in human bone marrow transplantation. Human donor bone is treated outside the body with an anti-T cell IT to reduce donor T cells and thereby prevent the occurrence of morbid graft-versus-host disease in the transplant recipient.[2,3]

This paper will discuss the status of immunotoxins for *in vivo* therapy. Most of the discussion will focus on tumor irradication. However, other possibilities exist, such as modulation of immune system subsets in the treatment of autoimmune diseases. Today, I think we are overall in a good situation. The immunotoxin field is quite young. The concept of altering the receptor specificity of a protein toxin, which contains its own inherent translocation function as opposed to simply targeting a toxic drug, is only 10 years old.[4] Over the past 10 years, the variables affecting immunotoxin potency and efficacy have been explored and patterns are beginning to emerge that will direct our future progress.[a]

The early studies on the use of immunotoxins to eradicate tumors from experimental animals were disappointing. Efficacy could not be demonstrated. I will somewhat arbitrarily define efficacy as a reduction in tumor load by a factor of 10 or greater. A 10-fold reduction in tumor burden would probably be marginally clinically useful for slow growing tumors, especially those exhibiting multiple drug resistance. A perspective for such a reduction can be gained from several examples of experimental animal tumor systems. If 10^5 tumor cells are injected and after therapy this load is 10^4 cells, the tumor burden has been reduced by a factor of 10 or 1 logarithm. And likewise, if 100 cells are injected and therapy reduces the viable cells to 10 we have a 1 log reduction. And because ITs like other anti-cancer drugs kill by a single-hit process, the same dose will kill 90,000 cells when 100,000 cells are present as will kill 90 cells when 100 cells are present.[1] A 1 log reduction in tumor cells can cure a tumor only if the burden is 9 cells or less. However a log reduction could shrink a spherical tumor to one half its previous diameter. A 3 log reduction could shrink it to one tenth of its initial diameter, but only totally irradicate a tumor of 999 cells or less. Tumor burdens in man can reach 10^{11} cells.

[a]Exceptions to this statement may occur with ITs constructed with very high affinity antibodies. The *in vivo* concentration of IT may then drop as the tumor burden increases due to depletion caused by essentially irreversible binding.

In addition to the early animal tumor model studies, there are currently several phase I clinical trials of ITs as anti-tumor agents in progress. In the only published report, treatment of T cell leukemia with a ricin A chain IT, efficacy could not be demonstrated.[5] As far as the other trials go, optimism has not been voiced. Although details are scanty, it appears that the current phase I clinical trials are using ITs of a design type already found non-efficacious in the early animal studies.

The good news is that in the past 18 months, two rigorous animal model studies have appeared which document IT-induced tumor log kills of over 3 logs or better.[6,7]

In the following pages, I will outline what we and others believe are the critical variables responsible for getting ITs to work *in vivo*. I will discuss where I think the promising advances will be made over the next several years. I will also briefly review the distinction in what we mean by potency and efficacy and how these distinctions relate to successes or failures in therapy with targeted drugs that utilize receptor-mediated transport systems to gain access to targeted cells.

Before all this I will give a very short review of what immunotoxins are, how ITs are made, and how ITs kill cells.

Immunotoxins are made by linking immunoglobulins directed at target cells to protein toxins or fragments of protein toxins. Diphtheria toxin is a prototype of the protein toxins. The toxin, a 535 residue protein, is a multi-domain structure and the domains are associated with unique functions. The enzymatic activity of the toxin, a transferase activity, lies at the amino terminus and is separated from the other domains by a tryptic-sensitive bond so that the toxin is functionally a two-chain structure. A single disulfide bond spans the tryptic-sensitive region tying the two chains known as the A chain (transferase) and the B chain together. The transferase activity takes ADP ribose from endogenase NAD and transfers it to elongation factor 2, a necessary factor for protein synthesis, and renders elongation factor 2 inactive. Since the substrate for the enzyme lies within the cytosol compartment the toxin catalytic site must reach this compartment.[8]

THE TOXIN INTOXICATION PATHWAY

The toxin gains entrance to cells by a receptor-mediated process and the binding domain is located at the carboxyl terminus of the protein. The middle of the toxin contains a very hydrophobic rich domain and this is believed to be associated with the translocation function. The translocation function and the binding region appear to overlap each other. Although considerable effort has gone into separating these two structural and functional regions, no one has yet been able to accomplish this.[8] We think that the evidence is compelling that the toxin binding site must be functional within an intracellular compartment for efficient membrane translocation to take place.[1,7]

Diphtheria toxin passes through many cellular compartments before it reaches the cytosol compartment where its enzymatic activity results in cell death. As cartooned in FIGURE 1, the receptor first binds to the B chain binding site, the toxin is endocytosed into a vesicle, and we know that these vesicles undergo acidification. For the toxin, acidification is an obligatory step and considerable evidence points to the fact that the toxin is in some way processed in an acidic compartment and this processing is necessary for translocation to occur.[9,10] Sometime subsequent to this acidification step, a bolus of toxin crosses the vesicular membrane to the cytosol compartment.[11,12] Just how this is achieved is uncertain. Possibilities are that the vesicle is lysed or that the vesicle fuses with the external plasma membrane and the resulting potential gradient change initiate toxin translocation.[13]

Although one molecule of toxin injected into the cytosol compartment can kill a cell in 48 hours,[14] the intoxication process that proceeds from the cell membrane imparts a bolus of toxin molecules into the cytosol. This bolus size is between 20 and 80 molecules.[11,12] This quantal event results in the death of a cell. The passage of toxin through the various compartments of the cell may be thought of as the sequential interaction of the three domains of the toxin with different cellular components.

The toxin then is an example of a targeting agent developed by nature and this

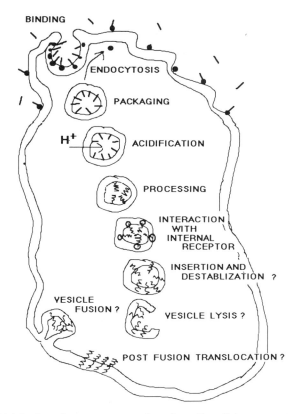

FIGURE 1. Diphtheria toxin traverses a number of specific cellular compartments and undergoes specific cellular initiated processing before the A chain is translocated to the cytosol resulting in cell death. A DT-based immunotoxin would enter target cells via a different receptor portal, but the IT is likely to be most efficient if the remaining route overlaps the parental toxin route.

targeting agent contains its binding function to the appropriate target as well as its own entry function, which lies in the translocation domain. The appeal of using the protein toxins as the toxic arm mediated by a monoclonal antibody is that the protein toxins contain their own membrane translocation function, which is highly efficient.[15] It is our desire to utilize as far as possible the efficient toxin translocation function for immunotoxins and to have immunotoxins parallel the same internal cellular route as the parent toxin to achieve the most efficacious targeted cell killing.[16–18]

VARIABLES IN IMMUNOTOXIN CONSTRUCTION

Immunotoxins are made by coupling monoclonal antibodies directed at the targeted cells to the toxin or a toxin subunit. The coupling procedures generally utilize the amino groups on both the toxin and the immunoglobulin. The couplings may be formed by imidate esters, which form amadine bonds, or by N-hydroxysuccinimide esters, which form amide bonds. Often a sulfur is involved in the central coupling as either a disulfide or as a thioether.[19] When immunoglobulins are coupled only to a toxin A chain, which lacks the translocation function, as is the case with diphtheria toxin A chain, the conjugate efficacy is markedly reduced.[21] However, the A chain of ricin has some degree of translocating function[21] and efficacy can be enhanced in certain circumstances[22,23] by NH_4Cl, carboxylic acid ionophores, and other agents affecting cell vesicle trafficking.[23] With such enhancing agents, the degree of efficacy appears to be highly dependent on the targeted surface antigen[22,24] and perhaps the level of ricin B chain contamination.[24] It is likely that when the translocation efficiency is reduced, routing becomes highly important. Any scheme that prolongs the lifetime of the conjugate in a non-degradative vesicular compartment will be advantageous. There is also a group of plant proteins called ribosomal-inactivating proteins that have properties similar to ricin A chain (e.g., gelonin,[25] saporin,[6] and pokeweed antiviral protein[26]). These proteins are similar to the A chain of ricin in that they do not contain a binding receptor on the surface of cells, but exhibit some degree of translocation function.

When high translocation efficiency is desired, immunoglobulins are coupled to the intact toxin (holo-immunotoxins).[27,28] This results in an immunotoxin with two binding moieties. The immunoglobulin is chosen to have a high affinity constant to the target cell, and the ricin B chain binding site has a lower affinity binding to all non-target cells. To reduce the binding of the conjugate to non-target cells, a competitor is added to block the cell surface galactose binding site of the ricin (FIGURE 2).[27,28] This competitor is usually lactose and is thought to be extruded from the internal vesicle compartment where the ricin B chain binding site participates in enhancing translocation.[19] The scheme is not efficacious *in vivo* because of the low concentration of lactose that can be achieved. However, we believe that future research will center on ways of covalently blocking the toxin binding site of holo-immunotoxins by a bond that is labile once the immunotoxin has been transported into the cell via the antibody moiety. Possible mechanisms to use in order to reverse a covalent blockade would be the 2 pH unit drop between the extracellular compartment and the acidified intracellular vesicle compartment. Enzymatic differences within the internal vesicle compartments could also be exploited. This type of scheme would maintain the native high efficiency toxin translocation machinery but eliminate interaction of the immunotoxin with non-target cells through the blockaded toxin binding site. One might ask, why would anyone want to get this complicated? The answer to this question is to improve the efficacy of immunotoxins.

ANALYSIS OF POTENCY AND EFFICACY IN RECEPTOR-MEDIATED PROCESSES

Most toxic agents kill by single-hit processes. Single-hit processes are described by an exponential relationship between the toxic dose and the fraction of survivors. If the fraction of survivors is S, the relationship is $S = e^{-kc}$, where k is some constant describing the efficiency of killing and c is the concentration of the toxin. In the usual dose-response plot, we plot percent survivors on the vertical axis versus the logarithm of the toxin concentration. Two different toxins or ITs, which differ in potency by a factor of 10, display two curves that are separated at every point by one log unit. The potency is determined by the concentration at which the first effect is noted. However, a plot like this tells little about efficacy, particularly efficacy of ridding an animal of a tumor load. (Most animal studies indicate that a successful anti-tumor therapy must eliminate all viable tumor cells.[29,30]) To look at efficacy, we change the plot and plot the fraction of survivors on the log axis versus dose on the linear axis. Then we see exponential decreases in survivors with increasing dose and the slopes are now different by a factor of 10 for two different ITs having two different potencies. This type of data plot requires an assay that will reach down to the level of survivors one is interested in. These types of assays are clonogenic assays or kinetic assays where the slopes of inactivation of protein synthesis measured at early times are extrapolated over the time period of the IT action to give the final value of survivors.

In many cases, potency and the efficacy of toxic agents are linearly related. The most potent agent also produces the most efficacious cell killing. However, protein toxins and immunotoxins intoxicate cells by a receptor-mediated process and the concentration of toxin in the external medium is not the relevant variable. Rather, the

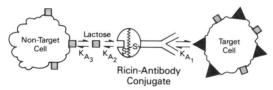

FIGURE 2. Schematic representation of an immunotoxin made with intact ricin and utilizing lactose to reduce nontarget cell toxicity due to the affinity, K_{A3} of ricin for its galactose-containing receptors present on all vertebrate cells. (From Neville.[1] With permission from CRC Press, Inc.)

number of occupied receptors is the relevant variable so we can change the formula $S = e^{-kc}$ by replacing c by a binding isotherm, that is, that the amount bound (B) is equal to the number of receptors (n) times the affinity constant (K_a) times the free concentration (F) divided by $1 + K_aF$.[31] Now, this does not change the apparent shape appreciably of the dose-response curve in many cases. FIGURE 3(a) shows curves generated with affinity of 10^{-11} M^{-1} and 10^8 receptors on the cell and the rate constant is arbitrary. But this is the kind of data that one often runs into and since the data down to the 10% protein synthesis level are not too good, one would not really be aware that this was very much different than a hyperbolic dose-response curve. However, if we take and plot the same data now as the log fraction of surviving cells we see what happens where saturation occurs (FIGURE 3b). We observe a plateau in efficacy and we can not go below a certain fraction of survivors. In the example in FIGURE 3, affinities of 10^{11} M^{-1} and 10^{10} M^{-1} are compared. The lower affinity IT provides a 4 log kill while at $K_a = 10^{11}$ M^{-1} the log kill does not extend below 1 log. (Note that the receptor occupancy below saturation dictated by nK_a has been held constant by changing n.) In the case where one-half saturation occurs at 10^{-11} M, one sees a situation where efficacy and potency are only related over a very narrow range ($<10^{-12}$ M). One sees that this is a potent agent but is unable to reduce the tumor burden below 90% of the initial number of cells. The failure to utilize these types of plots and the failure to utilize assays that will read out down to 5 and 6 log kill is one of the reasons that we

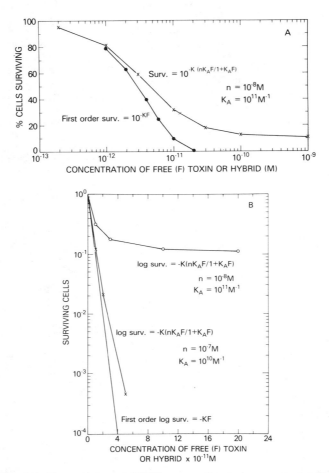

FIGURE 3(a and b). Theoretical curves of killing versus free toxin concentration illustrating the effect of a saturable process imposed between the medium and the killing process. The saturable process curves in A ($\times$ - $\times$) and B (O - O, $\times$ - $\times$) show deviations from first-order killing curves (referenced to the medium concentration), which are more pronounced when plotted over 4 logs of survivors as in (B). Immunotoxins exhibiting properties of the upper curve in (B) would not be capable of eradicating tumor loads of greater than 10 cells.

The first order curves presume that the concentration of toxin, c, which appears in the first order equation $S = e^{-kc}$ is directly proportional to the concentration of free toxin in the medium, F, so that $S = e^{-kf}$. Curves exhibiting saturation presume that the concentration of toxin, which appears in the first-order equation differs from the medium-free toxin concentration by a factor that describes a saturable process of n sites with an affinity constant K_A so that $S = e^{-k(nK_AF/1+K_AF)}$. The values for the first-order constant k differ in the two examples being 10^8 in the case of the non-saturable process, and 10^{11} for the saturable process, the difference, 10^3, being equal to nK_A, which appears in the equation for saturation. (From Neville & Youle.[31] With permission from publisher.)

have so many immunotoxins considered to "work" *in vitro* but won't "work" *in vivo*. The *in vitro* assay has been simply done as a dose-response curve and immunotoxin is shown to be much more potent than the parent toxin. This is because the affinity of the immunotoxin is greater than that of the present toxin. However, many of these immunotoxins are so inefficient that even when all the receptors are occupied over the duration of full toxin action, only 90% of the cells are inactivated. In FIGURE 4, we take an example from actual data in the literature that shows three different conjugates all

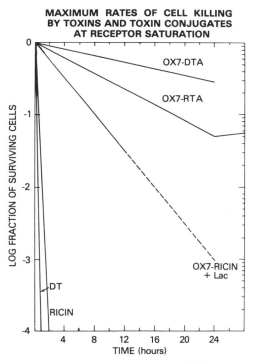

MAXIMUM RATES OF CELL KILLING BY TOXINS AND TOXIN CONJUGATES AT RECEPTOR SATURATION

FIGURE 4. The kinetics of toxin and immunotoxin action following the lag period at >90% receptor saturation. All data except diphtheria toxin, DT, are from AKR cells. DTA, immunotoxin with diphtheria toxin A chain. RTA, immunotoxin with ricin A chain. Dashed line is an extrapolation. (From Neville.[1] With permission from CRC Press, Inc.)

with the same antibody, Ox7 (anti-Thy 1.1) and in this case these are all directed against the same cell type.[1] The A chain of diphtheria toxin is rather inefficient. Immunotoxins using the A chain of ricin are more efficient but still can only achieve a 1 log kill in 24 hours. By utilizing intact ricin blockaded with lactose we achieve a log kill of 1 in about 8 hours and the assays we have used extrapolate to about a 3 log kill in 24 hours. Note, however, that none of these conjugates is nearly as active as the parent toxins. These toxins easily achieve log kills of 6 in clonogenic assays but their potential is much greater as extrapolated from the kinetic data and they show log kills up to 6 logs per hour. The killing rate occurs out to 15–20 hours at lower toxin concentrations.[1]

ANALYSIS OF *IN VIVO* EFFICACY

The methodologies just considered apply for tissue culture but what about assessing immunotoxin efficacy *in vivo?* A number of years ago, Skipper and co-workers[29] showed that by injecting different tumor doses into animals and determining the day of death, a relationship between these two was obtained and this was exponential. The relationship is shown by plotting the logarithm of injected cells on the vertical axis and the mean day of death on the horizontal axis (see Marsh and Neville in this volume). The log linear plot indicates that the tumor growth is exponential and the death occurs at a fixed tumor load. One can estimate this apparent lethal load by extrapolating this curve back to day zero and for murine leukemia the number comes out about 10^{10} cells. The plating efficiency of cells in the animal is determined by the minimum number of cells that will produce death and in the studies with murine leukemia this turned out often to be as low as 10 cells. The apparent lethal load should be divided by the *in vivo* plating efficiency to estimate the lethal tumor load. The advantage of this type of assay is that after injecting animals with a fixed number of cells and then treating with anti-tumor agent, if one observes the day of death then one can calculate the tumor load reduction of the agent.

The above methodology was used by Thorpe and co-workers at the Drug Targeting Laboratory in London and they reported a 1.7 log kill of murine leukemia cells by a ricin A chain immunotoxin and a 3 log kill with an immunotoxin made up of the $F(ab)_2$ pieces of Ox7[6] and the ribosomal-inactivating protein saporin. These assays were carried out in a peritoneal cavity nude mouse system. Even higher log kills up to 5 and 6 logs were obtained when the intact Ox7 antibody was used with saporin. This log kill was higher than that achieved *in vitro* by the same immunotoxin and suggests that there is an additive effect between the immunotoxin and the antibody moiety, particularly the Fc piece, which may activate some killer cells present in the nude mouse. Thus, there is a lack of correlation between *in vitro* cytotoxic data and *in vivo* cytotoxic data. Ox7-ricin A chain and Ox7-saporin exhibited equal cytotoxic activities in tissue culture yet the saporin conjugate was 1000 fold more efficacious *in vivo*.[6] Other examples of *in vivo* anti-tumor effects beyond that expected for the type of conjugate used based on tissue culture protein synthesis inhibition assays are in the literature. For example, a diphtheria toxin A chain immunotoxin was reported to induce a significant lag in tumor growth in a guinea pig model system.[32] Yet in our hands diphtheria toxin A chain conjugates provide at best a 0.5 log cell kill (FIGURE 4). It appears that *in vivo* certain A chain or RIP-based immunotoxins may induce anti-tumor effects beyond their ability *in vitro* to translocate to the cytosol and inhibit protein synthesis.[33] Sorting out these potentially useful interactions is important and will require rigorous *in vivo* models.

The saporin-Ox7 immunotoxin achieves the highest log kill *in vivo* yet to be reported. Thorpe and co-workers think that a considerable amount of the log kill they achieve over what others have reported in similar types of immunotoxins is due to the method of bonding between the toxin moiety and the Ox7. Blakey and co-workers have discussed evidence supportive of the hypothesis that certain cells may undergo mutations that lead to the production of enzymes that break down the amide bond of immunotoxins linked via amides.[34] If this is true, it indicates that routing is an extremely important variable for the constructing of high efficacy immunotoxins constructed with ribosomal-inactivating proteins or toxin A chains. These data would imply that for efficient killing the toxic fragment must stay associated with the antibody for some extended duration of time and this may represent the time taken to reach the compartment from which efficient translocation can occur.

Our own studies, conducted by Dr. Marsh, have achieved 3 log kills *in vivo* and have emphasized the importance of the B chain translocation function in immunotoxin constructed for *in vivo* use.[7]

In summary, I think that we have immunotoxins available today that have efficacy in certain *in vivo* model situations. It appears that major variables revolve around (1) the intracellular route the immunotoxin takes; (2) the stability of the bonds that holds the immunotoxin to the immunoglobulin; and (3) the presence of translocation functions either in the A chain of the immunotoxin or in the ribosomal-inactivating proteins or in the holo-immunotoxin. My colleagues and I think that in the next several years important contributions to the holo-immunotoxins field will be made by designing covalent blockade of the toxin binding site that can be reversed in an intracellular compartment.

REFERENCES

1. NEVILLE, D. M., JR. 1986. Immunotoxins: Current use and future prospects in bone marrow transplantation and cancer treatment. *In* CRC Critical Review in Therapeutic Drug Carrier Systems. **2:** 329–352. CRC Press, Inc. Boca Raton, FL.
2. VALLERA, D. A., R. C. ASH, E. D. ZANJANI, J. H. KERSEY, T. W. LEBEIN, P. C. L. BEVERLY, D. M. NEVILLE, JR. & R. J. YOULE. 1983. Anti-T-cell reagents for human bone marrow transplantation: Ricin linked to three monoclonal antibodies. Science **222:** 512–515.
3. FILIPOVICH, A. H., D. A. VALLERA, R. J. YOULE, D. M. NEVILLE, JR. & J. H. KERSEY. Transplantation Proc. **17:** 442–444.
4. CHANG, T. M. & D. M. NEVILLE, JR. 1977. J. Biol. Chem. **252:** 1505–1514.
5. LAURENT, G., J. PRIS, J. P. FARCET, P. CARAGON, H. BLYTHMAN, P. CASELLAS, P. PONCELET & F. K. JANSEN. 1986. Blood **67:** 1680–1687.
6. THORPE, P. E., A. N. F. BROWN, J. A. G. BREMNER, B. M. J. FOXWELL & F. STIRPE. 1985. J. Natl. Can. Inst. **75:** 151–159.
7. MARSH, J. W. & D. M. NEVILLE, JR. 1987. Ann. N.Y. Acad. Sci. (This volume.)
8. NEVILLE, D. M., JR. & T. H. HUDSON. 1986. Ann. Rev. Biochem. **55:** 195–224.
9. BOQUET, P., M. S. SILVERMAN, A. M. PAPPENHEIMER, JR. & W. B. VERNON. 1976. Proc. Natl. Acad. Sci. USA **73:** 4449–44453.
10. MARNELL, M. H., M. STOOKEY & R. K. DRAPER. 1982. J. Cell Biol. **93:** 57–62.
11. HUDSON, T. H. & D. M. NEVILLE, JR. 1985. J. Biol. Chem. **260:** 2675–2680.
12. HUDSON, T. H. & D. M. NEVILLE, JR. J. Biol. Chem. (In press.)
13. HUDSON, T. H. & D. M. NEVILLE, JR. (Submitted for publication.)
14. YAMAIZUMI, M., T. UCHIDA, E. MEKADA & Y. OKADA. 1979. Cell **18:** 1009–1014.
15. YOULE, R. J., G. J. MURRAY & D. M. NEVILLE, JR. 1981. Cell **23:** 551–559.
16. MARSH, J. W. & D. M. NEVILLE, JR. 1986. Biochem. **25:** 4461–4467.
17. MARSH, J. W., K. SRINIVASACHAR & D. M. NEVILLE, JR. Immunotoxin synthesis: Influence of chemical variables on efficacy. *In* Immunotoxins. A. Frankel, Ed. Martinos Nijhoff Publ. Boston.
18. MARSH, J. W. & D. M. NEVILLE, JR. (Submitted for publication.)
19. MARSH, J. W. & D. M. NEVILLE, JR. 1986. Immunotoxins: Chemical variables affecting cell killing efficiences. *In* Protein Tailoring and Reagents for Food and Medical Uses. Feeney & Whitaker, Eds.: 291–316. Marcel Dekker, Inc. New York.
20. MARSH, J. W., M. A. G. KIMAK & D. M. NEVILLE, JR. 1987. (Submitted for publication.)
21. ESWORTHY, R. S. & D. M. NEVILLE, JR. 1984. J. Biol. Chem. **259:** 11496–11504.
22. CASELLAS, P., B. J. P. BOURRIE, P. GROS & F. K. JANSEN. 1984. J. Biol. Chem. **259:** 9359–9364.
23. CHANG, T.-M. & D. W. KULLBERG. 1982. J. Biol. Chem. **257:** 12563–12572.

24. FULTON, R. J., D. C. BLAKEY, P. P. KNOWLES, J. W. UHR, P. E. THORPE & E. S. VITETTA. 1986. J. Biol. Chem. **261:** 5314–5319.
25. LAMBERT, J. M., P. D. SENTER, A. YAU-YOUNG, W. A. BLATTLER & V. S. GOLDMACHER. 1985. J. Biol. Chem. **260:** 12035–12041.
26. RAMAKRISHNAN, S. & L. L. HOUSTON. 1984. Cancer Res. **44:** 201–208.
27. YOULE, R. J. & D. M. NEVILLE, JR. 1980. Proc. Natl. Acad. Sci. USA **77:** 5483–5486.
28. NEVILLE, D. M., JR. & R. J. YOULE. 1982. Anti-Thy 1.2 monoclonal antibody-ricin hybrid utilized as a tumor suppressant. U.S. Patent 4,359,457.
29. SKIPPER, H. E., F. M. SCHABEL, JR. & W. S. WILCOX. 1965. Cancer Chemother. Rep. **45:** 5–28.
30. SINDELAR, W. F. & C. C. KURMAN. 1981. J. Natl. Cancer Inst. **67:** 1093–1102.
31. NEVILLE, D. M., JR. & R. J. YOULE. 1982. Immunol. Rev. **62:** 75–91.
32. BERNHARD, M. I., K. A. FOON, T. N. OELTMANN, M. E. KEY, K. M. HWANG, G. C. CLARKE, W. L. CHRISTENSEN, L. C. HOYER, M. G. HANNA & R. K. OLDHAM. 1983. Cancer Res. **43:** 4420–4428.
33. GREGG, E. O., S. H. BRIDGES, R. J. YOULE, D. L. LONGO, L. L. HOUSTON, M. J. GLENNIE, F. K. STEVENSON & I. GREEN. 1987. J. Immunol. (In press.)
34. BLAKEY, P. C., E. J. WAWRZYNCZAK, F. STIRPE & P. E. THORPE. *In* Membrane-mediated Cytotoxicity. B. Bonavida & R. J. Collier, Eds. UCLA Symp. on Mol. Cell. Biol. (In press).

Development of an Immunotoxin
with *in Vivo* Efficacy for Murine Systems

JON W. MARSH AND DAVID M. NEVILLE, JR.

Laboratory of Molecular Biology
National Institute of Mental Health
Bethesda, Maryland 20892

INTRODUCTION

Native protein toxins, such as the plant toxin ricin or the bacterial diphtheria toxin, possess three functions that give them their remarkable ability to kill cells.[1] These functions are generally ascribed to one of the toxin's two subunits, designated A and B. One function is the enzymatic activity, found in the A subunit, that is capable of inhibiting the cell's protein synthesizing machinery. The second function, a B chain function, is the ability to bind to a plasma membrane receptor(s). The binding of the toxin to the cell surface results in its internalization, through an endocytotic process. Although the toxin is internalized, it remains in the cellular vesicle/organelle system and is not accessible to the target (enzymatic substrate) macromolecule in the cytosol. The third function, the translocation function, which is generally ascribed to the B subunit, facilitates the transmembrane delivery of the toxin's enzymatic activity to the cytosolic compartment where protein synthesis is inhibited.

In constructing an immunotoxin, one would like to incorporate a toxin that possesses an efficient translocation function, but lacks the active toxin binding site of the B subunit. Experimentally, separation of the translocation function from the binding site has been difficult, and evidence suggests, at least with ricin, that the binding site is closely associated with the translocation function.[2] However, one can block the binding site of the toxin in some reversible way and this will not diminish the conjugate's ability to kill the cell. Although the toxin moiety must be internalized (this can occur through the conjugation to an antibody, and thus through the internalization of the antigen) interaction of the toxin moiety with a cell surface receptor is non-essential.

There is evidence in the literature that toxins do not have to bind to their normal plasma membrane receptor to enter into the cytosolic compartment, as long as they are internalized through some other means, such as through the conjugation to an antibody. That is, the productive (lethal) receptor is intracellular. Two reports involve cell lines that through mutation have gained resistance to ricin. This resistance is imparted by an aberrantly high sialyltransferase activity. The toxin binds to terminal galactosyl residues of complex carbohydrates on the cell surface, and the elevated transferase activity blocks these binding sites through the addition of neuraminic acid. In one report,[3] exposure of the cell to neuraminidase restored ricin binding, but the cells maintained a resistance to the toxin. In the second report,[4] a normally ricin-sensitive cell and its ricin-resistance variant (again through decreased ricin binding) were both found to be sensitive to a ricin-antibody conjugate directed against a common cell surface antigen.

CHARACTERIZATION OF A DIPHTHERIA TOXIN CONJUGATE

Another demonstration that the productive receptor is intracellular concerns diphtheria toxin. Mice, rats, and their isolated cells are approximately 10^4 times less sensitive to the toxin than sensitive species.[5] Murine cells bind, internalize, and degrade labeled diphtheria toxin.[5-10] In addition, murine EF_2 is fully susceptible to the enzymatic inactivation of the toxin's A chain.[5] Thus, it appears that murine cells lack a productive surface receptor or some processing event. So diphtheria toxin is not a productive (lethal) toxin with murine cells. Two recent reports have demonstrated, however, that if the toxin is chemically coupled to an alternative ligand, such transferrin[11] or concanavalin A,[12] a 10^4 and 10^3 increase in potency results, respectively. We have found that the conjugation of the toxin to an anti-murine T-cell

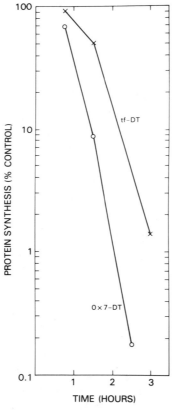

FIGURE 1. Kinetic study of protien synthesis inhibition by two diphtheria toxin conjugates. Murine leukemic AKR SL2 cells were incubated with 1,000 ng/ml of either the anti-Thy1.1 (Ox7) or transferring (tf) toxin conjugate. Protein synthesis was determined by pulsing the cell with radiolabeled leucine, and is expressed as percent of control, which has not been exposed to toxin.

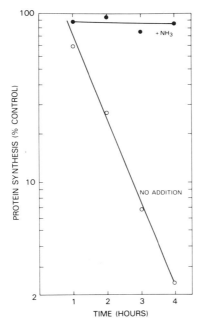

FIGURE 2. Protection of antibody-DT conjugate intoxication by ammonia. AKR cells were exposed to 500 ng/ml of the Ox7-DT in the presence (10 mM) or absense of ammonium chloride. Protein synthesis was determined as in FIGURE 1.

antibody (anti-Thy 1.1, Ox7[13]) also results in a highly efficacious agent. FIGURE 1 is a kinetic examination of this conjugate and a transferrin-diphtheria toxin conjugate and demonstrates the capacity of both of these conjugates to cause an exponential decline in protein synthesis. That this pseudo-first order inactivation of cellular protein synthesis preceded by a lag period is typical of the intoxication of sensitive (non-murine) cells by the native, unconjugated toxin.[14] Prior to intoxication of a sensitive cell, diphtheria toxin requires intravesicular acidification. Thus, the addition of lipophilic amines, such as ammonia, will protect a sensitive cell from exposure to the native toxin.[15] The addition of ammonia also protects murine cells from the intoxication process of the toxin-antibody conjugate (FIGURE 2). This result suggests that the toxin moiety of the conjugate may go through a similar sequence of events when compared to the intoxication of non-murine cells with the native toxin.

That the toxicity is specific for the antibody binding is demonstrated in FIGURE 3. The native toxin or the anti-Thy 1.1 antibody-diphtheria toxin conjugate (both at 500 ng/ml) were incubated with either the Thy-positive AKR-SL2 or the Thy-negative AKR-K36 cell lines. The ability of the cells to synthesize proteins was then followed as a function of time. The Thy-negative cells displayed no intoxication at this concentration, while the target cells (Thy-positive) were intoxicated only by the conjugate. If varied levels of the native toxin or conjugate were incubated with the two cell lines for 18 hours (FIGURE 4), we find that the two cell lines display similar sensitivities to the native toxin. However, there is a 3.6 log difference in the conjugate potency on the target versus non-target cell lines.

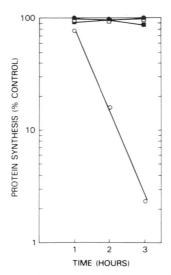

FIGURE 3. Intoxication of target and non-target cells by native and conjugated diphtheria toxin. Diphtheria toxin (500 ng/ml) was incubated with either Thy 1.1-positive ARK SL2 cells (open squares) or Thy 1.1-negative AKR K36 cells (closed squares). The anti-Thy 1.1 antibody-diphtheria toxin conjugate (also at 500 ng/ml) was likewise incubated with either the SL2 (open circles) or K36 (closed circles) cells. The loss of cellular ability to synthesize protein was followed kinetically as in FIGURE 1.

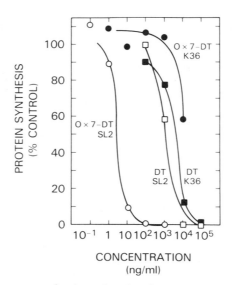

FIGURE 4. Dose-reponse curve of native toxin and conjugate on target and non-target cells. The cells (as in FIGURE 3) and varied levels of conjugate and toxin were incubated and protein synthesis was determined after 18 hours.

AN EFFICACIOUS *IN VIVO* AGENT

The native toxin or its conjugates exist as impotent and inefficacious toxins with non-target cells. Once internalized through an alternative ligand, as on target cells, the ineffective toxin moiety is converted to an active form. The nature of the toxin moiety interaction with murine cells, perhaps best described as a protoxin, suggests that the toxin-antibody conjugate may function as an *in vivo* agent. The toxin moiety does not contain productive binding activity, as transferrin or the antibody can supply, but does possess a translocation function, as demonstrated by the high rate of intoxication (FIGURE 1).

If 10^5 Thy 1.1 cells are injected into AKR/cum Thy 1.2 mice, the survival curve for those mice is that depicted in FIGURE 5. No further deaths (due to injected cells) were

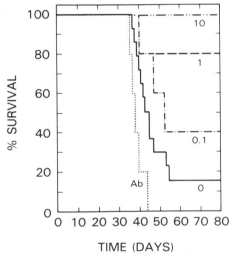

FIGURE 5. Survival curves of AKR/cum Thy 1.2 mice after introduction of AKR SL2 Thy 1.1 lymphoma cells. On day zero, 10^5 cells were injected intraperitoneally into groups of 5 to 15 mice. After 24 hours (day 1) varying levels of Ox7-DT conjugate (0, 0.1, 1.0, and 10 μg per mouse) were injected intraperitoneally, and the percent of survivors was determined daily. A control group receiving 7 μg native Ox7 antibody is designated as Ab (dotted curve) on the plot.

noted beyond 80 days. By increasing injected levels (0.1, 1, and 10 μg per mouse) of the Ox7-diphtheria toxin conjugate 24 hours after the introduction of the leukemic cells, increasing levels of cure were obtained. By comparison, injection of Ox7 antibody (or native toxin, data not shown) at 7 μg per mouse, the equivalent of 10 μg immunotoxin, lacks any positive therapy. Under the circumstances of this experiment, between one and two logs of cells had to be killed to bring about cure.

Utilizing the life span analysis plot developed by Howard Skipper and co-workers,[16] one can determine the efficacy of this conjugate in this particular tumor system. Groups of Thy 1.2 mice are injected with varied levels (10^4 to 10^7 cells per mouse) of Thy 1.1 leukemic cells, designated on the y-axis of FIGURE 6. The mean life span is then determined for each group of mice as plotted on the x-axis as days following injection of cells. The linearity of the semi-log plot indicated exponential growth through the observed range and that death occurred at a defined tumor burden. The injection of 10^7 leukemic cells (mean life span: 24.6 days) followed 24 hours later by 5 μg of the conjugate resulted in a 9.2 day extension of life (indicated by the first arrow in FIGURE 6), and is equivalent to a two log kill. Note that the 33.8 day value (mean life span of treated mice) on the x-axis approximates the life span for injection of 10^5 cells. Injection of 10^6 cells, followed by 5 μg immunotoxin 24 hours later, resulted in the cure of all treated mice. This result surpassed the limits of our assay system, but approached a three log kill. A similar log kill has been achieved by using Thy 1.1 AKR mice.[17]

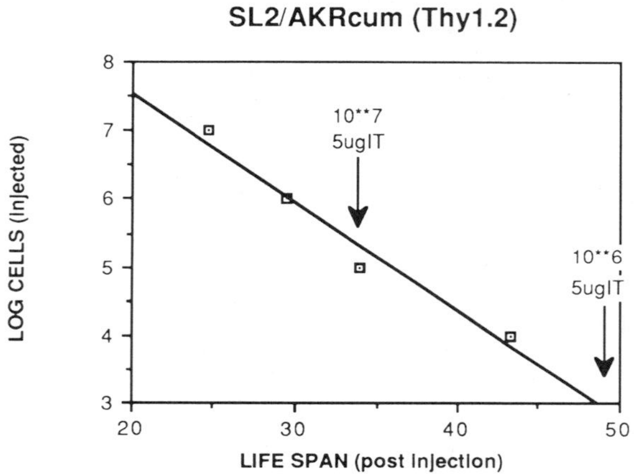

SL2/AKRcum (Thy1.2)

FIGURE 6. Relationship between lymphoma inoculant size and average life span. AKR/cum Thy 1.2 mice were injected (FIGURE 5) with varying levels of Thy 1.1 AKR cells. The average life span was then determined for each group. Mice, which received 10^7 cells on day zero, followed by 5 μg Ox7-DT conjugate 24 hours later, had extended life spans with a mean value indicated by the position of the first arrow. Mice receiving 10^6 cells followed by 5 μg conjugate one day later were all cured.

CONCLUSIONS

To bring this level of log kill into perspective, a comparison of the ability of chemical agents to reduce tumor burden can be made. The following examples were taken from the work of Skipper et al.[17] and involved determining the reduction of lymphoma cells in the thymus of AKR mice. The folic acid analogue, methotrexate, at a single dose equivalent to 0.5 LD_{10} resulted in a 1 log reduction in cells. At similar singular doses (~0.5 LD_{10}) the alkylating agent, cyclophosphamide, and the alkaloid, vincristine, both resulted in a 4 log reduction. The antibiotic daunomycin resulted in a 3 log kill. Thus, a single dose of the immunotoxin results in a similar cell kill compared to these chemical agents. A point worth mentioning is that these agents typically are efficacious only with rapidly growing cells. There is presently no reason to believe that immunotoxins are limited in that sense.

Immunotoxins do possess limitations, however, and this is the topic of a companion paper,[18] as well as previous reviews.[19,20] The murine immunotoxin system described here should assist us in studying the variables of *in vivo* conjugate action. Our approach permits a reproducible quantitation of cell kill, and thus optimization of chemical and physiological variables will be possible.

REFERENCES

1. NEVILLE, D. M., JR. & T. H. HUDSON. 1986. Ann. Rev. Biochem. **55:** 195–224.
2. MARSH, J. W. & D. M. NEVILLE, JR. Unpublished results.
3. GOTTLIEB, C. & S. KORNFELD. 1976. J. Biol. Chem. **251:** 7761–7768.
4. LEONARD, J. E., M. L. COLLINS, L. E. TANNEY & I. ROYSTON. 1985. Fed. Proc. **44:** 7466.
5. MOEHRING, J. M. & T. J. MOEHRING. 1976. Infect. Immun. **13:** 221–228.
6. CHANG, T. M. & D. M. NEVILLE, JR. 1977. J. Biol. Chem. **253:** 6866–6871.
7. HEAGY, W. E. & D. M. NEVILLE, JR. 1981. J. Biol. Chem. **256:** 12788–12792.
8. KEEN, J. H., F. R. MAXFIELD, M. C. HARDEGREE & W. H. HABIG. 1982. Proc. Natl. Acad. Sci. USA **79:** 2912–2916.
9. BONVENTRE, P. F., C. B. SAELINGER, B. IVINS, C. WOSCINSKI & M. AMORINI. 1975. Infec. Immun. **11:** 675–684.
10. BOQUET, P. & A. M. PAPPENHEIMER, JR. 1976. J. Biol. Chem. **251:** 5770–5778.
11. O'KEEFE, D. O. & R. K. DRAPER. 1985. J. Biol. Chem. **260:** 932–937.
12. GUILLEMOT, J. C., A. SUNDAN, S. OLSNES & K. SANDVIG. 1985. **122:** 193–199.
13. MASON, D. W. & A. F. WILLIAMS. 1980. Biochem. J. **187:** 1–20.
14. UCHIDA, T., A. M. PAPPENHEIMER, JR. & A. A. HARPER. 1973. J. Biol. Chem. **248:** 3845–3850.
15. KIM, K. & N. B. GROMAN. 1985. J. Bacteriol. **90:** 1552–1556.
16. SKIPPER, H. E., F. M. SCHABEL, JR., M. W. TRADER, W. R. LASTER, JR., L. SIMPSON-HERREN & H. H. LLOYD. 1972. Cancer Chemother. Rep **56:** 273–314.
17. MARSH, J. W. Unpublished resutls.
18. NEVILLE, D. M., JR. This volume.
19. NEVILLE, D. M. JR. 1986. Immunotoxins: Current use and future prospects in bone marrow transplantation and cancer treatment. *In* CRC Critical Review in Therapeutic Drug Carrier Systems. **2:** 329–352. CRC Press, Inc. Boca Raton, FL.
20. MARSH, J. W. & D. M. NEVILLE, JR. 1986. Immunotoxins: Chemical variables affecting cell killing efficiences. *In* Protein Tailoring and Reagents for Food and Medical Uses. R. E. Fenney & J. R. Whitaker, Eds.: 291–316. Marcel Dekker, Inc. New York.

Intracellular Pathways
of Ricin A Chain Cytotoxins[a]

VIC RASO, SIMON C. WATKINS, HENRY SLAYTER, AND
CATHERINE FEHRMANN

Department of Pathology
Dana-Farber Cancer Institue
Harvard Medical School
Boston, Massachusetts 02115

INTRODUCTION

Ricin, a toxic protein isolated from castor beans, is composed of two disulfide-linked subunits, the A chain and B chain. Its B chain is the binding moiety that allows this toxin to attach to cell surface galactose sites and eventually to enter cells by endocytosis. Once inside, the A chain manages to access the cytosol, perhaps with the assistance of B chain. Here it catalytically inactivates ribosomes at the rate of 1,500/min[1] and thereby effectively kills the cell by shutting down protein synthesis. The *in vitro* cytotoxic activity of ricin can be blocked by adding a high concentration of lactose to the culture medium. This sugar prevents the toxin from attaching to the cell surface by filling the binding site on B chain. In the absence of cell binding, the A chain cannot enter to reach the ribosomes so the cells are spared. Similarly, when the disulfide linkage connecting the A and B chains is severed by reduction with mercaptoethanol,[2] the toxin loses activity since the A chain on its own has no effective means for attaching to cells and penetrating into the cytosol. The isolated A chain however, retains its inherent enzymatic activity and this can be demonstrated in a cell-free protein synthesis system where the A chain comes into direct contact with ribosomes to inhibit their action.

Ricin is an indiscriminately lethal toxin since virtually all cells possess the membrane-situated galactose sites to which it can bind. The observation that isolated A chain has full cytotoxic potential has led to the strategy of replacing the B moiety with alternative carriers having more selective binding characteristics. Thus, purified A chain has been covalently coupled to a variety of antibodies and receptor ligands to produce an array of very specific site-directed toxic conjugates (FIGURE 1). The great diversity in expression of cell membrane receptors and antigenic determinants could conceivably be exploited through the use of such agents to recognize and efficiently kill defined classes of cells both *in vitro* and *in vivo*.

A variety of these derivative toxins have been synthesized by methods that have retained full carrier binding function as well as the enzymatic activity of its toxic moiety. Such toxin derivatives, however, have not all displayed equivalent cytotoxic effectiveness but rather activity has shown a dependence upon a number of related factors. The specific cell surface receptor or determinant chosen as a target, its density of expression, and affiliated internalization pathway all serve a primary function in determining the final potency. The origin of a toxic moiety can play a role and analogous conjugates built, for example, with ricin A or diphtheria A coupled to

[a]Supported by National Cancer Institute grant CA29039.

identical carriers may display differing cytotoxic activity.[3] Chemical linkage is also a determining factor, with disulfide-bonded conjugate toxins providing much greater cell kill than those formed with alternative connections. In addition, a number of exogenous agents have been found to greatly improve the potency of A chain toxins apparently by altering intracellular trafficking. These include such diverse substances as chloroquine, viruses, NH_4Cl, toxin B chains, and carboxylic ionophores. Clearly, toxic activity is ultimately governed by the efficiency and speed with which active A chain gains access to the cytosol where it inactivates components needed for protein synthesis. This underlines the importance for gaining a better understanding of how these derivative toxins get into cells and what they do once inside. Such information would not only assist in designing toxins with maximal activity but should also provide a better understanding of the basic cellular processes that allow access to the cytosolic compartment.

To study the introduction of toxic ricin A chain into cells, we have used the transferrin iron delivery pathway because this route of entry proceeds by several well defined and easily measurable steps (FIGURE 2).[4-6] Thus, transferrin, an 80 Kd serum glycoprotein, binds two ferric ions and attaches to specific receptors on the cell surface. This complex is taken into cells by receptor-mediated endocytosis, involving coated pits and coated vesicles and quickly enters the acidic environment of low density endosomes. The reduced pH within these vesicles induces transferrin to release iron so that it can enter the cytosol where it is utilized or stored. The receptor-ligand complex does not dissociate under these conditions and neither element enters the lysosomes. Instead they return to the cell surface where, at neutral pH, the iron-depleted apo-transferrin separates from its receptor. In this way, both components evade intracellular degradation and can be reutilized for multiple rounds of iron delivery.

RESULTS AND DISCUSSION

Lethal Action of Transferrin Receptor Directed Toxins

Ricin A chain has been targeted to the transferrin receptor by coupling it either to transferrin, its natural ligand, or to monoclonal antibodies reactive with various epitopes on the receptor (FIGURE 1).[7,8] The potent cytotoxic action displayed by these distinct conjugate forms has indicated that each can deliver active A chain to ribosomes in the cytosol. By monitoring the time course of inhibition of cellular protein synthesis, the speed at which this A chain is conveyed to its target can be determined. For human leukemia CEM cells, receptor-saturating levels of either transferrin-A chain (Tf-A) or anti-transferrin receptor-A chain (TfR-A) produced linear inactivation kinetics with a $t_{1/2} = 300$ min (FIGURE 3). Although ultimately effective, this rate of cell kill is slow compared to the average time of 15 min required for an occupied transferrin receptor to complete its cycle through the cell.[4,6] Apparently passage of active A chain into the cytosol was slow or occurred only occasionally during the cycling process. Therefore, a number of known cytoactive agents were tested concomitantly with the derivative toxins to accelerate their action. It was anticipated that these might alter normal intracellular pathways or modify any physical barriers to A chain translocation. Monensin, a carboxylic ionophore and one of the most efficient potentiators found,[9] radically changed the kinetics profile for protein synthesis inhibition produced by both Tf-A and TfR-A (FIGURE 3). Cells treated with these toxins in the presence of 10^{-7} M monensin displayed a 30–40 min lag phase followed by a sharp linear inactivation phase with $t_{1/2} = 15$ min. This lag period was not reduced by pretreatment of cells for 1 hour with either monensin alone or toxin alone before initiating the kinetics experiment by adding the second complementary agent. This indicated that they must act in conjunction rather than sequentially to produce the rapid kinetics.

A biphasic kinetics profile was not exclusively linked to monensin treatment but also appeared associated with B chain activity since almost indentical lag and $t_{1/2}$ parameters were observed upon treatment of CEM cells with whole ricin in the absence of ionophore. Moreover, this same characteristic pattern was obtained when a disulfide-coupled transferrin–whole ricin conjugate was tested with lactose to block B chain binding and ensure that toxin entered via the transferrin pathway (data not shown). These kinetics results can be accommodated to a simple compartment model. This scheme assumes that $t_{1/2} = 300$ min reflects the rate of toxin penetration into the cytosol from one cellular compartment and that $t_{1/2} = 15$ min represents the rate out of a second distinct compartment, which becomes accessible to toxin when monensin or B chain is present. The 30-min lag would represent the time required for monensin or B chain–mediated transfer of toxin into this second compartment.

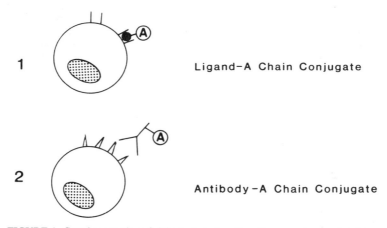

FIGURE 1. Specfic targeting of ricin A chain to cell surface receptors and antigens.

Perhaps the best way to appreciate the significance of improved inhibition kinetics is to measure its ultimate effect upon the extent of cell kill using a clonogenic assay (FIGURE 4).[10] Greater than 99.9995% cytoreduction resulted when 5×10^5 CEM cells were treated simultaneously with Tf-A and monensin for 3 hr before adding excess native transferrin to terminate further action. In accord with the slow kinetics of Tf-A by itself (FIGURE 3), neither agent alone showed high toxic potency under these abbreviated incubation conditions. The rapid elimination of more than 5 logs of cells by the combined action of Tf-A plus monensin was receptor specific since it could be totally blocked by prior exposure of the cells to excess transferrin (FIGURE 4). This high potency, quick action, and sharp specificity are desirable characteristics if one envisions using these derivative toxins for eventual *in vivo* therapeutics.

Synthesis and Characterization of [125]*I-labeled A Chain Toxins*

Given the toxic activity of Tf-A and TfR-A plus the potentiating influence of agents such as monensin, it was important to determine how closely these derivatives

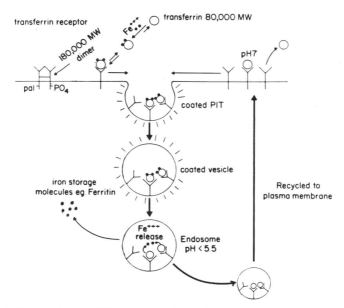

FIGURE 2. Scheme for the delivery of iron into cells by receptor-mediated endocytosis of transferrin.

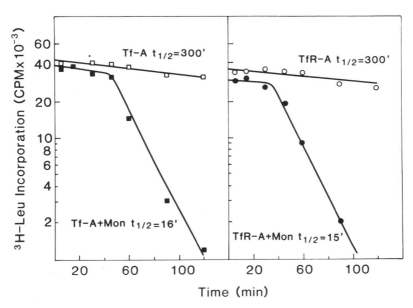

FIGURE 3. Kinetics of inhibition of protein synthesis with and without monensin. Tf-A, anti-TfR-A, and monensin all at 10^{-7} M. CEM cells were incubated with the designated components at 37°C in microtiter wells for the times noted and then were pulse-labeled with ^{3}H-leu for 30 min before harvesting and measuring incorporation.[7] All points were run in quadruplicate.

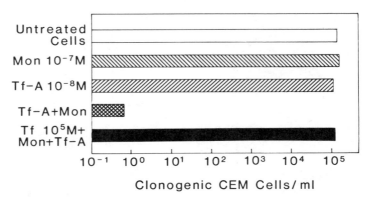

FIGURE 4. Elimination of clonogenic CEM cells by combined treatment with Tf-A and monensin. CEM cells 5×10^5/ml were either untreated or treated with Tf-A (10^{-8} M), monensin (10^{-7} M), and human transferrin (10^{-5} M) for 3 hr. They were washed, plated in media plus transferrin, and clonogenic cells were evaluated 2 weeks later as described in Bregni et al.[10]

followed the natural transferrin internalization pathway (FIGURE 2) and where they deviated from it to inactivate ribosomes. To accomplish this, conjugates were constructed with ^{125}I-labeled ricin A chain. This exclusive positioning ensured that intracellular trafficking of the toxin moiety could be monitored in an unambiguous manner. Ellman's reagent was used to protect the free sulfhydryl of isolated A chain during its iodination with ^{125}I using Iodogen. The deblocked radioiodinated A chain was then disulfide coupled to N-succinimidyl-3-(2-pyridyldithio)propionate derivatized human transferrin or mouse monoclonal anti-transferrin receptor antibodies. The resulting conjugates were purified on molecular sizing columns and the position of the radiolabel was verified by autoradiographic analysis following SDS-PAGE under reducing and non-reducing conditions. Whereas all of the radioactivity banded in the high molecular weight region characteristic for authentic Tf-A or TfR-A before disulfide cleavage, after breaking this bond, the radioactivity shifted to the 30K position of free A chain.

Receptor Binding and Cellular Uptake of ^{125}I-labeled A Chain Toxins

Cell-associated Tf-A and TfR-A was determined after incubation of 2×10^7 CEM cells with 4×10^5 cpm of the ^{125}I-labeled conjugates for 45 min at either 0°C or 37°C and then washing two times with PBS to remove unbound counts (FIGURE 5). Dissociation of transferrin from exposed surface receptors can be achieved by acid treatment[5] so that a brief 15-sec exposure of washed cells to 0.25 M acetic acid/0.5 M NaCl was used to distinguish external from internalized ^{125}I]Tf-A. By these criteria, it was easy to show that binding at 0°C was predominantly to surface receptors while at 37°C an additional internalized fraction was also present. This acid-resistant population of Tf-A molecules comprised ~70% of the total bound counts (FIGURE 5) and its temperature dependence was consistent with energy-requiring endocytotic uptake.

[125]I]TfR-A bound to CEM cells both at 0°C and 37°C, however, this interaction was not disrupted by a brief acid treatment (FIGURE 5). The extent of binding was four-fold higher than that of ligand-A chain even though reaction conditions and

specific activities were the same. Thus, the number of available receptor epitopes[11] appeared to exceed the active ligand binding sites on these CEM cells.

Structural Analysis of Intracellular [125I]-labeled A Chain Conjugates

Most protein ligands taken into cells by receptor-mediated endocytosis are delivered into lysosomes and degraded. Native transferrin is an exception to this norm (FIGURE 2), but it was important to determine if the A chain–modified species, Tf-A and TfR-A, also survived lysosomal degradation. Moreover, it was of interest to try to detect evidence for disulfide cleavage of these conjugates within the cell since it has been suspected that such separation might be required for toxicity to ensue.

Anti-A chain (anti-A) and anti-transferrin (anti-T) affinity columns were used to analyze [125I]Tf-A both before and after its incorporation into cells. Greater than 90% of the counts applied to the columns in PBS were retained, verifying the radiochemical purity of this [125I]Tf-A preparation (FIGURE 6). However, after splitting the connecting disulfide bond with mercaptoethanol, counts were bound only to the anti-A column. This finding not only showed that all of the label was located in the A chain half but also demonstrated the feasibility of using dual column analysis for detecting reductive cleavage.

[125I]Tf-A was allowed to react with CEM cells for 2 hr either at 37°C or 0°C to compare the fate of internalized versus receptor-bound molecules. These cells were washed with PBS and then lysed using 0.1% Triton X-100 to release the associated radioactivity for analysis on the affinity columns. The structural integrity of [125I]Tf-A was maintained regardless of whether it remained on the cell surface at 0°C or was incorporated into cells at 37°C, since in both instances greater than 90% of the applied counts was retained by the anti-A and anti-T columns (FIGURE 6). There was no indication of disulfide cleavage or free A chain because equivalent counts bound to each column. A small percent of breakdown, however, might have escaped detection in this system.

The composite toxin and monoclonal antibody halves of TfR-A were also found to be greatly preserved after interaction with cells as judged by analysis of anti-A and anti-mouse IgG affinity columns (FIGURE 6). An indication of a low level of catabolic

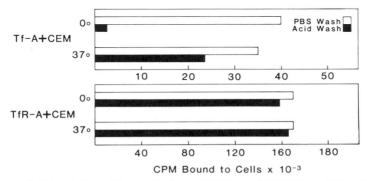

FIGURE 5. Cellular binding and internalization of [125I]Tf-A and [125I]TfR-A. CEM cells at 2 × 10⁷/ml were incubated with 4 × 10⁵ cpm of [125I]Tf-A or [125I]TfR-A for 45 min at the designated temperature. Cells were then washed twice with PBS and counted. They were then exposed to 0.25 M acetic acid/0.5 M NaCl for 15 sec, neutralized, washed with PBS, and recounted.

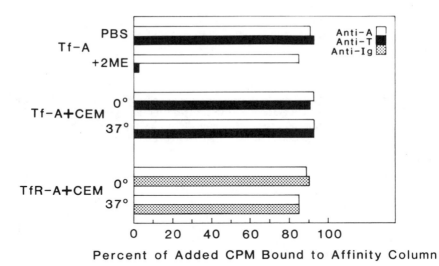

FIGURE 6. Binding of [125I]-A chain toxins to affinity columns. [[125I]]Tf-A (5,000 cpm) was applied to the anti-ricin A chain, anti-human transferrin, or control matrix columns (~0.5 ml packed gel). Where designated, mercaptoethanol (2 ME) at 0.1 M was used to split the disulfide linkage before dilution and application to affinity columns. CEM cells were incubated with radiolabeled conjugates for 2 hr at the designated temperature, washed, and lysed with 0.1% Triton X-100. After clearing by centrifugation, lysates were applied to the affinity columns.

activity was given by the 5% reduced levels of column-retained counts seen for lysates from the cells maintained at 37°C compared to 0°C.

Distribution of Tf-A and TfR-A Within Subcellular Compartments

A series of vesicle compartments and membrane networks are encountered during the transport of materials into cells via receptor-mediated endocytosis (FIGURE 2). Transferrin has been identified in several of these structures including coated pits, coated vesicles, endosomes, CURL (compartment for uncoupling receptor and ligand), and Golgi but apparently does not enter the lysosomes.[5] The absence of cellular degradation of Tf-A and TfR-A (FIGURE 6) suggested that these toxin derivatives also bypassed the lysosomal compartment. To test this further, CEM cells were incubated at 37°C for 2 hr with each of the [125I]-labeled A chain conjugates, freed of unbound counts by washing, and then disrupted mechanically to release their subcellular components.[5] The post-nuclear fraction was suspended in 15% Percoll and the mixture was then centrifuged to establish a density gradient. Fractions were collected to monitor separation of the different cytoplasmic components along with any labeled toxin that had become associated with them. The distribution profile shows that most of the radioactive Tf-A and TfR-A co-migrated to the top of the gradient along with the low-density subcellular elements (FIGURE 7). No substantial accumulation occurred at the high-density region at the bottom of these gradients where the lysosomal marker enzyme β-hexosaminidase was found. Thus, neither Tf-A nor TfR-A appeared to enter lysosomes but like the natural ligand transferrin, was restricted to low-density vesicles.[5]

$^{59}Fe^{3+}$ *Tf-A as a Probe of the Cellular Environment*

Transferrin releases its two ferric ions when it encounters acid conditions within endosomes (FIGURE 2).[5,6] Perhaps the most critical test for judging if Tf-A follows the same pathway would determine if the toxin retained a functional capacity for delivering iron into cells. To achieve this, Tf-A was freed of its constituent iron and then reconstituted with radioactive $^{59}Fe^{3+}$.[5] The capacity of >90% of applied radioactivity to bind to the specific anti-A and anti-T affinity columns established the radiochemical identity of this preparation (FIGURE 8). $^{59}Fe^{3+}$ Tf-A was allowed to react with CEM cells at either 0°C or 37°C, and the amount bound was determined after washing away any free radioactivity. Cells at 37°C, which could internalize toxin, incorporated five times as many counts as those maintained at 0°C, where interaction is restricted to receptor binding. To test the status of the cell-associated ^{59}Fe, cells were lysed with 0.1% of Triton X-100 and the lysate was applied to the affinity columns. The $^{59}Fe^{3+}$ from cells at 0°C was still bound to Tf-A as witnessed by its 70–90% retention on the anti-A and anti-T columns (FIGURE 8). In contrast, only 15% of $^{59}Fe^{3+}$ from cells incubated at 37°C remained associated with the toxin. This temperature-dependent cellular accumulation and uncoupling of iron from $^{59}Fe^{3+}$ Tf-A is strong evidence that this toxin does follow the *bona fide* transferrin pathway and enters the low pH environment of the endosomes.

Carboxylic ionophores catalyze the transfer of protons and monovalent cations across membrane barriers. This can result in the neutralization of acid conditions within vesicle compartments.[12] It was of interest to determine whether such an effect might account for the enhancing influence that these ionophores provide for the

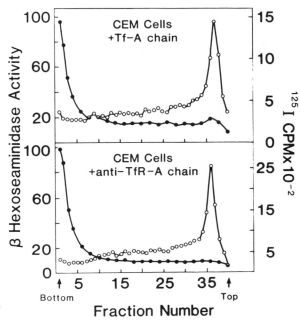

FIGURE 7. Percoll density gradient fractionation. Subcellular distribution of ^{125}I-Tf-A or ^{125}I-TfR-A (O— —O) and a lysosomal marker enzyme (●— —●) on 15% Percoll gradients.[5]

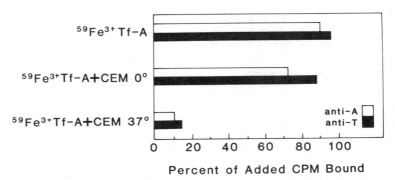

FIGURE 8. Binding of $^{59}Fe^{3+}$ Tf-A to affinity columns before and after interaction with CEM cells. Following interaction with $^{59}Fe^{3+}$ Tf-A for 3 hr at either 0°C or 37°C cells were lysed with 0.1% Triton X-100, cleared by centrifugation, and the lysate was applied to the affinity columns.

kinetics (FIGURE 3) and extent of cell kill (FIGURE 4) shown by A chain toxins. $^{59}Fe^{3+}$ Tf-A serves as a self-contained probe of its immediate environment and was therefore used to test this possibility. The labeled toxin was incubated for 3 hr at 37°C with cells in media alone or in media plus monensin. The accumulation of $^{59}Fe^{3+}$ by cells was measured and they were then lysed to determine the extent of iron dissociation from toxin (FIGURE 9). Levels of monensin, which produced maximal potentiating action (10^{-7} M), neither diminished the uptake of iron by cells nor prevented its acid-dependent uncoupling from Tf-A.

Cycling of Tf-A Out of Cells

After relinquishing its iron load into acidic endosomes, apo-transferrin remains bound to receptor and both are cycled back to the cell surface (FIGURE 2). The elevated pH on the outside causes this complex to dissociate, allowing reutilization of both receptor and transferrin.[6] Continued ligand uptake and efflux is maintained by the formation of new complexes on the surface.[4] Exocytosis of Tf-A from cells would be counterproductive in terms of its toxic activity so that this important aspect was closely

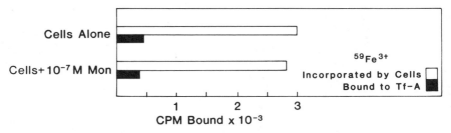

FIGURE 9. Influence of monensin on cellular uptake and uncoupling of $^{59}Fe^{3+}$ Tf-A. Radioactivity bound to cells was measured after incubation for 3 hr either with or without 10^{-7} M monensin and washing twice with PBS. Cells were then lysed with 0.1% Trition X-100 to release radioactivity for analysis on the anti-T column.

examined. It was of particular interest to determine if the release of internalized toxin could be modulated by native transferrin or monensin.

[^{125}I]Tf-A was incubated with CEM cells at 37°C for 30 min in media alone or media-containing 10^{-7} M monensin. The amount of radiolabeled toxin taken up by these cells was measured after washing away any unassociated toxin with PBS at 0°C. The [^{125}I]Tf-A loaded cells were then resuspended in media alone, media plus 10^{-5} M transferrin, media plus 10^{-7} M monensin, or media containing both agents. Exocytosis was allowed to proceed for 1 hr at 37°C before the cells were washed to determine how much [^{125}I]Tf-A was retained. The data in FIGURE 10 show that a substantial amount of the [^{125}I]Tf-A initially taken into the cells had been released into the fresh media. Moreover, clearance of toxin from cells was more extensive when transferrin was included during the incubation. This finding substantiates the notion that Tf-A and transferrin cycle via the same pathway and further suggests that most toxin molecules remain intact and receptor-bound during their journey through the cell and back out into the media. The presence of monensin appeared to produce no significant effect on the loading of cells with Tf-A nor on its subsequent exocytosis (FIGURE 10). If this ionophore enhances toxin activity by altering its pathway, then this action must by very

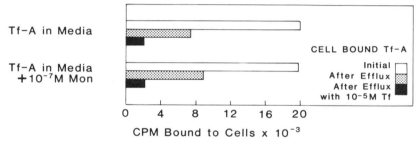

FIGURE 10. Efflux of ^{125}I-Tf-A from cells. CEM cells were incubated with ^{125}I-Tf-A ± monensin at 10^{-7} M for 30 min and then washed ± monensin to measure the amount initially bound. They were then transferred and incubated at 37°C in 1 ml of fresh media ± monensin and ± transferrin (10^{-5} M) for an additional hour before washing and measuring bound counts.

subtle, perhaps involving only a very small fraction of the total molecules taken up by cells.

Immunogold-Labeling of A Chain Conjugates in Ultrathin Cryosections

Antigenic determinants are preserved and accessible in ultrathin cryosections of cells so that biological molecules can be located using electron microscopy in conjunction with colloidal gold–labeled antibody probes.[13] This methodology was used to visualize the disposition of A chain toxins within cells, without interfering with their intracellular cycling since all labeling steps were performed afterwards on the frozen sections. Thus, Tf-A and TfR-A were allowed to enter CEM cells at 37°C for varying time periods and then these cells were fixed, frozen, and sectioned. Localization of the toxins was then accomplished using affinity-purified rabbit anti-ricin A chain antibodies followed by a 5 nm colloidal gold–labeled anti-rabbit IgG reagent.

A series of micrographs is shown to confirm the presence of Tf-A (FIGURE 11, A, B,

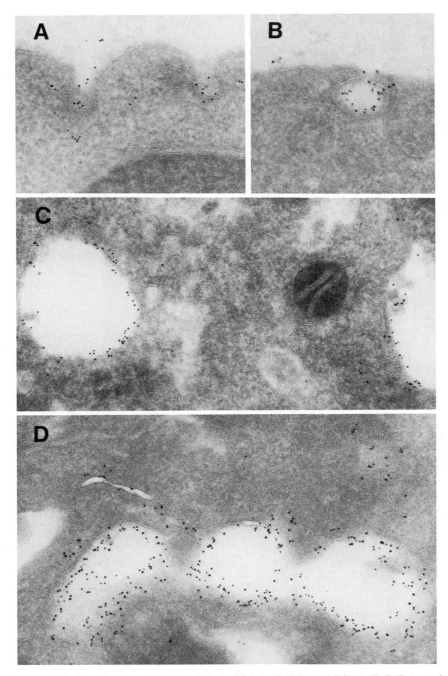

FIGURE 11. Identification of ricin A chain in Tf-A (A,B,C,G) and TfR-A (D,E,F) treated CEM cells. Cryosections were treated consecutively with affinity-purified rabbit anti-ricin A chain antibodies and a 5 nm colloidal gold labeled anti-rabbit IgG probe. (C) at 61,000×, all others at 77,000×.

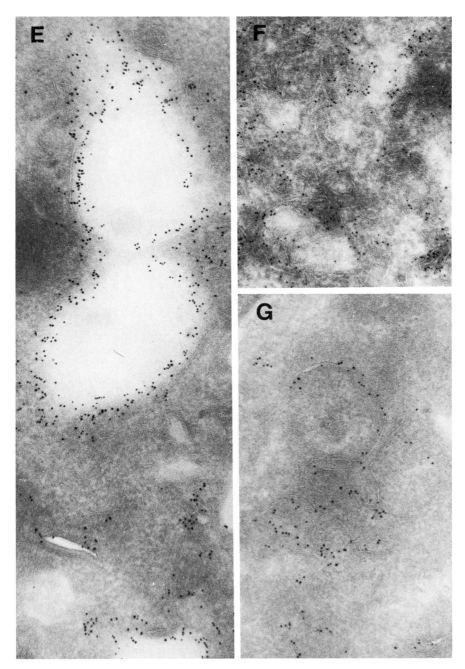

FIGURE 11. Continued

C, and G) and TfR-A (FIGURE 11, D, E, and F) within the structural elements associated with receptor-mediated endocytosis. Immunoreactive A chain was found on the cell surface, in coated pits and small vesicles (FIGURE 11, A and B), as well as within larger endosomes (FIGURE 11, C, D and E). The proximity of gold particles to the inner surface of such vesicles rather than being free in the lumen, suggests that the toxins remained bound to membrane-associated receptors. A substantial amount of gold label was also found in a network of smooth-surfaced tubules, which might correspond to the trans-Golgi reticulum or CURL regions of the cell.[14] In general, the intensity of labeling of intracellular compartments was more intense for cells treated with TfR-A than Tf-A. This correlates with the four-fold greater cell uptake of $[^{125}I]TfR$-A versus $[^{125}I]Tf$-A (FIGURE 5).

Reversal of Tf-A Intoxication

Radiotracer and immuno-ultrastructural techniques by necessity monitor the course taken by a majority of toxin molecules within the cell. To rely solely on such

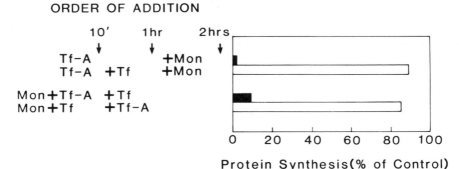

FIGURE 12. Rescue of cells from the lethal action of Tf-A. CEM cells were incubated for the designated time intervals with the indicated additions. Monensin was at 10^{-7} M, Tf-A at 10^{-7} M, and transferrin at 10^{-5} M. Experiments were run in quadruplicate and protein synthesis was measured with [^{3}H]leu as described.[7]

methods for defining toxic pathways therefore entails a danger since those molecules destined to kill a cell may follow a minor deviant route. In fact, the preceding findings showed that a substantial portion of Tf-A simply exited from cells (FIGURE 10) and this fraction presumably caused no damage. It was essential therefore to establish whether or not those toxin molecules that ultimately contact and damage ribosomes do indeed emanate from the normal transferrin cycle. If a common pathway is shared for a finite interval before divergence, then cells that have incorporated a lethal dose of Tf-A might be rescued by using transferrin to rapidly clear toxin from cells (FIGURE 10).

A series of toxicity experiments were performed in which the timing sequence and order of addition of Tf-A, transferrin, and monensin were varied to determine if rescue could be affected (FIGURE 12). In the first part of this experiment, Tf-A was added to cells at 10^{-7} M and left to cycle undisturbed for 1 hr before adding monensin (10^{-7} M) for 2 hr. Cells were then pulsed with [^{3}H]leucine to determine its incorporation into protein.[7] Toxin had clearly gained access to ribosomes since the capacity of these cells to synthesize protein was reduced to less than 10% that of untreated control cells. For the second part of the experiment, incorporation of Tf-A into cells was allowed to proceed for a 10-min interval, after which 10^{-5} M transferrin was added so that both components could cycle through cells during the 1 hr period before adding monensin. Most of the pre-internalized toxin had clearly been purged from cells by this maneuver since protein synthesis remained at 90% of the control level. Confinement of Tf-A within the transferrin pathway was transient since the ability to rescue cells was lost as the interval between the addition of this toxin and excess transferrin was increased. Cytotoxic Tf-A became resistant to clearance by excess transferrin in a log-linear manner as a function of time with its $t_{1/2} = 88$ min indicating the rate at which toxin diverged from the transferrin cycle.

When cells were treated simultaneously with Tf-A plus monensin for 10 min before adding excess transferrin, no rescue was achieved, since protein synthesis was <10% of control (FIGURE 12, part 3). This finding indicates that when monensin was present concurrently, cytotoxic Tf-A molecules were shunted from the transferrin cycle much more rapidly. Subsequent addition of excess transferrin was therefore too late to prevent lethal action. An inability to circumvent toxicity by subsequent clearance with transferrin was similarly encountered when cells were treated with the transferrin–whole ricin conjugate plus lactose even though no monensin was present (data not shown). This observation reinforces the interchangeability of monensin and B chain for their effect upon the kinetics of action of Tf-A. The last part of the experiment shown in FIGURE 12 serves as a control and illustrates that excess transferrin when added prior to Tf-A plus monensin prevented their combined action on cells by blocking receptor sites and protein synthesis levels remained normal.

SUMMARY

Ricin A chain, a potent ribosomal poison, was disulfide linked either to the iron transport protein, transferrin, or to anti-transferrin receptor antibodies to produce highly specific derivative toxins, Tf-A and TfR-A, respectively. The ability of these agents to gain access to and damage ribosomes within the cell was accelerated in the presence of carboxylic ionophores. Their effectiveness for killing clonogenic target cells was correspondingly enhanced by 5 logs after a brief treatment with Tf-A plus ionophore. Intracellular trafficking of Tf-A and TfR-A was monitored by a variety of methods to better understand their mechanism of action. Data obtained with ^{125}I-labeled A chain and $^{59}Fe^{3+}$-labeled toxin probes indicated that the natural iron delivery pathway was initially followed. This was characterized by specific attachment to surface receptors, internalization, entry into low-density acidic vesicles, uncoupling of iron, an absence of lysosomal degradation, and sustained cycling. Ultrastructural studies using a colloidal gold–labeled anti-A chain probe confirmed the presence of these toxins within the structural elements associated with endocytosis. Toxic Tf-A molecules, however, diverged from this pathway ($t_{1/2} = 88$ min) to eventually kill cells as witnessed by a gradual loss in the ability to rescue cells using excess transferrin. Potentiating agents, such as carboxylic ionophores or B chain, seem to act by speeding the divergence of Tf-A and TfR-A from the normal endocytotoic cycle.

REFERENCES

1. OLSNES, S., C. FERNANDEZ-PUENTES, L. CARRASCO & D. VAZQUEZ. 1975. Ribosome inactivation by the toxic lectins abrin and ricin. Kinetics of enzymic activities of toxin A-chains. Eur. J. Biochem. **60**: 281–288.

2. OLSNES, S. & A. PIHL. 1973. Different biological properties of the two constituent peptide chains of ricin. A toxic protein inhibiting protein synthesis. Biochemistry **12:** 3121–3126.
3. CAWLEY, D. B., H. R. HERSCHMAN, D. G. GILLILAND & R. J. COLLIER. 1980. Epidermal growth factor-toxin A chain conjugates: EGF-ricin A is a potent toxin while EGF-diphtheria fragment A is non-toxic. Cell **22:** 563–570.
4. KLAUSNER, R. D., J. VAN RENSWOUDE, G. ASHWELL, C. KEMPF, A. N. SCHECHTER, A. DEAN & K. R. BRIDGES. 1983. Receptor-mediated endocytosis of transferrin in K562 cells. J. Biol. Chem. **258:** 4715–4724.
5. VAN RENSWOUDE, J., K. R. BRIDGES, J. B. HARFORD & R. D. KLAUSNER. 1982. Receptor-mediated endocytosis of transferrin and uptake of Fe in K562 cells. Identification of a nonlysosomal acidic compartment. Proc. Natl. Acad. Sci. USA **79:** 6186–6190.
6. DAUTRY-VARSAT, A., A. CIECHANOVER & H. F. LODISH. 1983. pH and the recycling of transferrin during receptor-mediated endocytosis. Proc. Natl. Acad. Sci. USA **80:** 2258–2262.
7. RASO, V. & M. BASALA. 1984. A highly cytotoxic human transferrin-ricin A chain conjugate used to select receptor-modified cells. J. Biol. Chem. **259:** 1143–1149.
8. TROWBRIDGE, I. S. & D. L. DOMINGO. 1981. Anti-transferrin receptor monoclonal antibody and toxin-antibody conjugates affect growth of human tumor cells. Nature **29:** 171–173.
9. RASO, V. & J. LAWRENCE. 1984. Carboxylic ionophores enhance the cytotoxic potency of ligand- and antibody delivered ricin A chain. J. Exp. Med. **160:** 1234–1240.
10. BREGNI, M., P. DEFABRITIS, V. RASO, J. GREENBERGER, L. LIPTON, L. NADLER, L. ROTHSTEIN, J. RITZ & R. C. BAST JR. 1986. Elimination of clonogenic tumor cells from human bone marrow using a combination of monoclonal antibody: ricin A chain conjugates. Cancer Res. **46:** 1208–1213.
11. SCHNEIDER, C., R. SUTHERLAND, R. NEWMAN & M. GREAVES. 1982. Structural features of the cell surface receptor for transferrin that is recognized by the monoclonal antibody OKT9. J. Biol. Chem. **257:** 8516–8522.
12. PRESSMAN, B. C. 1976. Biological applications of ionophores. Ann. Rev. Biochem. **45:** 501–530.
13. TOKUYASU, K. T., P. A. MAHLER & S. Y. SINGER. 1985. Distributions of vimentin and desmin in developing chick myotubes in vivo. II. Immunoelectron microscopic study. J. Cell Biol. **100:** 1157–1166.
14. GEUZE, H. J., J. W. SLOT, G. J. A. M. STROUS, A. HASILIK & K. VON FIGURA. 1985. Possible pathways for lysosomal enzyme delivery. J. Cell Biol. **101:** 2253–2262.

Genetically Engineered Antibody Molecules and Their Application

SHERIE L. MORRISON, LETITIA WIMS,
SUSAN WALLICK, LEE TAN, AND VERNON T. OI[a]

Department of Microbiology
Columbia University College of Physicians and Surgeons
New York, New York 10032
and
[a]*Becton Dickinson Monoclonal Center*
Mountain View, California 94043

INTRODUCTION

Antibodies have long been recognized for their remarkable specificity. Indeed, the classical studies by Landsteiner demonstrated that antibodies are able to distinguish between *ortho, meta,* and *para* forms of the same haptenic group.[1] Antibodies have therefore seemed ideal candidates for the so-called magic bullet, which could with exquisite specificity identify and destroy an undesirable substance or cell. Antibodies also seem to be a potential means to deliver a drug to a defined target, provided that an antibody specific for the unique chemical differences inherent in that target can be produced.

Originally, the source of antibodies was antisera, which by their nature are limited in quantity and heterogeneous in quality. After the development of hybridomas,[2] a potentially unlimited quantity of antibodies with precisely defined specificities became available. A more recent source of antibodies has been genetically engineered antibodies produced by transfectomas.[3–6] With transfectomas, one is not limited by the specificity and isotype that happens to result following fusion to a normal spleen cell; both of these can be changed by the appropriate genetic manipulation. Transfectomas can be used to isotype switch both within[7] and between species.

Chimeric antibodies in which the specificity derived from a mouse myeloma or hybridoma is joined to human constant region have been produced.[4,8,9] These molecules in part overcome the species limitations inherent in monoclonal antibodies. It has become relatively easy to produce mouse monoclonals of a desired specificity; it has proven much more difficult to produce human monoclonals with the desired properties. Human monoclonals would be preferable for many applications, especially *in vivo* diagnosis and therapy.

The ability to express antibody molecules following gene transfection provides additional advantages. Using *in vitro* mutagenesis, it is possible to make alterations in the variable region of the molecule that alter the binding specificity. It is also possible to express antigen binding domains covalently associated with non-Ig sequences.[10] Such molecules may be useful in delivering protein drugs, such as some toxins to specific cells. In addition, it is possible to make covalent changes in the constant region that facilitate drug delivery; these might include changes in size, effector function, and changes to facilitate the covalent attachment of a drug without altering the binding affinity of the antibody.

Vectors for Transfection

Gene transfection is an inefficient process, with usually $<10^{-4}$ of treated cells going on to become stably transfected. Therefore, there must be a method to select the rare transfected cells from the many non-transfected cells.

The most commonly used vectors are based on those developed by Berg and co-workers.[11–13] These have several essential features. Firstly, they contain a plasmid origin of replication and a marker selectible in prokaryotes. This makes it relatively easy to obtain large quantities of DNA and facilitates their genetic manipulation. Secondly, they contain a marker expressible and selectible in eukaryotes. This consists of a eukaryotic transcription unit with an SV40 promoter, splice, and poly A addition site. Into this eukaryotic transcription unit is placed a dominant selectible marker derived from prokaryotes. One of these, *neo,* derived from the Tn5 transposon, encodes a phosphotransferase that inactivates the kanamycin-like antibiotic G418, an inhibitor of protein synthesis. A second selectible gene, *gpt,* (xanthine-guanine phosphoribosyl-transferase) provides resistance to mycophenolic acid, an inhibitor of purine biosynthesis. It is important that both of these are dominant selectible markers so they can be used with cell lines that have not been drug marked; in addition, they select against entirely different biochemical pathways, hence they can be used simultaneously to generate double drug resistance lines. This is important when selecting for the expression of two different transfected genes (see below).

Production of a functional antibody molecule requires the synthesis of both heavy and light chains. Initial experiments[4] took advantage of the availability of the two independent, dominant selectible markers. The H chain was first introduced using pSV2-gpt and mycophenolic acid selection; using pSV2-neo L chain was subsequently introduced into the H chain producing transfectants and transfectants resistant to both mycophenolic acid and G418 and producing both heavy and light chains selected. This approach is workable, but it requires two steps.

More recently an approach has been developed in which double drug resistant lines can be selected in one step.[14] The original vectors used the pBR origin of replication. A second series of vector was constructed using the origin of replication from pACYC; pBR and pACYC are compatible plasmids and so both can non-competitively replicate within a bacterium. The pACYC vector contains the prokaryotic selectible marker Cm® while the pBR vector contains Amp®. Into one vector is placed a heavy chain and the *gpt* gene; into the other vector is placed the L chain gene and the selectible marker *neo.* When transfection is by protoplast fusion (see below), both vectors can be simultaneously transferred and selected in a recipient cell.

Methods of Gene Transfer

A common procedure for DNA transfer is to make calcium phosphate precipitates of the DNA.[15,16] However, this method does not work very well for lymphoid cells. It is possible to achieve transfection using this method, but only at low frequencies.[3,17]

Protoplast fusion has proven to be an effective way of transfecting lymphoid cells.[18] Using protoplast fusion, frequencies of $>10^{-3}$ can be achieved using the optimal vectors and recipient cell line, J558L.[19] A reduced transfection frequency is seen with other myeloma lines. Recent minor modifications of the basic protoplast fusion procedure have resulted in an increased transfection frequency. This increased frequency is especially important when dealing with cell lines with low transfection frequencies.

For the modified protoplast fusion procedure, protoplasts are prepared essentially as previously described except they are diluted into DME + 10% sucrose + 10 mM MgCl$_2$.[14] For fusion, 4×10^6 cells that had been washed once in DME are mixed with 5 ml of protoplasts (fewer cells are used for cell lines with a high transfection frequency). The cells and protoplasts are pelleted together, and medium removed by aspiration. The pellet is resuspended in 0.5 ml of 41.7% PEG, 12.5% DMSO, 100 mM Tris, pH 8.0 in DME at 37°C, and gently agitated for 1 min. The pellet is then diluted with 0.5 ml of 50% PEG, 100 mM Tris, pH 8.0 in DME at 37°C and gently agitated for 2 min. The pellet is then disrupted with 10 ml of warm DME (37°C), repelleted by centrifugation at room temperature, and resuspended in complete growth medium. Cells are plated into microtiter dishes at a concentration of 4×10^4 cells/well. Selective medium is added after 48 hr.

Representative data from protoplast fusion experiments are shown in TABLE 1. When bacteria with two compatible plasmids are used and selection is made with one drug, frequencies $>10^{-5}$ are achieved with the two non-producing myelomas, SP2/0 and P$_3$X63Ag8.653. Other cell lines (J558L, EL4) will give frequencies more than tenfold higher. However, when clones are simultaneously selected with both selective

TABLE 1. Transfection by Protoplast Fusion

	P$_3$X63Ag8.653		SP2/0	
Selective Medium	Wells with Surviving Clones	Approximate Transfection Frequency	Wells with Surviving Clones	Approximate Transfection Frequency
Mycophenolic acid	504/612	2×10^{-5}	282/622	1×10^{-5}
G418 + Mycophenolic acid	100/580	4×10^{-6}	56/586	2×10^{-6}

P$_3$X63Ag8.653 or SP2/0 cells were fused with bacteria containing compatible plasmids bearing either a *gpt* or *neo* gene and then plated into microtiter dishes (4×10^4 cells/well). After 48 hours, clones were either singly selected (mycophenolic acid) or doubly detected (mycophenolic acid + G418). The plasmids used were pSV2gpt with a chimeric heavy chain gene and pACYCneo with a chimeric light chain gene.

drugs, the frequency of stable transfectants drops about fivefold. It is not clear at this time if this reduced frequency results because only 20% of the cells integrate and express both markers, or if the drop is a consequence of the inherent toxicity of double selection.

Electroporation has also proven to be an efficient method of transfecting lymphoid cells. For electroporation, cells are pelleted and resuspended at a concentration of 10^6/ml in ice-cold PBS. Cells (0.8 ml) are placed along with 8 μg of linearized DNA from each plasmid into an electroporation cuvette (Biorad). A pulse of 200 V, 960 μF is delivered using a Biorad Gene Pulser. After the pulse, cells are removed from the cuvette, washed once in cold DME +10% horse serum, resuspended in complete medium, and plated into microtiter dishes at a concentration of approximately 1.6×10^4 cells/well. Selective medium is applied after 48 hr. Results from a representative experiment are shown in TABLE 2. In this experiment, cells were simultaneously transfected with two different plasmids bearing two different selectible markers. When selected for expression of one or the other, a frequency of $>10^{-5}$ was achieved, very similar to what is observed with protoplasts. With double selection, the frequency drops by a factor of 10–20. Therefore, for double selection under these conditions, electroporation is less efficient than using compatible vectors and protoplast fusion, but it is

TABLE 2. Transfection by Electroporation

Selective Medium	Wells with Surviving Clones	Approximate Transfection Frequency
Mycophenolic acid	14/48	1.8×10^{-5}
G418	24/48	3×10^{-5}
Mycophenolic acid + G418	1/48	1.3×10^{-6}

SP2/0 cells transfected by electroporation were plated into microtiter dishes at a concentration of 1.6×10^4 cells/well. Selective medium was added 48 hours after plating. The plasmids used were pSV2gpt with a chimeric heavy chain gene and pACYCneo with a chimeric light chain gene.

feasible. It is also possible that modifications of the conditions used for electroporation will improve the frequency.

Methods of Cloning Immunoglobulin Genes

The immunoglobulin (Ig) expression vectors that we have employed all use rearranged Ig genes driven by their own promoters and with their own regulatory sequences. The rationale for this approach is that Igs are expressed at high levels in plasma cells; therefore, if we can achieve comparable expression after transfection we will have high levels of protein available for functional studies.

In order for the approach of gene transfection to be broadly applicable, it must be feasible to clone the variable regions for the specificities of interest. The characteristics of Ig, the locus, facilitate this cloning. V regions must be rearranged to be expressed; expressed V regions are juxtaposed to J regions while unexpressed V regions are not. Therefore it is possible to use J region probes to identify restriction fragments bearing rearranged V's. Thus one does not need to know the exact characteristics of a rearranged V or its sequence to be able to clone it. A complication inherent in this approach is that hybridomas often contain aberrant rearrangements, some of which may be transcribed. Therefore, a frequent problem is the positive identification of the correct rearrangement.

Recently, we have also demonstrated the feasibility of reconstructing expressed V regions from cDNA clones. cDNA clones usually are easier to make than genomic clones, especially since the use of constant region primers enables one to selectively prime for Ig transcripts. The method we used to express the cDNAs took advantage of the fact that we had an expression vector with a variable region that shared restriction sites at the 5' end of V and at J with the cDNA of interest. In this case, the expression vector (MPC-11)[20] and the anti-dextran cDNAs[21,22] we used belong to the very large J558 family. Members of this family are homologous and share many features. At amino acid four in V, there is a common *Pvu*II site; in J_3, present in both, is a *Pst*I site. Replacement of the *Pvu*II-*Pst*I fragment of MPC-11 with the same fragment from the cDNA, leads to the insertion of the anti-dextran variable region into the expression vector. The leader sequence and the first four amino acids of V are from MPC-11; however since these four amino acids are identical in MPC-11 and the anti-dextrans there is no alteration in specificity. The total V until J_3 is from the anti-dextran hybridoma. After J, the splice signals and regulatory sequences are derived from MPC-11 (FIG. 1). When this reconstructed variable region was joined to a constant region and transfected into a light chain–producing cell line (J558L), it was seen to direct the synthesis of an intact H chain, which assembled with the L chain and was secreted (FIG. 2).

The general expression vector systems we employ have several important properties. Firstly, H chains and L chains are on separate plasmids. Although it is feasible to include both H and L on the same plasmid and there is no inherent size limitation in these vectors, it becomes much more difficult to genetically manipulate large plasmids because of the paucity of novel restriction sites. Therefore, smaller plasmids are preferable if the objective is to be able to genetically engineer antibodies. A second feature is the presence of unique sites within the vectors that were introduced using linkers.[4] These sites facilitate transferring variable regions between plasmids; therefore once a variable region has been cloned into one expression vector, it becomes much simpler to then express it associated with different constant regions.

Production of Novel Proteins

In order to be able to use gene transfection to produce novel Ig molecules, the Ig produced must be a faithful representation of the Ig genes used. In the initial experiments using the S107A kappa light chain, it was shown that the gene expressed

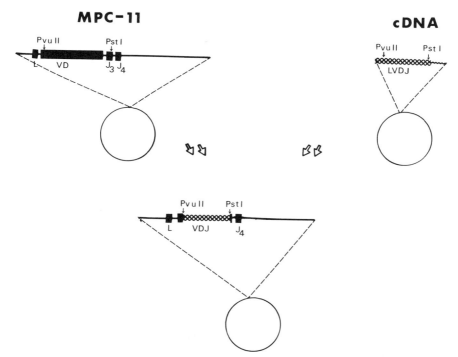

FIGURE 1. Construction of a vector capable of expressing a heavy chain cDNA. The coding sequences from the MPC-11 myeloma are shown as a solid black line. The coding sequences of the cDNA are indicated as a hatched area. The synthesis of the cDNA was initiated using an isotype-specific primer, which primed at the 5' side of CH_1. To exchange the variable regions both the cDNA and MPC-11 plasmids were cleaved with *Pvu*II and *Pst*I. The *Pvu*II-*Pst*I fragment from the cDNA was then ligated into *Pvu*II-*Pst*I cleaved MPC-11. The reconstructed variable region was then inserted 5' of a constant region in a complete H chain expression vector. The drawing is not to scale and all restriction sites are not shown.

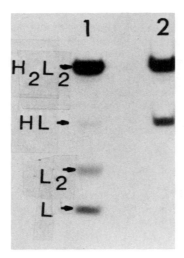

FIGURE 2. Synthesis, assembly, and secretion of an anti-dextran heavy chain constructed from a cDNA following transfection into the J558L (produces only λ light chains) myeloma. The anti-dextran variable region is joined to human γ_4 constant region. Cells were labeled with [^{35}S]methionine for 3 hours, secretions prepared, and immunoglobulin specifically immunoprecipitated and analyzed on SDS-PAGE. The reconstructed heavy chain gene directs the synthesis of a complete H chain that assembles with the λ light chain of the myeloma and is secreted as H_2L_2 molecules. Position of bands in marker proteins are indicated. Lane 1, myeloma (MPC-11); Lane 2, secreted Ig from the transfectant.

after transfection had the same apparent molecular weight and isoelectric point as the kappa light chain produced by the S107 myeloma.[3] In addition, the kappa light chain produced following transfection was like the kappa light chain produced by the parental myeloma in that it was secreted only when associated with a heavy chain.

When chimeric mouse-human Igs were produced using gene transfection, these proteins were also shown to exhibit the expected specificity and properties. Antiphosphocholine specific chimeric proteins were shown to assemble into H_2L_2 molecules, to bind antigen, and to be recognized by anti-idiotypic antibodies specific for the original mouse myeloma protein; the anti-idiotypic antibodies were either specific for the heavy chain alone or required the proper assembly of heavy and light chain to generate the antigenic determinant.[4] Similarly, anti-DNP specific, chimeric proteins exhibited the expected specificity.[9]

Subsequent experiments have reinforced the concept that chimeric Igs exhibit the expected binding specificity. Additional anti-hapten antibodies have been produced.[7,8] Chimeric antibodies binding tumor-associated antigen have been shown to exhibit reactivity patterns identical to the starting hybridoma.[23,24] Recently, chimeric Igs specific for the T cell antigen Leu3/T4 have also been shown to have the predicted reactivity.[25] All of these experiments demonstrate the feasibility of producing specific antibodies using gene transfection.

The first reports of chimeric Ig used human constant regions of the μ, ϵ, γ_1, or γ_2 isotypes.[4,9,8] Subsequently, the γ_3 and γ_4 isotypes have been produced.[26] More recently, it has been feasible to express human IgA. The dansyl-specific variable region was ligated 5′ of the human α_1 constant region gene (gift of Dr. Greg Hollis) in the pSV2-gpt vector. The resulting construct was transfected into J558L cells and stable transfectants isolated. The chimeric α chain assembled with the endogenous λ light chain; H_2L_2 and higher polymers were present in the secretions (FIGURE 3). Thus, all isotypes of human Ig except δ have been expressed as chimeric proteins.

One potential application of transfectomas is to study structure-function relationships in antibody molecules. Human γ_3 has an extended hinge region consisting of four exons; human γ_4 exhibits quite different properties in spite of extensive sequence similarities (> 90% identical in CH_2 and CH_3) in their constant regions. It is now possible to define precisely the contribution of the hinge region to the properties of the molecules. IgG_3 genes have been constructed, expressed, and the proteins isolated that have one, two, three, or four (wild type) hinge exons (FIGURE 4); notice the change in molecular weight of the heavy chains with the subsequent hinge deletions. In addition, the γ_3 hinge has been placed in the γ_4 constant region and *vice versa*. These proteins will now be used to investigate the properties of the Ig, including its ability to fix complement and the segmental flexibility of the molecules. This example provides just one illustration of the potential uses of genetically engineered antibody molecules.

In order to maximize the usefulness of genetically engineered antibodies for such applications as drug delivery, it must be possible to make alterations in the antibody. The limitations are that the antibodies must be assembled and secreted and must retain their ability to specifically bind antigen.

To determine if we could define an upper limit on the size of an antibody molecule that could be produced, we constructed an IgG_3 heavy chain in which CH_1 and the hinge region were duplicated; in a second construct CH_1, hinge, and CH_2 were

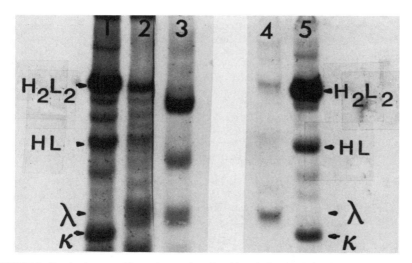

FIGURE 3. Synthesis, assembly, and secretion of a chimeric heavy chain with a human alpha 1 constant region. The anti-dansyl variable region was joined to human alpha 1 heavy chain and transfected into the J558L myeloma. Transfectants synthesizing the chimeric heavy chains were labeled with [^{35}S]methionine for 3 hours, cytoplasmic lysates and secretions prepared and immunoprecipitated. The immunoprecipitates were analyzed using SDS-PAGE. The chimeric alpha heavy chain assembles into H_2L_2 molecules; these are secreted both as monomers and polymers. Lanes 1 and 5, MPC-11 myeloma; Lane 2, cytoplasmic chimeric IgA; Lane 3, BALB/c mouse IgA; and Lane 4, secreted chimeric IgA.

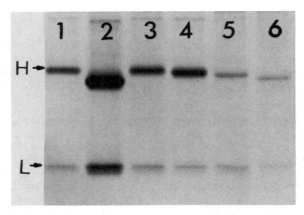

FIGURE 4. Synthesis of chimeric immunoglobulins with alterations in their hinge regions. Chimeric heavy chain genes were cotransfected with a chimeric light chain gene (mouse anti-dansyl with human kappa) into a non-producing myeloma. Transfectants producing immunoglobulin were labeled for 3 hours with [^{35}S]methionine, cytoplasmic lysates prepared and immunoprecipitated. The immunoprecipitates were analyzed on SDS-PAGE following treatment with β-mercaptoethanol. Lane 1, γ_4 with the complete hinge of γ_3; Lane 2, γ_4; Lane 3, γ_3 with an intact hinge; Lane 4, γ_3 lacking hinge exon 4; Lane 5, γ_3 lacking hinge exons 3 and 4; and Lane 6, γ_3 lacking hinge exons 2, 3, and 4.

duplicated. When the gene with CH_1 and the hinge duplicated was used for transfection a greatly reduced transfection frequency was seen; when the surviving transfectants were analyzed, none produced any detectable heavy chain protein. These results suggest, but do not prove conclusively, that the heavy chain encoded by this construct was toxic to the cells. Such heavy chain toxicity has been postulated by many groups;[27,28] indeed variants producing only heavy chains could be isolated from the MPC-11 myeloma only after a deletion was introduced into the heavy chain, which permitted its secretion in the absence of a light chain.[29]

In contrast, the gene encoding a heavy chain in which CH_1, hinge, and CH_2 are duplicated is expressed following transfection. It assembles with a mouse λ light chain and is secreted (FIGURE 5). These experiments suggest there will be limitations in the Ig molecules that can be produced, but that these limitations are not inherently related to size.

In another series of experiments, we set out to determine how deletions of various domains will affect the ability of Ig molecules to assemble, to be secreted, and to function. IgG_3 heavy chain genes encoding proteins with deletions of CH_2, hinge + CH_2, CH_1 + hinge and CH_1 + hinge + CH_2 were constructed and transfected into myeloma cells.

When the gene with the deletion of CH_2 was used, it was found to direct the synthesis of a protein of the expected molecular weight. This shortened heavy chain assembled with either mouse λ light chain or chimeric V-DNS-human κ light chain into an H_2L_2 molecule that was secreted (FIGURE 6).

When the hinge + CH_2 were deleted, the heavy chain apparently assembled into HL half molecules, which were secreted (FIGURE 7). However, it is impossible to say conclusively that these are not H_2. However, when CH_1 + the hinge were deleted, no assembly of the heavy chain with either other heavy chains or with L chain occurred. This is not surprising since the free cysteine that forms the interchain disulfide bonds is present in CH_1. However, even in the absence of interchain disulfide bonds, the shortened heavy chain is secreted.

It is also possible to produce a heavy chain in which the variable region is directly joined to CH_3. This heavy chain is secreted when cotransfected with a chimeric light chain into a non-producing myeloma. It does not form covalent bonds with either light chain or another heavy chain.

DISCUSSION AND PROSPECTS

The feasibility of producing genetically engineered antibody molecules has now been demonstrated in many laboratories. The experiments reported here show that it is possible to produce immunoglobulin with greatly altered structures. Somewhat surprisingly, secretion of these structurally altered Igs generally seems to occur, so it is possible to obtain them in adequate quantities for study. The usefulness of these molecules will be determined by their biologic properties.

The potential application of antibody molecules is determined not only by their specificity, but also by their effector functions. That is, their serum half-life, tissue distribution, and then ability to fix complement and participate in antibody-dependent cellular cytotoxicity, will, among other things, determine their *in vivo* function. Antibodies have evolved to perform many different functions. With genetic engineer-

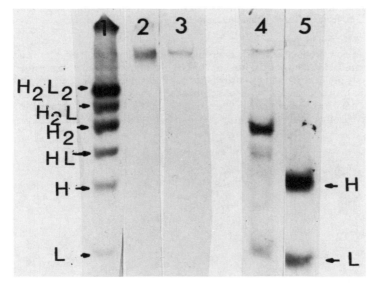

FIGURE 5. Synthesis, assembly, and secretion of a chimeric heavy chain gene in which the CH_1 hinge, CH_2 region has been duplicated. J558L cells were transfected with the chimeric gene and transfectomas synthesizing the heavy chain isolated. Cells were labeled for 3 hours using [^{35}S]methionine, cytoplasm and secretions prepared, the immunoglobulin immunoprecipitated with an anti-heavy chain antiserum, and analyzed by SDS-PAGE. Lane 1, MPC-11; Lane 2, cytoplasm from the transfectant; Lane 3, secretion from the transfectant; Lane 4, cytoplasmic Ig from transfectant treated with β-mercaptoethanol; and Lane 5, MPC-11 treated with β-mercaptoethanol. Arrows mark the positions of the marker Ig in MPC-11.

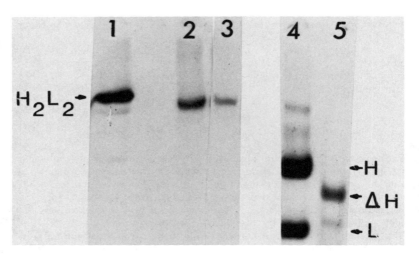

FIGURE 6. Synthesis of a chimeric heavy chain in which CH_2 has been deleted. J558L was transfected with the chimeric heavy chain gene and transfectants synthesizing protein were isolated. Transfectants were labeled for 3 hours using [^{35}S]methionine and cytoplasmic and secreted Ig prepared by immunoprecipitating with anti-heavy chain. The immunoprecipitates were analyzed by SDS-PAGE. Lane 1, MPC-11; Lane 2, cytoplasmic Ig of transfectant; Lane 3, secreted Ig of transfectant; Lane 4, MPC-11 treated with β-mercaptoethanol; Lane 5, cytoplasmic Ig of transfectant treated with β-mercaptoethanol.

ing we can now produce antibody molecules in which the desired effector function has been maximized and unwanted function has been eliminated. It is also possible to make an antibody molecule in which a drug is part of the molecule (e.g., a chimeric antibody ricin gene). Antibodies can also be modified so as to facilitate their *in vitro* manipulation. Antibodies could be altered so that it is easier to add more molecules of a radioactive isotope without changing their binding specificity.

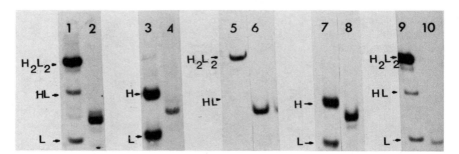

FIGURE 7. Secretions from cells transfected with heavy chains bearing domain deletions. Cells were labeled with [^{35}S]methionine for 3 hours, secretions prepared, and immunoprecipitated. The immunoprecipitated proteins were analyzed by SDS-PAGE. Lane 1, MPC-11; Lane 2, γ_3 with CH_1 and hinge deleted; Lane 3, MPC-11 treated with β-mercaptoethanol; Lane 4, CH_1 and hinge deleted protein treated with β-mercaptoethanol; Lane 5, MPC-11; Lane 6, γ_3 with hinge and CH_2 deletion; Lane 7, MPC-11 treated wtih β-mercaptoethanol; Lane 8, hinge and CH_2 deleted protein treated with β-mercaptoethanol; Lane 9, MPC-11; and Lane 10, γ_3 with CH_1, hinge and CH_2 deleted.

The specificity of antibody molecules can also be manipulated using genetic engineering. In certain cases, antibodies with either higher or lower affinities are desirable; *in vitro* mutagenesis of the variable regions can be used to change the binding specificity or affinity of the antibody.

Modern techniques permit us to make antibody molecules with virtually any structure. The challenge now is to determine what structures correlate with optimal function.

SUMMARY

Immunoglobulin genes can be efficiently expressed following transfection into myeloma cells. Using protoplast fusion, transfection frequencies greater than 10^{-3} can be achieved. Compatible plasmids containing two different selectible markers are used to simultaneously deliver heavy and light chain genes to the same cell. To produce molecules with differing specificities the rearranged and expressed variable regions can be cloned from the appropriate hybridoma. In some cases, variable regions from cDNAs can be inserted into the expression vectors. It is possible to manipulate the immunoglobulin genes and produce novel antibody molecules. Antibodies have been produced in which the variable regions from mouse antibodies have been joined to human constant regions. In addition, antibodies with altered constant regions have been produced. These genetically engineered antibodies provide a unique set of reagents to study structure-function relationships within the molecule. They also can potentially be used in the diagnosis and therapy of human disease.

REFERENCES

1. LANDSTEINER, K. 1945. The Specificity of Serological Reactions. Harvard University Press. Cambridge, MA.
2. KOHLER, G. & C. MILSTEIN. 1974. Continuous cultures of fused cells secreting antibody of predefined specificty. Nature (London) **256:** 495–497.
3. OI, V. T., S. L. MORRISON, L. A. HERZENBERG & P. A. BERG. 1983. Immunoglobulin gene expression in transformed lymphoid cells. Proc. Natl. Acad. Sci. USA **80:** 825–829.
4. MORRISON, S. L., M. J. JOHNSON, L. A HERZENBERG & V. T. OI. 1984. Chimeric human antibody molecules: mouse antigen-binding domains with human constant region domains. Proc. Natl. Acad. Sci. USA **81:** 6851–6855.
5. OCHI, A., R. G. HAWLEY, T. HAWLEY, M. J. SCHULMAN, A. TRAUNECKER, G. KOHLER & N. HOZUMI. 1983. Functional immunoglobulin M production after transfection of cloned immunoglobulin heavy and light chain genes into lymphoid cells. Proc. Natl. Acad. Sci. USA **80:** 6351–6355.
6. OCHI, A., R. G. HAWLEY, M. J. SHULMAN & H. HOZUMI. 1983. Transfer of a cloned Ig-light chain gene to mutant hybridoma cells restores specific antibody production. Nature (London) **302:** 340–342.
7. DANGL, J., T. WENSEL, L. STRYER, S. L. MORRISON, L. A. HERZENBERG & V. T. OI. Manuscript in preparation.
8. NEUBERGER, M. S., G. T. WILLIAMS, E. B. MITCHELL, S. S. JOUHAL, J. G. FLANAGAN & T. H. RABBITT. 1985. A hapten-specific chimaeric IgE antibody with human physiological effector function. Nature (London) **314:** 268–270.
9. BOUHANNE, G. L., N. HOZUMI & M. J. SHULMAN. 1984. Production of functional chimeric mouse/human antibody. Nature (London) **312:** 643–646.
10. NEUBERGER, M. S., G. T. WILLIAMS & R. O. FOX. 1984. Recombinant antibodies possessing novel effector functions. Nature (London) **312:** 604–608.
11. MULLIGAN, R. C. & P. BERG. 1980. Expression of a bacterial gene in mammalian cells. Science **209:** 1422–1427.

ANNALS NEW YORK ACADEMY OF SCIENCES

12. MULLIGAN, R. C. & P. BERG. 1981. Selection for animal cells that express the *Escherichia coli* gene coding for xanthine-guanine phosphoribosyltransferase. Proc. Natl. Acad. Sci. USA **78**: 2072–2076.
13. SOUTHERN, P. J. & P. BERG. 1982. Transformation of mammalian cells to antibiotic resistance with a bacterial gene under control of the SV40 early region promoter. J. Molec. Appl. Genet. **1**: 327–341.
14. OI, V. T. & S. L. MORRISON. 1986. Chimeric antibodies. BioTechnique **4**: 214–221.
15. GRAHAM, F. L. & A. J. VAN DER EB. 1973. A new technique for the assay of infectivity of human adenovirus sDNA. Virology **52**: 456–467.
16. CHU, G. & P. A. SHARP. 1981. SV40 DNA transfection of cells in suspension: analysis of the efficiency of transcription and translation of T-antigen. Gene **13**: 197–202.
17. RICE, D. & D. BALTIMORE. 1982. Regulated expression of an immunoglobulin kappa gene introduced into a mouse lymphoid cell line. Proc. Natl. Acad. Sci. USA **79**: 7862–7865.
18. SANDRI-GOLDIN, R. M., A. L. GOLDIN, M. LEVINE & J. C. GLORIOSO. 1981. High frequency transfer of cloned herpes simplex virus type I sequences to mammalian cells by protoplast fusion. Molec. Cell. Biol. **1**: 743–752.
19. GILLIES, S. D., S. L. MORRISON, V. T. OI & S. TONEGAWA. 1983. A tissue specific transcription enhancer element is located in the major intron of a rearranged immunoglobulin heavy chain gene. Cell **33**: 717–728.
20. KOBRIN, B. J., C. MILCAREK & S. L. MORRISON. 1986. Sequence near the 3′ secretion-specific polyadenylation site influence levels of secretion-specific and membrane-specific IgG$_{2b}$ mRNA in myeloma cells. Molec. Cell. Biol. **6**: 1687–1697.
21. SIKDER, S. K., P. N. ALKOLKAR, P. M. KALADAS, S. L. MORRISON & E. A. KABAT. 1985. Sequences of the variable regions of hybridoma antibodies to $\alpha(1\rightarrow6)$ dextran in BALB/c and C57B1/6 mice. J Immunol. **135**: 4215–4221.
22. ALKOLKAR, P. N., S. K. SIKDER, S. B. BHATTACHARYA, J. LIAO, F. GRUEZO, S. L. MORRISON & E. A. KABART. 1988. Different V$_L$ and V$_H$ germ line genes are used to produce similar combining sites with sepcificity for $\alpha(1\rightarrow6)$ dextrans. Submitted for publication.
23. SAHAGAN, B. G., H. DORAI, J. SALTZGABER-MULLER, F. TONEGUZZO, C. GUINDON, S. P. LILLY, K. W. McDONALD, D. V. MORRISSEY, B. A. STONE, G. L. DAVIS, P. K. McINTOSH & G. P. MOORE. 1986. A genetically engineered murine/human chimeric antibody retains specificity for human tumor-associated antigen. J. Immunol. **137**: 1066–1074.
24. SUN, L. K., P. CURTIS, E. RAKOWICZ-SZULCZYNSKA, J. GHRAYEB, S. L. MORRISON, N. CHANG & H. KOPROWSKI. 1986. Chimeric antibodies with 17-1A-derived variable and human contant regions. Hybridoma **5** (Suppl. 1): S17–S20.
25. OI, V. T., N. FEDERSPIEL, P. HINTON, M. McNALLY, L. ROARK & V. WATERS. Manuscript in preparation.
26. OI, V. T. & S. L. MORRISON. Unpublished data.
27. KOHLER, G. 1980. Immunoglobulin chain loss in hybridoma lines. Proc. Natl. Acad. Sci. USA. **77**: 2197–2199.
28. WILDE, C. D. & C. MILSTEIN. 1980. Analysis of immunoglobulin chain secretion using hybrid myelomas. Eur. J. Immunol. **10**: 462–467.
29. MORRISON, S. L. 1978. Murine heavy chain disease. Eur. J. Immunol. **8**: 194–199.

The Pharmacology of Monoclonal Antibodies[a]

J. N. WEINSTEIN,[b] R. R. EGER,[b] D. G. COVELL,[b]
C. D. V. BLACK,[b] J. MULSHINE,[c] J. A. CARRASQUILLO,[d]
S. M. LARSON,[d] AND A. M. KEENAN[d]

[b]National Cancer Institute
[c]NCI-Navy Medical Oncology Branch
Naval Hospital
and
[d]Clinical Center
National Institutes of Health
Bethesda, Maryland 20892

INTRODUCTION

We are entering an era in which biological macromolecules can be designed to order and genetically or synthetically produced. If the experience with classical low molecular weight drugs is any guide, it will be possible — in fact, easy — to produce many more such agents than can be tested for effect in animals, let alone in humans. Predictive criteria are required for the process of rational design, and these must be based on an understanding of fundamental physiological and pharmacological principles.

Monoclonal antibodies illustrate the point. Hundreds of new monoclonal reagents with possible clinical use are being developed every year. Each of them could be administered as whole antibody, F(ab′)₂, or Fab. Each could be conjugated to a toxin, a drug, a radionuclide, or a liposome containing one of those agents. Each could be class-switched to change effector functions or could be mutated in its binding site. As noted previously,[1] the combinatorial aspects of trying every possibility are out of the question even before one has considered such current and likely future developments as (1) chimeric molecules combining mouse variable and human constant domains; (2) Fv (variable domain) fragments; (3) recombinants consisting of murine hypervariable segments and human variable domain framework; (4) conjugates formed by genetically grafting a linker peptide onto the molecule; and (5) enzyme-antibody or toxin-antibody chimeras. At the end of this developmental process will be ligand molecules consisting of antibody-derived binding sites grafted onto molecules designed *de novo*.

A predictive pharmacology of biologicals must be based on theoretical and experimental information from several hierarchical levels: global (whole body), regional, local, cellular, and molecular. Here we will focus on one study of whole body pharmacokinetics, one development in regional delivery, and one issue at the local, or tissue, level.

[a]The work of R.R.E. was supported by a gift from Hybritech, Inc. to the Cancer Immunotherapy Fund. The opinions and assertions contained herein are the private views of the authors and are not to be construed as being official or reflecting the views of the Department of the Navy, Department of Defense, or Department of Health and Human Services.

PHARMACOKINETICS OF AN [111]IN-LABELED MONOCLONAL ANTIBODY IN HUMANS

Our work on the global pharmacology of monoclonals in animals has been described in detail elsewhere.[2-4] In brief, we have developed pharmacokinetic models for IgG biodistribution and have compared whole IgG, $F(ab')_2$ fragments, and Fab' fragments of an anti-B-cell antibody and an isotype-matched control. In the setting of clinical trials, less experimental information is available, since we cannot sample all organs. Hence, the kinetic model to be described below (FIGURE 1) was developed on the basis of data from blood and urine coupled with quantitative analysis of gamma scintigraphy.

Using data from twelve patients, we have analyzed the pharmacokinetics of [111]In-9.2.27, an antimelanoma murine IgG_{2a}, infused i.v. over 2 hr at a total dose of 1, 50, or 100 mg.[5] The experimental results have been presented *in extenso* by Carrasquillo *et al.*[6] The patients had disseminated melanoma, but images indicated that the tumor load was not sufficient to perturb global pharmacokinetics significantly. Hence, the model was taken to represent [111]In-9.2.27 in the absence of binding sites on tumor.

Plasma data (FIGURE 2) and gamma camera images (FIGURE 3) indicated dose-dependent kinetics. Based on these observations and known features of IgG kinetics, we formulated a nonlinear compartmental model for the [111]In-9.2.27 and associated low molecular weight ^{111}In species. The model, shown in FIGURE 1, included (1) three compartments representing intact [111]In-9.2.27 ("plasma," "nonsaturable,"

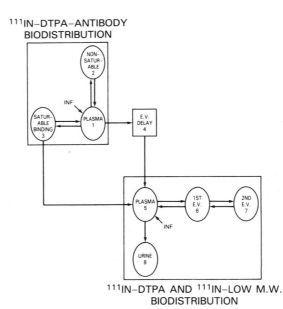

FIGURE 1. Model of [111]In-9.2.27 IgG2a pharmacokinetics in humans. Top-left: ^{111}In-DTPA-9.2.27 distribution. Bottom-right: ^{111}In-DTPA and ^{111}In-labeled metabolite biodistribution, from the model of Houston *et al.*[32] for In-DTPA. Infusions into plasma take place via compartments 1 and 5. E.V., extravascular; M.W., molecular weight. (From Eger *et al.*[5] With permission from *Cancer Research.*)

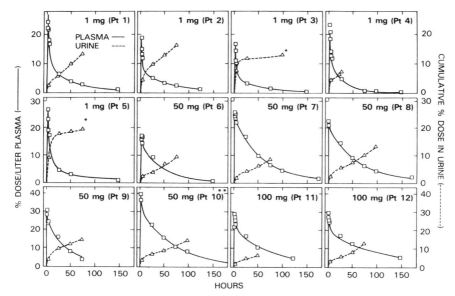

FIGURE 2. Plasma (squares) and cumulative urine (triangles) measurements for each patient receiving [111]In-9.2.27. Curves are weighted least-squares fits of the model to the data for each patient. Displayed urine values for patients 3 and 5 are 0.5 times actual values. (From Eger *et al.*[5] With permission from *Cancer Research.*)

and "saturable binding" compartments); (2) four compartments representing ^{111}In-diethylenetriaminepentaacetic acid (^{111}In-DTPA) and other low molecular weight ^{111}In species; and (3) one compartment representing ^{111}In in undetermined chemical forms ("extravascular delay" compartment). Between 4 and 30% of the ^{111}In, depending on the preparation, was injected as free ^{111}In-DTPA, hence the model accounted for the fact that label was being injected simultaneously into compartments 1 and 5. Analysis of the urinary data suggested catabolism of antibody or release of label in the saturable compartment and also in either the plasma or the nonsaturable compartment. The model indicated that the saturable compartment fills very rapidly, and can contain approximately 0.5 mg. A dose of 3.5 mg would maintain saturation for 200 hr. Thus, nonspecific background arising from the saturable compartment could be minimized by injecting a dose greater than about 5 mg or else by a "cold loading" dose of unlabeled antibody injected prior to administration of the radiolabeled antibody.[5]

Computer integration of gamma camera counts over the spleen showed a clear saturable component of uptake, whereas integration over the liver failed to show such a pattern. The model had initially been developed without reference to the imaging, but imaging data from the liver and spleen were then fitted by summing fractions of model simulations of each compartment. This analysis confirmed the presence of a saturable uptake by the spleen (21% of the saturable binding compartment). More interesting, it uncovered a quantitatively important component of saturation in the liver (35% of the saturable binding compartment) that had not been obvious from inspection of the images or quantitative counts. In terms of concentration, the spleen contained 247% of the saturable compartment per kg, whereas the liver accounted for 25%/kg. As indicated by comparing the images of patient 3 and patient 11 in FIGURE 3, the bone marrow also showed saturable uptake. We hypothesize that the 1,000 Å openings characteristic of sinusoidal blood vessels in the liver, spleen, and bone marrow permit rapid access of antibody to "sites" of binding and/or uptake. These "sites" might recognize all murine IgG, subclasses of murine IgG, or idiotypic determinants. Alternatively, they might reflect antigenic cross-reactivity of 9.2.27 with endothelium or basal lamina. Such cross-reaction has been identified by histochemistry on cut sections.[7,8] Comparison with data on other antibodies at similar doses will be required to decide the issue. The distribution of an ^{131}I-labeled antibody has been analyzed in

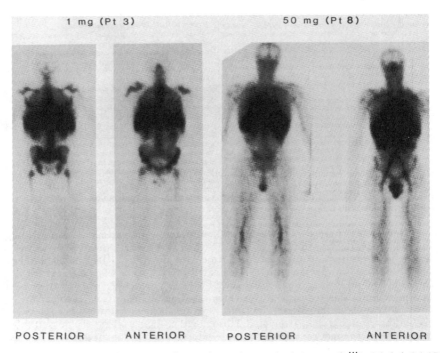

FIGURE 3. Whole body images of a patient who received 1 mg of ^{111}In-labeled 9.2.27 anti-melanoma antibody and a patient who received 50 mg. The images were taken 24 hr after a 2-hr infusion. The images showed high levels of radioactivity in liver, spleen, and marrow at the 1-mg level and less in these organs at 50 mg. This difference reflected a component of saturable binding. (From Eger *et al.*[5] With permission from *Cancer Research*.)

terms of a compartmental model by Koizumi *et al.*[9] The points of similarity and difference with respect to our analysis of the ^{111}In-labeled reagent are under study.

REGIONAL PHARMACOLOGY: THE LYMPHATICS

For gamma camera imaging, monoclonal antibodies have generally been given i.v. However, regional delivery can be considered when the location of the target is known.

If the target is a malignant or normal cell type within lymph nodes, delivery by way of the lymphatic vessels may be very efficient.

The following calculation[10] indicates the rationale for regional delivery: Consider a 1 g tumor in a 70 kg human. If the blood flow per gram of tumor were taken to equal the average blood flow per gram to other tissues in the body, a given antibody molecule injected i.v. would pass through the tumor capillaries only once every 49 days. Much more rarely would it enter the extravascular space of the tumor. Therefore, only small fractions of a percent of dose can accumulate in tumor after i.v injection, regardless of the binding properties. This same "dilutional" effect pertains to low molecular weight drugs as well, but with macromolecules, regional localization is much more often possible.

If a low molecular weight, water-soluble substance is injected s.c., almost all of it passes into blood capillaries. Macromolecules, on the other hand, are cleared largely via the lymphatics. After entering lymphatic capillaries, injected antibody passes with the lymph into larger and larger vessels under the impetus of intrinsic smooth muscle action, extrinsic skeletal muscle action, and hydrostatic pressure differences, with the aid of a one-way valve system. Upon reaching a lymph node, lymph flows into the subcapsular space, then through sinusoids in the cortex and medulla. Antibody in the lymph may bind to normal or malignant cells in the node or else it may pass to additional nodes in the chain. If not removed from the lymph, it passes into the systemic circulation.

Lymphatic Delivery of Antibody in Animals

The work of our laboratory on lymphatic delivery began with antibodies directed against histocompatibility antigens and lymphocyte markers in the mouse.[11-14] This work defined the essential pharmacology of lymphatic delivery and provided background for studies on lymphoma and on modulation of immune cell subsets. Studies with a metastatic tumor model in the guinea pig then demonstrated the feasibility of the lymphatic route for detecting early lymph node metastases of solid tumors.[15]

An extension of the technique was developed to reach lymph node groups not readily accessed from sites of s.c. injection. To reach the nodes to which lung cancers metastasize, antibody is injected through the bronchial wall in the area of a primary tumor using a cytology needle and fiberoptic bronchoscope. The antibody is expected to follow the drainage pathways, as do metastasizing cells, to nodes of the lung and mediastinum. We showed the technical feasibility of this approach in dogs using a murine monoclonal IgG reactive with mouse I-E^k.[16] The anti-I-E^k was known to cross-react with determinants on antigen-presenting cells in a number of species, including the dog.[17] Uptake in hilar and carinal nodes showed antigen-specificity and was approximately 100 fold greater than in distant nodes. Analogous techniques might, in principle, be applied to colorectal carcinoma. The status of regional nodes in patients with low rectal carcinoma can determine whether the anal sphincter is saved at surgery or the patient requires a permanent colostomy.

Clinical Studies of Lymphatic Delivery

In 1975, Order *et al.*[18,19] reported case studies using the polyclonal gamma globulin fraction of an antiserum raised against ferritin, a "tumor-associated" antigen. Patients with Hodgkin's disease were injected directly into cannulated lymphatic vessels. In 1980, DeLand *et al.*[20,21] reported on a series of patients injected subcutaneously with polyclonal IgG directed against carcinoembryonic antigen. Cancerous nodes were detected, but the investigators suggested the possibility that specific uptake related to shed antigen rather than to the presence of malignant cells in the nodes. Thompson *et al.*[22] injected a murine IgM monoclonal antibody in the finger webs of patients with breast cancer to image axillary nodes. A study of 9 patients showed generally positive correlation between antibody accumulation and the presence of metastases. The findings suggested specificity of localization, but the authors emphasized that they did not have surgical specimens for verification.

At the National Institutes of Health, we have used several different antimelanoma antibodies in an attempt to image metastases in patients with stage II melanoma. A preliminary report[23] gives some scattered suggestions of selective uptake but no reliable localization in cancerous nodes and no clinically useful imaging. Similar studies by Nelp *et al.*[24] have, likewise, yielded no consistent, clinically useful imaging. We do not know at present whether optimal reagents, labels, and methods of administration would change the picture. Lymph node metastases of melanoma may simply grow in such a way as to preclude effective access to (or "percolation" into) the cancerous nodes. These may be rather general problems with respect to metastases of solid tumors.

For T-cell lymphoma, the results are much better, as we have reported elsewhere.[25] T101 is a mouse IgG_{2a} directed against the T65 antigen on cells of chronic lymphocytic leukemia and cutaneous T-cell lymphoma (CTCL). T65 is also expressed on normal T-cells. ^{111}In-labeled T101 was injected in the toe webs of patients with CTCL. Serial scans showed highly efficient uptake of label in the inguinal-femoral and iliac nodes within 3 hr. Activity in the nodes plateaued within 24–48 hr and then declined. FIGURE 4 shows the first two patients imaged. The first had minimal involvement (LN 2) of the nodes, and the regional nodes took up 24% of the ^{111}In dose; the second had bulky disease in the nodes, which took up 36% of dose. Additional patients have shown similarly efficient uptake, and injection of an isotype-matched control antibody in the same patients has demonstrated that the uptake of T101 is largely antigen-specific. However, T101 reacts with normal T-cells, hence the uptake cannot be called "tumor specific."

LOCAL PHARMACOLOGY: THE "PERCOLATION" PROBLEM

As noted in the introduction, i.v. administration introduces an inherent inefficiency of delivery to any given site in the body. There are also local (tissue-level) barriers to efficient delivery. Therapy of solid tumors with antibodies is limited by difficulty of penetration from the source of supply —a blood vessel, a lymph sinusoid, or the edge of a dense nodule of cells. If passage across an endothelial layer or basement membrane is the rate-limited step in penetration, then one confronts a classical problem in the physiology of the microvasculature. Despite several generations of concerted effort, there is still not general agreement about the mechanisms or pathways by which macromolecules, including immunoglobulins, cross capillary walls.[26]

Alternatively, the overall rate at which antibody reaches antigenic sites may be limited by the rate of transport through the tumor substance itself, rather than the capillary wall. We first encountered this issue experimentally in studies of lymphatic delivery to large lymph node metastases of a solid tumor in guinea pigs.[15] However, the problem is general and pertains to any route of delivery. We addressed this "percolation" problem by formulating the convection-diffusion-reaction equations for protein flux in the presence of uniformly distributed binding sites, with or without metabolic sinks.[1,27] The equations were solved numerically by a collocation method and, in some cases, analytically. The aim was to test the sensitivity of penetration to changes in characteristics of the antibody and properties of the extravascular space. Since the time of the initial calculations, immunohistochemical and autoradiographic studies

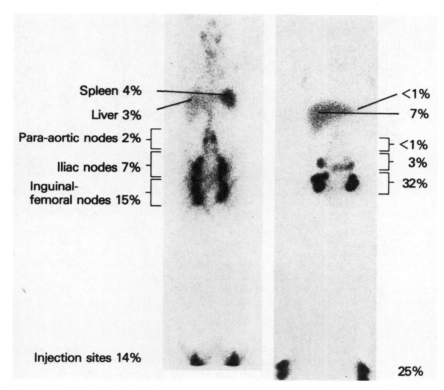

FIGURE 4. Anterior whole body scintigrams 2 to 3 days after administration of ^{111}In-labeled T101 in the toe webs of both feet in patients with cutaneous T-cell lymphoma. Numbers indicate percentages of injected activity in organs, nodes, and injection sites. Values for iliac and inguinal-femoral nodes represent the means of those obtained separately for left and right sides. The lefthand patient had minimal disease in the nodes. The patient on the right had bulky disease. Double foci in the feet of the righthand patient resulted from dorsiflexion and plantar flexion during imaging. The efficiencies of lymph node imaging were orders of magnitude higher than after i.v. injection. (From Keenan *et al.*[25] With permission from *Journal of Nuclear Medicine.*)

from several laboratories[28-30] have shown non-uniform distribution of antibody within tumors.

Convection is probably the most important process in flux of macromolecules through macroscopic distances in tumors,[31] but the rate-determining mechanism for movement across microscopic distances into densely packed cellular areas is unclear.

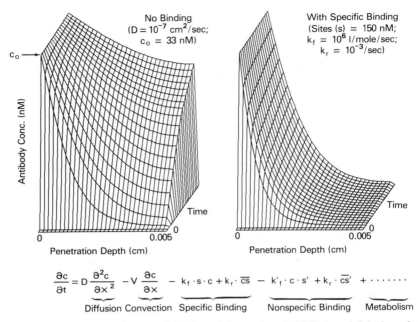

$$\frac{\partial c}{\partial t} = D \frac{\partial^2 c}{\partial x^2} - V \frac{\partial c}{\partial x} \underbrace{- k_f \cdot s \cdot c + k_r \cdot \overline{cs}}_{\text{Specific Binding}} \underbrace{- k'_f \cdot c \cdot s' + k_r \cdot \overline{cs'}}_{\text{Nonspecific Binding}} \underbrace{+ \cdots\cdots}_{\text{Metabolism}}$$

Diffusion   Convection

FIGURE 5. Simulations of the partial differential equations for diffusion of Fab through the substance of a tumor, with and without saturable binding. The lefthand boundary could correspond either to the surface of a nodule of tumor cells or to the outer surface of a capillary. The concentration of Fab at that boundary is considered to be held constant. These calculations were part of a sensitivity analysis. The emphasis here is on the qualitative finding: under the given wenditions, binding slows down penetration and renders it less uniform. (Modified from Weinstein et al.[1])

At least in some cases, the pattern of penetration suggests diffusion. We decided to concentrate first on diffusion and to use a one-dimensional Cartesian geometry. FIGURE 5 shows one part of a sensitivity analysis. Addition of saturable antigenic sites (righthand panel) delays penetration and renders it less uniform.

FIGURE 6 illustrates the result when equations for local penetration are combined with those for a global pharmacokinetic model of antibody distribution. The lefthand boundary in each panel represents Fab concentration adjacent to a capillary. That boundary concentration is zero at the time of injection, rises to a maximum over a matter of hours as Fab leaks across the blood vessel, and then follows plasma levels down. The most striking prediction from the sensitivity analysis is this: Raising the forward rate constant for binding (k_f) will retard penetration. The same is qualitatively true for reductions in the reverse rate constant for binding (k_r). Since the affinity is k_f/k_r, we conclude that whichever way the affinity is increased, penetration will be retarded. Hence, if uniform binding is desired for therapy, a lower-affinity antibody may be preferable to an equivalent higher affinity one. The retardation could be alleviated by increasing the dose of antibody to the point at which it swamped available binding sites rapidly, but this would concomitantly reduce the effective selectivity for tumor. If the therapeutic aim were to concentrate antibody near the blood vessels (for example, to destroy them with a conjugated drug, toxin, or α-emitter), then high affinity would presumably be best. The qualitative predictions from this analysis are expected to hold whether the mechanism of transport is diffusive or convective.

Both numerical solution and analytical manipulation of the equations led to a second interesting conclusion: In the absence of metabolic sinks, the total "area under the curve" (i.e., concentration × time) exposure of each point in the tumor carried out to infinite time would be the same as that for any other point in the tumor, regardless of the binding properties of the antibody. On the other hand, the calculations predict a spatial gradient of exposures in the presence of a metabolic sink.

These calculations can be made more complex in a variety of ways. Convection and diffusion can be considered simultaneously. Cylindrical geometries can be introduced to represent more accurately the case of a blood vessel and its surroundings. Additional spatial dimensions, partitioning into gel-like regions of the interstitium, monovalent-bivalent binding models, heterogeneity of binding sites, or histological heterogeneity could be introduced. We expect, however, that many of the qualitative features of the behavior would remain unchanged.

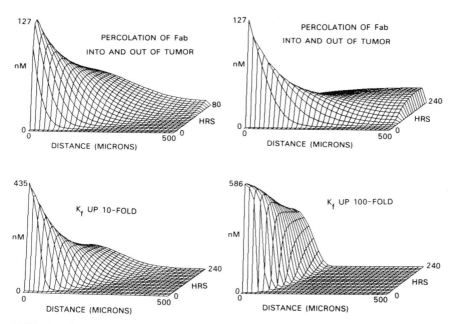

FIGURE 6. Sensitivity analysis of Fab diffusion through a tumor with different assumed forward rate constants (k_f) for binding to antigen. The lefthand boundary could correspond either to the surface of a nodule of tumor cells or to the outer surface of a capillary. Fab concentration at that boundary rises from zero and then falls again as a function of time after injection. The top two panels are the same except for a change in the time axis (the righthand panel shows longer time evolution of the distribution). The bottom panels show the effects of increasing k_f. The distribution of Fab throughout the tumor becomes less uniform as k_f increases, indicating that a lower k_f (and lower affinity of binding) might be preferable for some therapeutic applications of monoclonal antibodies. On the other hand, high k_f might be desirable if the objective of therapy were to damage tumor vasculature. (From Weinstein *et al.*[1] With permission from Alan R. Liss.)

CONCLUSION

In principle, imaging with monoclonal antibodies can be much more sensitive than current techniques for detection of tumors, as the following calculation (based on a similar calculation in Weinstein *et al.*[13]) makes clear. Consider an antigenic tumor that binds 200,000 antibody molecules at saturation. If the antibody is labeled with [131]I (not an ideal isotope) to a specific activity of 10 mCi/mg, there will be 1.1 dpm per cell. A gamma camera capable of showing a point source of 100,000 dpm in reasonable time against spontaneous background would then, in principle, be able to detect 100,000 tumor cells (i.e., 0.1 mg). That represents an improvement of several orders of magnitude over techniques such as standard X-ray, computerized tomography, clinical examination, and magnetic resonance imaging. Detection of 100,000 cells after i.v administration of antibody is not currently feasible (though it may not be out of the question for lymphatic delivery). In fact, the smallest metastases detected with monoclonal antibodies in most clinical studies to date are on the order of 1 g. The calculation is meant to point out, however, that diagnostic imaging is not limited by intrinsic sensitivity. Rather, the practical limits of detection are largely determined by pharmacologic factors — how much antibody can be delivered and bound selectively to the tumor and how much the nonspecific background can be reduced.

ACKNOWLEDGMENTS

We gratefully acknowledge the contributions of the many other investigators involved in the preclinical and clinical studies described here.

REFERENCES

1. WEINSTEIN, J. N., D. G. COVELL, J. BARBET, R. R. EGER, O. D. HOLTON III, M. J. TALLEY, R. J. PARKER & C. D. V. BLACK. 1987. Local and cellular factors in the pharmacology of monoclonal antibodies. *In* Membrane Mediated Cytotoxicity. B. Bonavida & R. J. Collier, Eds.: 279–289. Alan R. Liss, New York.
2. COVELL, D. G., J. BARBET, O. D. HOLTON III, C. D. V. BLACK & J. N. WEINSTEIN. 1986. The pharmacokinetics of monoclonal IgG1, F(ab')$_2$ and Fab' in mice. Cancer Res. **46:** 3969–3978.
3. COVELL, D. G., M. A. STELLER, R. J. PARKER & J. N. WEINSTEIN. 1985. Delivery of monoclonal antibodies through the lymphatics: Characterization by compartmental modeling. Computer Appl. Med. Care **10:** 884–888.
4. HOLTON, O. D. III, C. D. V. BLACK, R. J. PARKER, D. G. COVELL, J. BARBET, S. M. SIEBER, M. J. TALLEY & J. N. WEINSTEIN. 1987. Biodistribution of monoclonal IgG$_1$, F(ab')$_2$, and Fab' in mice after intravenous injection: A comparison between anti-B cell (anti-LyB8.2) and irelevant (MOPC-21) antibodies. J. Immunol.
5. EGER, R. R., D. G. COVELL, J. A. CARRASQUILLO, P. G. ABRAMS, K. A. FOON, J. C. REYNOLDS, R. W. SCHROFF, A. C. MORGAN, S. M. LARSON & J. N. WEINSTEIN. 1987. Kinetic model for the biodistribution of an ^{111}In-labeled monoclonal antibody in humans. Cancer Res. **47:** 3328–3336.
6. CARRASQUILLO, J. A., P. G. ABRAMS, R. W. SCHROFF, J. C. REYNOLDS, C. S. WOODHOUSE, A. C. MORGAN, A. M. KEENAN, K. A. FOON, P. PERENTESIS, S. MARSHALL, M. HOROWITZ, J. SZYMENDERA, R. K. OLDHAM & S. M. LARSON. 1988. Effect of [111]In 9.2.27 monoclonal antibody dose on the imaging of metastatic melanoma. J. Nucl. Med. (In press.)
7. MORGAN, A. C., C. S. WOODHOUSE, R. M. BARTHOLOMEW & R. W. SCHROFF. 1986.

Human melanoma-associated antigens: analysis of antigenic heterogeneity by molecular, serologic, and flow cytometric approaches. Mol. Immunol. **23**: 193–200.

8. STUHLMILLER, G. M., M. J. BOROWITZ, B. P. CROKER & H. F. SEIGLER. 1982. Multiple assay characterization of murine monoclonal anti-melanoma antibodies. Hybridoma **1**: 447–460.

9. KOIZUMI, K., G. L. DeNARDO, S. J. DeNARDO, M. T. HAYS, H. H. HINES, P. O. SCHEIBE, J. PENG, D. J. MACEY, N. TONAMI & K. HISADA. 1986. Multicompartmental analysis of the kinetics of radioiodinated monoclonal antibodies in patients with cancer. J. Nucl. Med. **27**: 1243–1254.

10. WEINSTEIN, J. N., O. D. HOLTON III, C. D. V. BLACK, A. M. KEENAN, D. G. COVELL, G. F. SPAULDING, J. BARBET, M. S. STELLER, S. M. SIEBER, M. J. TALLEY & R. J. PARKER. 1986. Regional delivery of monoclonal antitumor antibodies: Detection and possible treatment of lymph node metastases. *In* Cancer Metastasis: Experimental and Clinical Strategies. D. R. Welch, B. K. Bhuyan & L. A. Liotta, Eds.: 169–180. Alan R. Liss. New York.

11. WEINSTEIN, J. N., R. J. PARKER, A. M. KEENAN, S. K. DOWER, H. C. MORSE III & S. M. SIEBER. 1982. Monoclonal antibodies in the lymphatics: Toward the diagnosis and therapy of tumor metastases. Science **218**: 1334–1337.

12. WEINSTEIN, J. N., M. A. STELLER, D. G. COVELL, O. D. HOLTON III, A. M. KEENAN, S. M. SIEBER & R. J. PARKER. 1984. Monoclonal anti-tumor antibodies in the lymphatics. Cancer Treat. Rep. **68**: 257–264.

13. WEINSTEIN, J. N., R. J. PARKER, O. D. HOLTON III, A. M. KEENAN, D. G. COVELL, C. D. V. BLACK & S. M. SIEBER. 1985. Lymphatic delivery of monoclonal antibodies: Potential for detection and treatment of lymph node metastases. Cancer Invest. **3**: 85–95.

14. STELLER, M. A., R. J. PARKER, D. G. COVELL, O. D. HOLTON III, A. M. KEENAN, S. M. SIEBER & J. N. WEINSTEIN. 1986. Optimization of monoclonal antibody delivery via the lymphatics: The dose-dependence. Cancer Res. **46**: 1830–1834.

15. WEINSTEIN, J. N., M. A. STELLER, A. M. KEENAN, D. G. COVELL, M. E. KEY, S. M. SIEBER, R. K. OLDMAN, K. M. HWANG & R. J. PARKER. 1983. Monoclonal antibodies in the lymphatics: Selective delivery to lymph node metastases of a solid tumor. Science **222**: 423–426.

16. MULSHINE, J. L., A. M. KEENAN, J. A. CARRASQUILLO, T. WALSH, R. I. LINNOILA, O. D. HOLTON III, J. HARWELL, S. M. LARSON, P. A. BUNN & J. N. WEINSTEIN. 1987. Immunolymphoscintigraphy of pulmonary and mediastinal lymph nodes in dogs: A new approach to lung cancer imaging. Cancer Res. **47**: 3572–3576.

17. WATANABE, M., T. SUZUKI, M. TANIGUCHI & N. SHINOHARA. 1983. Monoclonal anti-Ia murine allo antibodies cross reactive with the Ia-homologies of other mammalian species including humans. Transplantation **36**: 712–718.

18. ORDER, S. E., W. D. BLOOMER, A. G. JONES, W. D. KAPLAN, M. A. DAVIS, S. J. ADELSTEIN & S. HELLMAN. 1975. Radionuclide immunoglobulin lymphangiography: A case report. Cancer **35**: 1487–1492.

19. ORDER, S. E. 1977. Immunospecific radionuclide immunoglobulin lymphography. *In* Clinical Lymphography. M. E. Clouse, Ed. **7**: 316–322. Williams and Wilkins. Baltimore.

20. DeLAND, F. H., E. E. KIM, R. L. CORGAN, S. CASPER, F. J. PRIMUS, E. SPREMULLI, N. ESTES & D. M. GOLDENBERG. 1979. Axillary lymphoscintigraphy by radioimmunodetection of carcinoembryonic antigen in breast cancer. J. Nucl. Med. **20**: 1243–1250.

21. DeLAND, F. H., E. E. KIM & D. M. GOLDENBERG. 1980. Lymphoscintigraphy with radionuclide-labeled antibodies to carcinoembryonic antigen. Cancer Res. **40**: 2997–3000.

22. THOMPSON, C. H., S. A. STACKER, N. SALEHI, M. LICHTENSTEIN, M. J. LEYDEN, J. T. ANDREWS & I. F. C. McKENZIE. 1984. Immunoscintigraphy for detection of lymph node metastases from breast cancer. Lancet (Dec. 1): 1245–1247.

23. LOTZE, M. T., J. A. CARRASQUILLO, J. N. WEINSTEIN, G. J. BRYANT, P. PERENTESIS, J. C. REYNOLDS, L. A. MATIS, R. R. EGER, A. M. KEENAN, I. HELLSTROM, K-E. HELLSTROM & S. M. LARSON. 1986. Ann. Surgery **204**: 223–235.

24. NELP, W. B., J. F. EARY, R. F. JONES, R. KISHORE, K. A. KROHN, P. L. BEAUMIER, K-E.

HELLSTROM & I. HELLSTROM. 1986. Preliminary studies of radiolabeled monoclonal antibody lymphoscintigraphy in malignant melanoma. J. Nucl. Med. **26**: 66.

25.   KEENAN, A. M., J. N. WEINSTEIN, J. L. MULSHINE, J. A. CARRASQUILLO, P. A. BUNN JR., J. C. REYNOLDS, K. A. FOON, P. PERENTESIS, B. GHOSH & S. M. LARSON. 1987. Evaluation of lymphoma by immunolymphoscintigraphy: Subcutaneous injection of indium-111-labeled T101 monoclonal antibody. J. Nucl. Med. **28**: 42–46.

26.   POZNANSKY, M. J. & R. L. JULIANO. 1984. Pharmac. Rev. **36**: 277–334.

27.   WEINSTEIN, J. N., C. D. V. BLACK, R. PARKER, R. R. EGER, S. M. SIEBER, B. MOZAYENI & D. G. COVELL. 1986. Selected issues in the pharmacology of monoclonal antibodies. *In* Site-specific Drug Delivery. E. Tomlinson & S. S. Davis, Eds.: 81–92. John Wiley. New York.

28.   MEEKER, T. C., J. LOWDER, D. G. MALONEY, R. A. MILLER, K. THIELEMANS, R. WARNKE & R. LEVY. 1985. A clinical trial of anti-idiotype therapy for B cell malignancies. Blood **65**: 1349–1363.

29.   ABRAMS, P. G. & R. K. OLDHAM. 1985. Monoclonal antibody therapy of solid tumors. *In* Monoclonal Antibody Therapy of Human Cancer. K. A. Foon & A. C. Morgan Jr., Eds.: 103. Martinus Nijhof. Boston.

30.   JONES, P. L., B. M. GALLAGHER & H. SANDS. 1986. Autoradiographic analysis of monoclonal antibody distribution in human colon and breast tumor xenografts. Cancer Immunol. Immunotherapy. **22**: 139–143.

31.   SWABB, E. A., J. WEI & M. GULLINO. 1974. Diffusion and convection in normal and neoplastic tissues. Cancer Res. **34**: 2814.

32.   HOUSTON, S. A., W. F. D. SAMPSON & M. A. A. MACLEOD. 1979. A compartmental model for the distribution of In-113m-DTPA and Tc-99m(Sn)DTPA in man following intravenous injection. Int. J. Nucl. Med. Biol. **6**: 85–95.

Targeting Enzyme Albumin Conjugates

Examining the Magic Bullet[a]

MARK J. POZNANSKY

Department of Physiology
University of Alberta
Edmonton, Alberta
Canada, T6J 2H7

INTRODUCTION

In his now famous statement, the great cell biologist, Paul Ehrlich predicted our current interest in "magic bullets" and the potential of site-specific delivery of drug molecules.[1] In a sense he foreshadowed this very meeting with his statement: ". . . bodies which possess a particular affinity for a certain organ . . . as a carrier by which to bring therapeutically active groups to the organ in question." This statement was made at a time in 1898 when antibodies had not yet been discovered. Unfortunately, Paul Ehrlich did not warn us of the many pitfalls and multiple barriers that exist to the successful use of such magic bullets in a system as complex as the human organism. Poznansky and Juliano in 1984 attempted a lengthy and critical review on the subject "Biological Approaches to the Controlled Delivery of Drugs."[2] In referring to 588 publications, they merely scratched the surface in terms of the published literature, which burgeoned between the late 1960s and the mid 1980s.

Earlier work (1965–1978) stressed the need for drug-carrier systems primarily to alter the pharmacokinetics of already proven drugs whose efficacy might be improved by altering the rates of metabolism in the liver or clearance by the kidneys. Some of these approaches also lead to the "slow release" technology, which allowed not only for altered pharmacokinetics but also varied means and frequency of administration. These approaches generally did little for the prospects of site-specific delivery; getting a cytotoxic drug to cancerous tissue while sparing other normal, though equally sensitive tissue.[3]

With the advances in "carrier technology" and the advantages some of these systems afford, attention has more recently been focused[4] on the questions of site-specific targeting or delivery of either individual drug molecules or entire carrier systems (e.g. liposomes, albumin, polyethylene glycol, etc.). Three targeting approaches seem to have dominated the approach; antibodies directed against specific cell surface antigens,[5] hormones functioning as specific ligands for receptors on specific targets,[6] and glycoconjugates also functioning as specific ligands for receptors on specific cells that recognize particular sugar residues.[7] In the following pages, we will demonstrate the use of the first two of these approaches for targeting: antibodies against cell surface antigens on tumor cells and ligands (insulin and Apo B) directed against either the insulin receptor or the LDL receptor on a number of different cell lines.

[a]Supported in part by the Medical Research Council of Canada.

211

ENZYME-ALBUMIN CONJUGATES

Some ten years ago, our laboratory became interested in the possibility of altering enzymes to make them more amenable for use in medicine.[8-11] While enzymes might be considered ideal drugs in some ways because of their high degree of specificity and their ability to function under normal physiological conditions, they suffer a number of serious limitations in their use as a result of (1) availability in pure form, (2) rapid biodegradation largely by proteolytic inactivation, (3) immunologic reactivity as a foreign protein, and (4) problems associated with the delivery of the enzyme to the appropriate site of action. The last limitation is especially important in considering enzyme replacement therapy for a number of disorders, such as lysosomal storage diseases, where it may be essential that the enzyme be delivered not only to a particular tissue but also to a specific intracellular site, such as the lysosome. Our solution at least to the first three of these limitations has been the production of enzyme-albumin conjugates, which appears to substantially decrease the sensitivity of the product to biodegradation and at the same time reducing or entirely eliminating the antigenic nature of the enzyme, presumably by either masking the antigenic sites or by inducing tolerance.[12] The albumin must, of course, be homologous.

The objective of this presentation is to describe our attempts (and dilemmas) with respect to the site-specific targeting or delivery of the enzyme. From this perspective, many of our objectives and the problems that we encounter are the same as those for any other drug-carrier system in terms of stability, plasma clearance, and access to particular sites. We might consider for a moment the multiple barriers that any drug delivery or carrier system is likely to have to contend with. If the system is introduced intravenously, then the system must be able to avoid capture by the reticuloendothelial system; phagocytic cells found in the blood, liver, spleen, bone marrow, etc., whose primary function is to search out and destroy just such foreign bodies. After avoiding the RES, the carrier must be able to pass the endothelial cell barrier in order to reach underlying target tissue (FIGURE 5) in addition to the basal lamina which underlie this organized cell barrier. Once the delivery system has reached its cellular target, then consideration must be given as to how it will cross the cell membrane and reach any specific intracellular organelle or site if indeed its ultimate target is within the cell. In the following pages, we will show how we have attempted to deal with these barriers in terms of our ability to target enzymes or enzyme-albumin conjugates. While these conjugates are usually on the large size (with molecular weights in the range of 500,000), these demonstrations may hold equally well for other-drug delivery systems that have been described by other authors.

TARGETING *IN VITRO* OR IN TISSUE CULTURE

In biomedical research, the use of model systems (frequently cells grown in tissue culture) often simplifies our work and makes incredibly complicated systems potentially understandable. Unfortunately, in the case of drug delivery systems, the simplicity of the tissue culture dish is deceptive in terms of the concepts of drug delivery and the multiple barriers found in considering an entire organism. The following data demonstrate our successful attempts to direct L-asparaginase to tumor cells (either a mouse tumor cell line or human pancreatic tumor cells) or cholesterol esterase to fibroblasts from a patient with cholesterol ester storage disease.

The first set of experiments demonstrate the L-asparaginase sensitivity of human pancreatic tumor cells (Panc-1), demonstrating the efficacy of using monoclonal antibodies (Mabs) directed against cell surface antigens to direct the enzyme.[10,11] These experiments, performed on Panc-1 cells in tissue culture, demonstrate that the site-specific antibody is able to maintain a level of L-asparaginase activity at the tumor cell site and thus inhibit growth of the cells, whereas the enzyme itself or bound to a non-specific antibody is less effective and likely to be lost following washing of the cells. The fact that the free enzyme becomes ineffective with time is an indication that the free form of the enzyme is more susceptible to proteolytic degradation than the enzyme in its conjugated form with albumin as previously demonstrated.[9,11] FIGURES 1 and 2 demonstrate the ease with which an enzyme can be targeted to a specific cell (at least in tissue culture) and exert its effect in a much more efficient manner than an

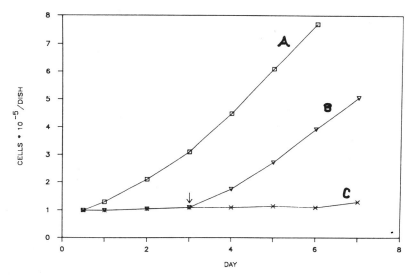

FIGURE 1. Panc-1 cells (human pancreatic tumor cells in continuous culture) were seeded on day 0 at 10^5 cells/dish in the presence of added albumin (A), L-asparaginase-albumin conjugates (B), or L-asparaginase-albumin-monoclonal antibodies (C). On day 3, cells receiving L-asparaginase-albumin conjugates (B) could be given a second dose of the conjugate (B) and the growth could be retarded as in (C). Conditions were as described previously.[10] When monoclonal antibodies were used that did not react with the surface of the Panc-1 cells then the growth curves demonstrated were as in (B).

equivalent amount of drug or enzyme in its free form. At this point we have no evidence to suggest that the Mab is doing anything but directing and binding the enzyme to the cell surface and maintaining a low asparagine level in the vicinity of the cell and thus retarding cell growth or division.

TABLES 1 and 2 demonstrate the possibility of correcting an enzyme deficiency disease (in tissue culture) in fibroblasts from a patient with a lysosomal storage disease. KC fibroblasts are cells from a patient with cholesterol ester storage disease (CESD).[14] In this instance, we know that adding the enzyme cholesterol esterase (from *Pseudomonas*) to the culture medium of the cells is without effect on the levels of stored cholesterol ester. Our approach here was to use insulin as targeting agent in the expectation that following binding to the insulin receptor on the cell surface, there is

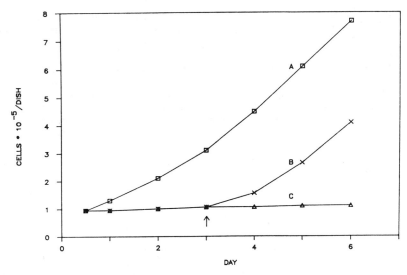

FIGURE 2. Panc-1 cells were grown and prepared as in FIGURE 1. Curve A represents the normal growth curve of the tumor cells. Cells in (B) received a dose of L-asparaginase-albumin-monoclonal antibody (non-specific) and cells in (C) received an equivalent amount of L-asparaginase-albumin-monoclonal antibody (specific) to the Panc-1 cells. All three sets of cells were washed with standard medium (minus additional enzyme) on day 3.

evidence that the complex undergoes internalization by a process resembling receptor-mediated endocytosis with the eventual deposition of the complex in the lysosomes.[6] Incubating KC cells with enzyme that has been conjugated with an excess of insulin (with or without the accompanying albumin) results in a very significant reduction in cholesterol ester and a concomitant increase in free cholesterol levels, best exemplified by the CE/C ratio (TABLE 1). For this reduction to take place, the enzyme must be covalently bound to the insulin, suggesting an obligatory uptake of the two compo-

TABLE 1.

	Cholesterol (C) (g/mg protein)	Cholesterol Ester (CE) (g/mg protein)	CE/C
Normal Fibroblasts	51.8	5.68	.110
+ Enzyme	53.2	5.80	.109
+ Enzyme-Insulin	53.9	5.83	.108
KC Fibroblasts (CESD)	49.8	32.65	.656
+ Enzyme	50.1	32.50	.649
+ Enzyme-Insulin	60.8	15.81	.260
+ Enzyme-Albumin	49.6	32.85	.662
+ Enzyme-Albumin-Insulin	61.2	16.10	.263
+ Enzyme-Insulin + 100× Excess Insulin	51.2	30.8	.602

KC is a 12-year-old patient with CESD (cholesterol ester storage disease) and an 80% deficiency in fibroblast or lymphocyte cholesterol ester specific acid lipase. Administered enzyme is cholesterol esterase from *Pseudomonas*.

nents. The fact that a 100-fold excess of free insulin is able to inhibit the effect of the enzyme-insulin conjugate (no reduction in CE/C) is strong evidence to suggest that the complex is indeed entering the cell and gaining access to the CE stored in the lysosome via the suggested pathway for the insulin and insulin receptor. It is not surprising that the enzyme-insulin is without effect on normal fibroblasts since the cholesterol ester levels present in these cells are low and thought not to represent lysosomal stores.

TABLE 2 represents data from a similar set of experiments using KC cells and normal fibroblasts, but here the apo B or LDL receptor is used in place of the insulin receptor. In these experiments, rather than using insulin-cholesterol esterase or insulin-albumin-cholesterol esterase conjugates, the cholesterol esterase has been introduced into an Apo B recombinant. The process involves the reconstitution of purified apoprotein B into phospholipid vesicles to mimic the LDL particle but in the possible total absence of either cholesterol or cholesterol ester. As expected, neither the apo B recombinant particle or the recombinant with enzyme are effective in reducing CE levels in normal fibroblasts. In KC cells, however, the apoB-enzyme recombinant is

TABLE 2.

	Cholesterol (C) (g/mg protein)	Cholesterol Ester (CE) (g/mg protein)	CE/C
Normal Fibroblasts[a]	51.6	3.60	.069
+ Apo B recombinant	50.9	3.55	.070
+ Apo B − enzyme recombinant	52.8	3.54	.067
KC Fibroblasts[a]	52.8	31.2	.591
+ Enzyme	53.1	30.5	.574
+ Apo B recombinant	51.2	29.6	.578
+ Apo B − enzyme recombinant	68.4	14.0	.205
KC Fibroblasts[b]	62.8	38.8	.618
+ Enzyme	64.1	37.1	.579
+ Apo B recombinant	61.9	37.8	.611
+ Apo B − enzyme	63.2	32.0	.506

[a]Normal and KC fibroblasts grown in lipoprotein deficient serum for 24 hr prior to experiment to promote expression of Apo B (LDL) receptors.
[b]KC Fibroblasts grown in 5% fetal calf serum to down-regulate LDL receptors.

effective in lowering CE levels to an extent similar to that seen when insulin was used as the delivery or targeting agent. The recombinant itself was without effect. These experiments were all done with cells whose LDL receptors had been unregulated by incubation for 24 hr in the absence of serum lipoproteins. When KC cells are not so treated and when the LDL receptors are either absent or are poorly expressed on the cell surface, then the apo B-enzyme recombinant particle is again without effect (or only minimal effect at best). As in the case for the use of insulin as the targeting agent, one might conclude that the cholesterol esterase in the recombinant particle is gaining access to stored cholesterol ester via receptor-mediated endocytosis utilizing the LDL or apo B receptor.

In terms of targeting efficacy and the possibility of directing enzymes in a site-specific manner, the experiments described in FIGURE 1 and 2 and in TABLES 1 and 2, albeit in tissue culture, are very exciting if not encouraging. Unfortunately the targeting strategy suffers a quite serious letdown when we progress to *in vivo* or whole animal experiments.

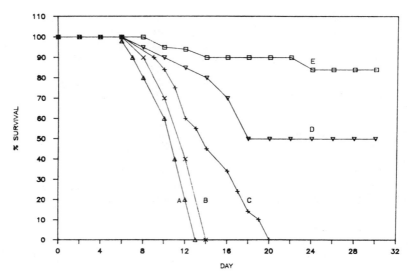

FIGURE 3. C3H/HeJ mice received 5×10^5 6C3HED tumor cells on day 0 via intraperitoneal injection. 24 hr later, groups of 10 mice received: (A) Intravenous albumin as control, (B) L-asparaginase-albumin anti-H2K monoclonal antibody given i.v., (C) L-asparaginase given i.v., (D) L-asparaginase given i.p., and (E) L-asparaginase-albumin-monoclonal antibody (anti H2K) given i.p. The survival rates are simply the % of animals surviving at a given date.

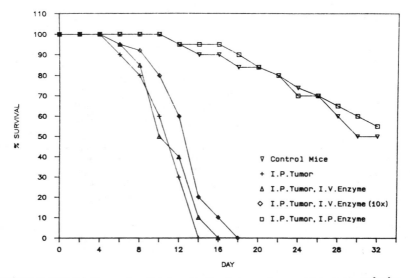

FIGURE 4. BALB/cCr were irradiated on day 0 and given subsequent injections of $5^2 10^5$ Panc-1 cells (the human pancreatic tumor cell line) at 6 hr. Enzyme-albumin-monoclonal antibody (specific to the Panc-1 cells) was administered at 24 hr either i.p. or i.v. The control mice (no tumor cells) have only a 50% survival rate at 32 days, presumably because they are immunoincompetent due to the radiation treatment. The mice had to be rendered immunoincompetent in order for the human Panc-1 cell to grow *in vivo*.

TARGETING IN THE WHOLE ANIMAL

FIGURES 3 and 4 demonstrate our attempts to use conjugates of L-asparaginase, albumin, and monoclonal antibodies in two tumor cell lines *in vivo;* a mouse tumor (CH3ED) grown in syngeneic CH3 mice and a human pancreatic tumor cell line (Panc-1) grown in irradiated BALB/cCr mice. The results shown in the two figures are very similar. When the tumor cells are administered intraperitoneally, followed by an intraperitoneal injection of the enzyme (24 hr later), the efficacy of the therapeutic agent is excellent with virtually complete suppression of tumor cell growth (survival rates equal to controls receiving no tumor). In the case of the human pancreatic tumor cells (FIGURE 4), the mice had to be irradiated prior to injection of the tumor cell line to retard the natural rejection of the foreign cell line by immune-competent mice. When the enzyme conjugated to albumin and to the monoclonal antibody was administered intravenously (even at 10 times the effective intraperitoneal dose), the enzyme was seen to be ineffective even compared to the mice receiving only tumor cells. We know

TABLE 3.

	α-Glucosidase[a]	α-Glucosidase-Albumin[b]	α-Glucosidase-Insulin[c]
Blood	12.2	52.1	21.1
Liver	48.5	22.9	42.4
Spleen	15.1	5.5	6.8
Kidneys	5.0	0.2	0.5
Urine	1.3	0.1	–
Thyroid	1.5	1.0	1.1
Heart	0.2	0.8	2.8[d]
Lungs	3.8	4.2	3.1
Peritoneum	1.6	0.3	0.9
Muscle (total mass)	0.4	0.1	2.9[d]
Bone (total mass)	1.1	1.4	1.8
RBCs	0.9	0.6	1.7

[a]$[^{125}I]$α-glucosidase distribution measured 1 hr after injection.
[b]$[^{125}I]$α-glucosidase-albumin distribution measured 4 hr after injection.
[c]$[^{125}I]$α-glucosidase-insulin distribution measured 1 hr after injection.
[d]Statistical analysis indicates these values differ from equivalent tissues using other enzyme preparations at the 0.01 level.

from experiments not described here that the L-asparaginase-albumin-Mab conjugate has a very respectable circulation (>4 hr) time and we conclude that the enzyme complex, while having a high affinity for the tumor cells is simply trapped within the circulation and never is able to find the appropriate target. We attribute this to the effectiveness of the endothelial cell barrier between the circulation and the peritoneal cavity. A similar limitation was seen (FIGURE 3) for the mouse tumor cell line and its growth in the peritoneal cavity. Here we demonstrate that the barrier exists for L-asparaginase alone to almost the same extent as it does with the conjugate utilizing a Mab directed against the tumor cell. In both cases i.p. introduction of conjugates even 24 hr following introduction of the tumor cells gave excellent results.

With these somewhat depressing results in mind, we sought to achieve enzyme targeting by the use of ligands know to leave the circulation. Our first attempt was with insulin. We had previously shown[6] (TABLE 1) that insulin can function as an effective targeting agent to introduce conjugated enzyme into cells via a mechanism reflecting receptor-mediated endocytosis. The question we asked was whether a similar mechanism could be used to target the enzyme out of the circulation, past the endothelial barrier to underlying target tissue. Because of our interest in glycogen storage disease (Pompe's) our enzyme was α-glucosidase and our target was muscle (especially cardiac and respiratory muscle). The results summarized in TABLE 3 are promising at best. Whereas no significant amount of [^{125}I]α-glucosidase can be detected in muscle tissue when the enzyme is administered either free or conjugated with albumin, a statistically significant amount (though still small) of the enzyme can be detected in both cardiac and total muscle mass when insulin is included in the conjugate. Perhaps more indicative of the effectiveness of the insulin-mediated targeting is the shift in the liver-to-spleen ratio seen for the enzyme-insulin conjugate (6.2) as compared to the free enzyme (3.2) or enzyme-albumin conjugate (4.2). Higher liver-to-spleen ratios generally represent higher levels of uptake by hepatocytes as opposed to the more phagocytic cells of the RES including the liver's Kupffer cells. Like the muscle cell

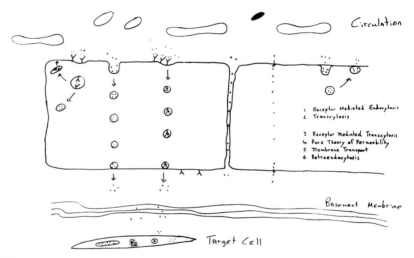

FIGURE 5. An amateur artist's rendering of the endothelial cell as a barrier to the movement of all or most peptide and polypeptide species. The various possible permeation routes are depicted. The evidence for the existence of route 3 is increasing and we have proposed[2] that drug delivery schemes (enzyme delivery in our case) might utilize a mechanism such as "receptor-mediated transcytosis" in order to pass the endothelial barrier and reach underlying target tissue following i.v. administration.

membrane, the hepatocyte plasma membrane is especially rich in insulin receptors although they are found in virtually all tissue including red blood cells. Nevertheless, the insulin appears to have effectively targeted the α-glucosidase to tissues to a much greater degree than it would have been delivered in the absence of the insulin. While perhaps some benefit in the targeting of such a non-toxic molecule as α-glucosidase, this level of specificity would not be acceptable to most targeting strategies.

CONCLUSION

A central question thus remains: How is a macromolecular particle designed as a drug delivery system introduced intravenously to recognize a particular endothelial barrier and cross it to reach the underlying target tissue. In 1984, we put forward the concept of "receptor-mediated transcytosis"[2] in expectation that it might be possible to target a delivery system to a particular endothelium to have it transported out of the circulation to the target by such a mechanism. At the time, the suggestion was put forward as mere speculation with little but circumstantial evidence. Since that time the concept that plasma borne peptides may cross the endothelial barrier by specific transport mechanism has been demonstrated for a number of different proteins including albumin,[15] insulin,[16] and LDL.[17] We have put forward the notion that specific receptors on the endothelial surface may determine the extent to which peptides arrive at underlying tissue. If this is correct then we should consider identifying such receptors and targeting to them in order to effect a tissue- or site-specific delivery of drugs. FIGURE 5 depicts such a scenario and the various routes that proteins may attempt to navigate.

REFERENCES

1. EHRLICH, P. 1906. *In* Collected Studies on Immunity. **2:** 442–447.
2. POZNANSKY, M. J. & R. L. JULIANO. 1984. Pharmacol. Rev. **36(4):** 277–336.
3. PAPAHADJOPOULOS, D., Ed. 1978. Liposomes and their Use in Biology and Medicine. Ann. N.Y. Acad. Sci. **308.**
4. POSTE, G. & R. KIRSH. 1983. Biotechnology **1:** 869–878.
5. MOOLTEN, F. L. & S. R. COOPERBRAND. 1970. Science **169:** 68–70.
6. POZNANSKY, M. J., R. SINGH, B. SINGH & G. FANTUS. 1984. Science **223:** 1304–1306.
7. ROGERS, J. C. & S. KORNFELD. 1971. Biochem. Biophys. Res. Commun. **45:** 622–629.
8. POZNANSKY, M. J. 1977. *In* Biomedical Applications of Immobilized Enzymes and Proteins. T. M. S. Chang, Ed **2:** 341–354. Plenum Press. New York.
9. POZNANSKY, M. J. & D. BHARDWAJ. 1981. Biochem. J. **196:** 89–93.
10. POZNANSKY, M. J. & M. SHANDLING, M. A. SALKIE, J. ELLIOTT & E. LAU. 1982. Cancer Res. **42:** 1020–1025.
11. POZNANSKY, M. J. 1983. Pharmac. Ther. **21:** 53–76.
12. POZNANSKY, M. J. 1986. *In* Protein Tailoring for Food and Medical Uses. R. E. Feeney & J. R. Whitaker, Eds.: 317–338. Marcel Dekker. New York.
13. WU, M-C, G. K. ARIMURA & A. A. YUNIS. 1978. Int. J. Cancer **22:** 728–733.
14. POZNANSKY, M. J. & K. HUTCHISON. 1987. Manuscript submitted for publication.
15. GHITESCU, L., A. FIXMAN, M. SIMIONESCU & N. SIMIONESCU. 1986. J. Cell Biol. **102:** 1304–1311.
16. KING, G. L. & S. M. JOHNSON. 1985. Science **227:** 1583–1586.
17. VASILE, E., M. SIMIONESCU & N. SIMIONESCU. 1983. J. Cell Biol. **96:** 1677–1689.

An Approach to Chemotherapy Based on Base Sequence Information and Nucleic Acid Chemistry

Matagen (Masking Tape for Gene Expression)

PAUL O. P. TS'O, PAUL S. MILLER, LAURE AURELIAN,
AKIRA MURAKAMI, CHERYL AGRIS,
KATHLEEN R. BLAKE, SHWU-BIN LIN, BOK L. LEE,
AND CYNTHIA C. SMITH

Division of Biophysics
School of Hygiene and Public Health
The Johns Hopkins University
Baltimore, Maryland 21205

INTRODUCTION

Advances in modern biological research reveal that the properties and behavior of living organisms are governed by their genes and the regulatory mechanisms involved in gene expression. Thus, DNA sequences and DNA sequences expressed in the form of RNA provide basic information about living organisms. Specific nucleotide sequences in DNA replication and transcription and RNA processing and translation provide key information about the operation and the specificity of these biochemical processes. During the past decade, increasing amounts of information have been collected concerning these sequences of genes, particularly viruses. For example, the complete nucleotide sequence of the human T-cell leukemia virus III (HTLV-III) has been elucidated recently.[1] More information on gene sequences will surely be collected rapidly in the future. This sequence information could be used to understand gene function and thus the biological properties of living organisms.

In addition to utilizing this information on genes and viruses in basic studies, can we develop a major innovative strategy for chemotherapy using our knowledge of base sequences? Can we utilize this information on sequences to block or control specifically the expression of the genes of an infectious foreign agent, such as a virus, or the undesirable expression of a gene in a pathological process, such as neoplasia?

How can we specifically block gene expression? For the gene or its corresponding mRNA to function properly the nucleotide sequences must exist at least transiently in an exposed, single-stranded state. If these exposed sequences were to base pair with a complementary nucleic acid analog, the expression of the gene could be masked and thus, controlled. In order to function within living cells, the nucleic acid analog should have the following properties:

(1) The nucleic acid analog must retain the absolute specificity of the Watson-Crick base pairing scheme. Therefore, no change in the structure of the bases should be made. If possible, the mutual interaction between the cellular target nucleic acid and the analogs should be increased without reducing base-pairing specificity. This can be achieved by the reduction of the repulsion force between the two strands in the helical duplex.

(2) The nucleic acid analog must be able to penetrate cellular membranes and enter the cell, and preferably the analog should be able to penetrate readily into the various organs of the body.

(3) The nucleic acid analog must be resistant to hydrolysis by cellular enzymes. In other words, the chemical structure of the analogs must be such that it is inherently resistant to nucleases.

(4) The nucleic acid analog must have a sequence complementary to a specifically targeted, single-stranded cellular nucleic acid so the function of the target nucleic acid will be under the specific control of the analog upon duplex formation.

This strategy for chemotherapy should function well for control of foreign nucleic acids, such as viral nucleic acids inside mammalian or human cells. Presumably, crucial nucleotide sequences of foreign pathogens will not be the same as those of the host. Therefore, once the crucial sequence of a virus has been determined, a nucleic acid analog complementary to that sequence would then be introduced into mammalian cells to control the replication or the pathogenesis of the virus.

A similar approach may be used to control oncogenes. Oncogenes have been recently implicated in the process of carcinogenesis. Over-expression of such genes, or overactivity of the oncogene product, can possibly lead to neoplasia. A variety of molecular events, including gene rearrangement, promoter insertion, gene amplification, point mutation, etc., could result in such over-expression or over-activity of the oncogenes. More specifically, point mutations can also result in activation of oncogenes in such a way that the activity of the gene product increases. An example of such activation is the mutation in the twelfth codon of the H-*ras* gene.[2]

Sequences of some oncogenes and even cellular proto-oncogenes have been determined from studies on oncogenic viruses. For example, the gene products of the *myc* gene, and therefore the gene sequence, have been elucidated.[3] It is still relatively difficult to study the precise function of these genes in the process of carcinogenesis or metastasis. It would be valuable to have a specific means to suppress the expression of these genes to determine their role in neoplasia. It should be kept in mind however, that many of these genes also exist in normal cells and may have vital functions. The hope we have is to suppress the mutated oncogene expression or to reduce the excessive expression of the normal oncogene appropriately.

From another viewpoint, heredity studies indicate that defects in certain genes are related to the development of cancer and that these defective genes function in a recessive manner. This is in contrast to oncogenes, which function in a dominant manner, at least in transfection experiments. Such defective genes have been termed "anti-oncogenes," suggesting that these genes are regulatory in nature; their normal function being to regulate or suppress the expression of the oncogenes. Thus, a defect in an anti-oncogene results in loss of regulation of oncogenes.[4] In this case, if the nucleotide sequence and the precise mode of action of anti-oncogenes can be understood, then we will have an obvious means to imitate the regulation of the oncogene.

Research done over the past 15 years in the Division of Biophysics, The Johns Hopkins University, School of Hygiene and Public Health, has led to the development of a family of oligonucleotide analogs that has the properties described above and can inhibit specific biological systems, including animal viruses in mammalian and human cells.

We have prepared two types of nonionic oligonucleotide analogs: oligonucleotide alkylphosphotriesters and oligonucleoside methylphosphonates (FIGURE 1). The latter analogs are also given the name Matagen (an acronym for Masking Tape for Gene Expression). FIGURE 2 compares the phosphodiester backbone of the deoxyoligonucleotides and methylphosphonate backbone of Matagen and outlines the differences in

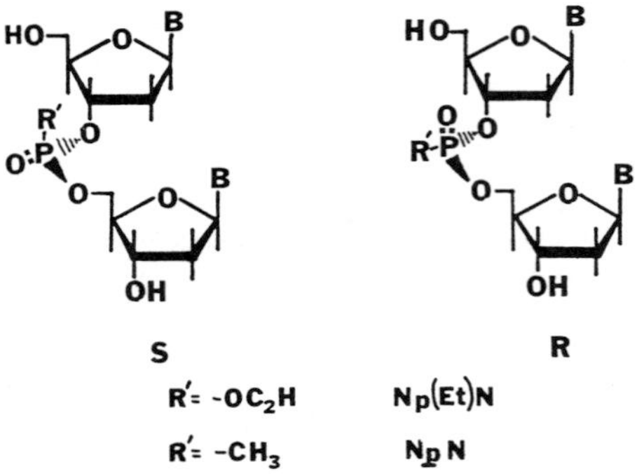

FIGURE 1. Diastereoisomers of a dinucleotide ethylphosphotriester. [d-Np(Et)N] and a dinucleoside methylphosphonate (d-NpN).

the physical, chemical, biochemical, and biological properties of the oligomers. The bases, sugar, and a portion of the sugar phosphate backbone of these analogs are identical to those of natural nucleic acids. However, the analogs are not charged due to the replacement of the negatively charged phosphodiester linkage with the nonionic methylphosphonate internucleotide bond. This type of modification allows the analogs to form complementary duplexes with single-stranded nucleic acids with a high degree of specificity. These analogs are resistant to nucleases and are taken up readily in intact form by mammalian and certain bacterial cells in culture.

The methylphosphonate modification results in the formation of a pair of diastereoisomers that differ in configuration about the phosphorus atom, as shown in FIGURE 1. These dideoxyribonucleoside methylphosphonate diastereoisomers can be separated by reversed phase high performance liquid chromatography. The configurations of the methylphosphonate linkage of one diastereoisomer of dApT have been determined by X-ray crystallographic studies,[5] whereas the diastereoisomer of dApA has been separated and individually assigned by NMR nuclear Overhauser enhancement experiments.[6] Studies on the interaction of dimers with complementary polynucleotides show that the two diastereoisomers (denoted as S or R, representing pseudo axial and pseudo equatorial configuration) form complexes of slightly different thermal stabilities. For example, the equatorial (R) isomer of d-ApA forms a less stable complex with poly U in the d-ApA:poly(U) system [(2A:1U) complex, T_m (melting temperature) = 15.4°C)] than does the axial (S) isomer (T_m = 19.8°C). Comparative studies on the thermal stability of complexes formed between the oligonucleoside methylphosphonates and complementary polynucleotides show that the T_m (melting temperature) of the nonionic oligonucleotide complex is usually higher than that of the complex formed between the naturally occurring oligonucleotides and their complementary polynucleotides. For instance, the poly dT · deoxy A_4 complex (2T:1A) has a T_m of 35.5°C, while the corresponding poly dT · deoxy A_4 analog has a T_m of 44.5°C under the same salt conditions.[7] Clearly, the removal of the negative charge from the oligonucleotide analog has increased the stability of the complexes.

Methods have been developed to synthesize and characterize oligodeoxyribonucleoside methylphosphonates. The base stacking patterns of both isomers of d-ApA are very similar to those of the dinucleoside monophosphate, d-ApA, with the stacking of the S isomer being identical to that of the diester.[6,8]

Methylphosphonate oligomers of defined sequence are readily prepared in good overall yields on insoluble polymer supports by stepwise additions of protected deoxyribonucleoside methylphosphonic imidazolides to the growing oligomer chain.[9] The 5'-hydroxyl groups of oligomers, which terminate with a nucleoside phosphodiester linkage, can be phosphorylated by polynucleotide kinase. The size of the oligomer can be determined by partial hydrolysis of the methylphosphonate linkages with piperidine followed by polyacrylamide gel electrophoresis, which separates the oligomers according to their chain lengths. The sequence of the oligomers can be determined by a modified Maxam-Gilbert procedure. Sequence-specific ^{32}P-labeled oligomers hybridize with mRNA in agarose gels. Since the oligomers serve as primers for reverse transcriptase, their binding position on mRNA can also be characterized.[10]

Two general strategies have been developed to utilize Matagen to block the expression of a gene in mammalian cells. The first approach is to block the translation of a targeted mRNA and the second approach is to inhibit the mRNA processing, particularly the splicing of pre-mRNA. These approaches are illustrated in FIGURE 3

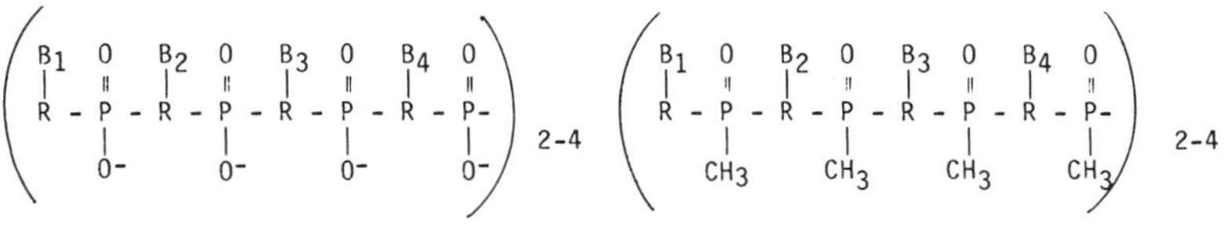

$$\left(\begin{array}{cccccccc} B_1 & O & B_2 & O & B_3 & O & B_4 & O \\ | & \| & | & \| & | & \| & | & \| \\ R & - & P & - & R & - & P & - & R & - & P & - & R & - & P- \\ | & & | & & | & & | \\ O^- & & O^- & & O^- & & O^- \end{array} \right)_{2-4}$$

oligodeoxyribonucleotides

$$\left(\begin{array}{cccccccc} B_1 & O & B_2 & O & B_3 & O & B_4 & O \\ | & \| & | & \| & | & \| & | & \| \\ R & - & P & - & R & - & P & - & R & - & P & - & R & - & P- \\ | & & | & & | & & | \\ CH_3 & & CH_3 & & CH_3 & & CH_3 \end{array} \right)_{2-4}$$

oligodeoxyriobnucleoside methylphosphonates (Matagen)

Negatively charged phosphodiester backbone	Nonionic methylphosphonate backbone
Forms duplexes with complementary polynucleotides	Forms duplexes with complementary polynucleotides. Stability of duplex higher than that of oligodeoxyribonucleotide duplexes.
Backbone readily hydrolyzed by nucleases	Backbone totally resistant to nuclease hydrolysis
Oligomer usually not taken up intact by cells	Oligomer taken up intact by cells by passive diffusion

Olidodeoxyribonucleoside methylphosphonates are active in the following cells:

Transformed Syrian Hamster Fibroblasts (BP-6)

Transformed Human Cells (HTB 1080)

Rabbit Reticulocytes

African Green Monkey Kidney Cells (BSC40)

Mouse L-Cells

FIGURE 2. Comparison of oligodeoxyribonucleotides and oligodeoxyribonucleoside methylphosphonates (Matagen).

Activity: Blocks specific sequences of critical single-stranded
            regions of cellular nucleic acids.

I.   Inhibition of translation of mRNA - Inhibition of translation
      by Matagen Complementary to the initiation codon region of mRNA

                        ————→ A U G ←————————

                        TpApCpNpNpNpNpN

    A.   Inhibition of rabbit globin synthesis in rabbit reticulocytes
          and lysates

    B.   Inhibition of vesicular stomatitis virus (VSV) protein
          synthesis in VSV-infected mouse L-cells

II.   Inhibition of Splicing of pre-mRNA - Inhibition of splicing by
      Matagen complementary to the splice junctions of pre-mRNA

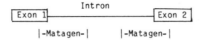

    A.   Inhibition of large T antigen synthesis in SV40-infected cells.

    B.   Inhibition of proteins encoded by immediate early mRNA 4 and 5
          in Herpes simplex virus type 1 and 2-infected cells.

FIGURE 3. Matagen (*Ma*sking *Ta*pe for *Gene Expression*).

α GLOBIN mRNA

    1   10   30   40   60   70
G^mPPP AmCmACUUCUGG ------AAGGAACCACCAUGGUGCUG----------------GACCAACAUCA ------------(A)N

                            TACC   GGTTGTAGT
                            TACCA
                            TACCACGT

β GLOBIN mRNA

    1   10   5U   60   70   80
G^mPPP AmCmACUUGCUUUU-----AAACAGACAGAAUGGUGCAUCUGUCCAGTGAGGAGAAG----------------------(A)N

     GAACGAAAA   TACC
                               TACCA
                               TACCACGT
                          TGTCTTAC
                      TGTCTGTCTTAC   GTCCTCCT

FIGURE 4. Partial nucleotide sequence of rabbit α-globin mRNA and rabbit β-globin mRNA. Below each mRNA are shown the sequences of the complementary oligodeoxyribonucleoside methylphosphonates. The underlined portion of each oligomer shows the position of the methylphosphonate internucleotide linkages. (From Blake *et al.*[12] With permission from *Biochemistry.*)

and are described in more detail in the following sections. In earlier experiments, we have also attempted to block the interaction between bacterial 16S rRNA and bacterial mRNA by sequence-specific Matagen.

SPECIFIC INHIBITION OF BACTERIAL PROTEIN SYNTHESIS

We have synthesized a Matagen with the sequence d-ApGpGpApGpGpT, which is complementary to the 16S rRNA of the Shine-Dalgarno sequence, -ACCUCCU-, which in turn is complementary to the initiation codon region of the bacterial mRNA. The Shine-Dalgarno sequence is absent in 18S ribosomal RNA of mammalian cells. This Matagen blocks the interaction between the 16S rRNA and the bacterial mRNA and thereby inhibits the translation of bacterial mRNA.[11] It does not inhibit translation of globin mRNA in a mammalian cell-free translation system. Since the *E. coli* cell wall prevents the uptake of Matagen, experiments were performed with an *E. coli* mutant that has an altered, more permeable cell wall. Experiments in a cell-free *E. coli* system and with the living *E. coli* mutant clearly demonstrated that the d-ApGpGpApGpGpT Matagen is a powerful, specific inhibitor of protein synthesis and bacterial growth, exerting little inhibitory effect in a mammalian translational system (globin synthesis in rabbit reticulocytes) or on growth of human cells (HT1080, human fibrosarcoma fibroblast). This set of early experiments demonstrates the strategy to control a class of pathogenic microorganisms that present no physical barrier to the entrance of Matagen and utilize a different mechanism for mRNA-ribosome recognition in protein synthesis.

MATAGEN DESIGNED TO INHIBIT PROTEIN SYNTHESIS BY MASKING mRNA TRANSLATION

Two systems were used to investigate the ability of sequence-specific Matagen to prevent translation of mRNA. In the first system, Matagens with sequences complementary to various regions of rabbit globin mRNA were tested as inhibitors of globin synthesis in rabbit reticulocyte lysates and cells.[12] In the second system, Matagens with sequences complementary to the initiation codon regions of selected vesicular stomatitis virus (VSV) mRNAs were studied for their effects on virus protein synthesis both in a cell-free system and in virus-infected cells.[13]

Inhibition of Globin mRNA Translation

Matagens were synthesized with sequences complementary to the 5' end, the initiation codon region or the coding region of rabbit globin mRNA. The sequences of these matagens and their binding sites on globin mRNA are shown in FIGURE 4. These Matagens were shown to interact appropriately with their target complementary mRNA binding sites by their ability to serve as primers for the enzyme reverse transcriptase. In several cases the priming efficiency of the Matagen was enhanced when the oligomer was first preannealed with the mRNA. The priming efficiency of each Matagen correlated with the predicted secondary structure of this particular Matagen binding site on globin mRNA. That is, Matagens whose binding sites are located in the hydrogen bonding stem region of the mRNA are less efficient primers than those whose binding sites are located in single-stranded loop regions.

Matagens inhibit translation of globin mRNA in a rabbit reticulocyte lysate system, as shown in TABLE 1. This inhibition is influenced by the sequence and the chain length of the Matagen, the location of the Matagen binding site on the mRNA, and finally, the presence or absence of secondary structure at the binding site. In general, oligomers that bind to the 5′ end and initiation codon regions of β-globin mRNA inhibit both α- and β-globin synthesis whereas oligomers that bind to the

TABLE 1. Inhibition of Rabbit Globin mRNA Translation by Oligodeoxyribonucleoside Methylphosphonates in a Rabbit Reticulocyte Lysate at 37°C

Oligomer	Binding Site	Concentration (μM)	% Inhibition α	β
5′-end				
d-ApAAAGCAAG	β 4–12	100	56	51
		100[a]	70	70
Initiation codon region				
d-CCAT	α 37–40	100	0	0
	β 54–57	200	28	42
d-ApCCAT	α 37–41	100	23	36
	β 54–58	200	67	67
d-TpGCACCAT	α 37–44	100	35	28
	β 54–61	200	73	70
d-CpATTCTGT	β 49–56	50	2	2
		100	0	7
		200	11	8
		100[a]	30	36
		200[a]	48	34
d-CpATTCTGTCTGT	β 45–56	25	17	14
		100	49	50
Coding region				
d-ApCAGATGC	β 59–66	25	5	−7
		50	5	4
		100	33	24
		100[a]	76	66
d-TpGATGTTGG	α 62–70	25	16	8
		50	24	9
		100	38	11
d-TpCCTCCTG	β 72–80	25	8	16
		100	15	36
Other				
d-ACAGACAT	none	25	7	−14
		100	19	8
d-TTTTTT	poly A tail	300	0	0

[a]Oligomer preannealed to mRNA before translation.
Data from Blake et al.[12]

coding region of α-globin mRNA or the coding region of β-globin mRNA inhibit translation of their target mRNA in a specific manner. Of particular interest is the Matagen d-CpATTCTGT whose nucleotide sequence is complementary to nucleotides 49–56 of β-globin mRNA. Under the usual conditions of the translation experiment, this Matagen has little or no inhibitory effect on either α- or β- globin synthesis, even at

TABLE 2. Effects of Oligodeoxyribonucleoside Methylphosphonates on Globin Synthesis in Rabbit Reticulocytes at 25°C

Oligomer	Concentration (μM)	% Inhibition α	% Inhibition β
d-Tp*GCACCAT*	200	42	29
d-Cp*ATTCTGT*	200	0	0
d-Cp*ATTCTGTCTGT*	200	21	17
d-Tp*GATGTTGG*	100	59	59

Data from Blake *et al.*[12]

oligomer concentrations up to 200 μM. However, if the oligomer is preannealed to the mRNA prior to translation inhibition as high as 35–50% is observed.

Matagens also effectively inhibit globin synthesis in rabbit reticulocytes at 25°C, as shown in TABLE 2. The effects of the oligomers on cellular globin synthesis are similar to those in the lysate system and suggest that the conformation of globin mRNA is the same in both systems during translation. For example, d-Cp*ATTCTGT,* which does not inhibit unless it is preannealed with mRNA, has no effect on reticulocyte globin synthesis. This observation strongly suggests that the secondary structure of globin mRNA inside the living reticulocytes is similar to that in the lysate and that the conformation of mRNAs in living cells may be probed by Matagen.

Inhibition of VSV Protein Synthesis

Matagens with sequences complementary to the initiation codon regions of N, NS, and G mRNA of VSV were synthesized (FIGURE 5). Although these Matagens are completely complementary only to their target mRNA, a computer search revealed that they do have varying degrees of complementarity with other VSV mRNAs (TABLE 3). The Matagens were tested for their ability to inhibit translation of VSV mRNA in a rabbit reticulocyte lysate translation system and in VSV-infected mouse L

N mRNA

```
1                10              20
GᵐpppAᵐACAGUAAUCAAAAUGUCUCUUACA--------(A)n
                         TACAGACAA
```

NS RNA

```
1                10              20
GᵐpppAᵐACAGAUAUCAUGGAUAAUCUCACA--------(A)n
                      TACCTATTA
```

G mRNA

```
1                10            30
GᵐpppAᵐACAGAGAUC-------CUAUGAAGUCG-------(A)n
                            TACTTCACG
```

FIGURE 5. Matagens complementary to VSV mRNA. (From Agris *et al.*[13] With permission from *Biochemistry*.)

TABLE 3. Complementarity between Oligodeoxyribonucleoside Methylphosphonates and VSV mRNA or Rabbit Globin mRNA

Oligonucleoside Methylphosphonate	Number of Contiguous Oligomer Bases	Number of Complementary Sites of VSV mRNA[a]								
		VSV mRNA						Globin mRNA		
		L	G	NS	N	M	Total	α	β	Total
d-Ap*ACAGACAT* (I)	9	0	0	0	1	0	1	0	0	0
	8	0	0	0	0	0	0	0	0	0
	7	2	0	0	0	0	0	0	0	0
	6	4	4	0 1[b]	1	0	9 1[b]	0	0	0
	5	16	1	2 1[b]	3	1 1[b]	23 2[b]	1 1[b]	3	4 1[b]
d-Ap*TTATCCAT* (II)	9	0	0	1	0	0	1	0	0	0
	8	1	0	0	0	0	1	0	0	0
	7	2	0	0	1	0	3	0	0	0
	6	8	1	0	2	0	11	0	0	0
	5	33	10	5 1[b]	6 1[b]	3	57 2[b]	0	1	1
d-Gp*CACTTCAT* (III)	9	0	1	0	0	0	1	0	0	0
	8	1	0	0	0	0	1	0	0	0
	7	1	1	0	0	0	2	0	0	0
	6	9	1	2	0	1	13	0	1[b]	1[b]
	5	40 2[b]	7 1[b]	8 2[b]	6 1[b]	6 1[c]	67 7[b]	0	1	1

[a]These values represent the number of nonoverlapping sites on the mRNA, which are complementary to 5 or more contiguous bases of the oligomer.
[b]Site is located in the 3'-noncoding region of the mRNA.
[c]Site is located in the 5'-noncoding region of the mRNA.
Data from Agris *et al.*[13]

TABLE 4. Effects of Oligodeoxyribonucleoside Methylphosphonates on VSV and Globin Protein Synthesis in a Rabbit Reticulocyte Lysate at 30°C[a]

Oligomer	Concentration (μM)	% Change[b]				
		NS	N	M	α globin	β globin
d-Ap*ACAGACAT* (I)	50	+7	−26	+20	−6	−9
	100	−7	−36	+12	−15	−9
	150	−38	−77	−43		
d-Ap*TTATCCAT* (II)	50	+5	−4	+7	+18	+14
	100	−15	−25	+2	+63	+50
	150	−24	−35	−18		
d-Gp*CACTTCAT* (III)	50	−4	−15	0	+26	+20
	100	+2	−16	+6	+40	+55

[a]Average of 2 or 3 experiments, with a range of ±6% (VSV) or ±4% (globin).
[b]Minus sign indicates inhibition of translation, while a plus sign indicates stimulation of translation.
Data from Agris *et al.*[13]

cells. In the lysate system, oligomers complementary to N and NS mRNAs inhibited translation of VSV N and NS mRNAs whereas the oligomer complementary to G mRNA had only a slight inhibitory effect on N protein synthesis (TABLE 4). The N-specific oligomer specifically inhibited N protein synthesis whereas the NS-specific oligomer inhibited both N and NS protein synthesis. This reduced specificity of inhibition may be due to formation of partial duplexes between the NS-specific oligomer and VSV N mRNA. The oligomers had little or no inhibitory effects on the synthesis of globin mRNA in the same lysate system (TABLE 4). All three oligomers specifically inhibited synthesis of all five viral proteins in VSV-infected cells in a concentration-dependent manner (TABLE 5). The oligomers had no effect on cellular protein synthesis in uninfected cells or on cell growth. As a control, an oligothymidylate, which forms only weak duplexes with poly(rA), was shown to have only a slight effect on VSV protein synthesis or yield of virus. It should be noted that all three oligomers have extensive partial complementarity with the coding regions of L mRNA (TABLE 3). The non-specific inhibition of viral protein synthesis in infected cells may

TABLE 5. Effects of Oligodeoxyribonucleoside Methylphosphonates on VSV Protein Synthesis in Mouse L Cells[a]

Oligonucleoside Methylphosphonate	Concentration (μM)	% Inhibition[b]				
		L	G	NS	N	M
d-Ap*ACAGACAT* (I)	50	4	+3	7	12	13
	100	12	2	12	9	27
	150	69	73	57	67	63
d-Ap*TTATCCAT* (II)	50	20	4	7	4	9
	100	38	31	26	29	38
	150	59	42	43	47	46
d-Gp*CACTTCAT* (III)	50	35	25	45	15	10
	100	94	88	90	80	63
	150	96	94	97	99	92
d-Tp*TTTTTTT* (IV)	50	14	10	9	20	5
	100	15	13	17	22	11
	150	16	30	8	25	15

[a]Average of 2 or 3 experiments with a range of ±5%.
[b]Plus sign indicates stimulation of protein synthesis.
Data from Agris *et al.*[13]

reflect the role of N, NS, and/or L proteins in the replication and transcription of viral RNA or result from duplex formation between the oligomers and complementary, plus-strand viral RNA. The oligomers also significantly inhibited VSV production in a manner corresponding to their effects on VSV protein synthesis as shown in TABLE 4. These results demonstrate that the Matagen can be used to study viral gene expression and to control virus production.

MATAGENS TARGETED AGAINST THE SPLICE JUNCTIONS OF PRE-mRNA

As discussed above, Matagens targeted against single-stranded regions of mRNA are more effective inhibitors of mRNA translation than those whose targeted binding sites are involved in secondary structure. Based on our current understanding of

SV40 LARGE T ANTIGEN RNA

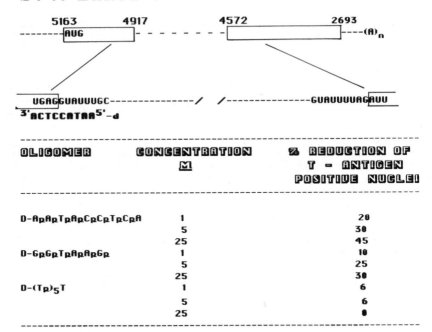

OLIGOMER	CONCENTRATION M	% REDUCTION OF T - ANTIGEN POSITIVE NUCLEI
D-ApApTpApCpCpTpCpA	1	20
	5	30
	25	45
D-GpGpTpApApGp	1	10
	5	25
	25	30
D-(Tp)$_5$T	1	6
	5	6
	25	0

FIGURE 6. Partial nucleotide sequence of the splice junctions of SV40 large T-antigen pre-mRNA. The sequence of the methylphosphonate oligomer complementary to the donor splice junction is shown below the pre-mRNA sequence. The table shows the effects of this oligomer and oligomers complementary to U$_1$ RNA on large T-antigen synthesis in SV40-infected BSC40 cells.

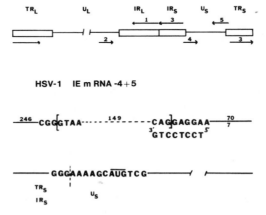

FIGURE 7. Location and direction of synthesis (arrows) of IE mRNAs 4 and 5. Open bars represent terminal (TR$_L$, TR$_S$) and inverted (IR$_L$ and IR$_S$) repeats bounding the unique long (U$_L$) and short (U$_S$) HSV-1 DNA sequences. Intervening nucleotides are numbered. Intron is bounded by brackets. The sequence of the oligomer is shown below the mRNA sequence. (From Smith *et al.*[14] With permission from the publisher.)

TABLE 6. Effects of Oligodeoxyribonucleoside Methylphosphonates on VSV Production[a]

Oligonucleoside	Concentration (μM)	Log reduction (pfu/ml)[b] Hours post-infection 6	24
d-Ap*ACAGACAT* (I)	50	0.07	0.07
	100	0.40	0.07
	150	1.08	0.62
d-Ap*TTATCCAT* (II)	50	0.08	0.10
	100	0.36	0.20
	150	0.52	0.39
d-Gp*CACTTCAT* (III)	50	0.40	+0.02
	100	1.18	0.79
	150	1.52	1.02
d-Tp*TTTTTTTT* (IV)	50	0.10	0.07
	100	0.12	0.09
	150	0.15	0.07

[a]Average of 2 or 3 experiments with a range of ±0.03 log reduction (pfu/ml).
[b]Plus sign indicates stimulation of VSV production.
Data from Agris *et al.*[13]

mRNA biosynthesis, it would appear that the splice junctions of pre-mRNAs would be ideal targets for Matagens. Recent experiments have demonstrated that the splice junctions interact with the RNAs of small ribonucleoproteins that mediate the splicing process. These observations suggest that the splice junctions are in a single-stranded form. We have prepared Matagens complementary to the splice junctions of two viral pre-mRNAs in order to test the possibility of controlling gene expression at the level of mRNA processing.

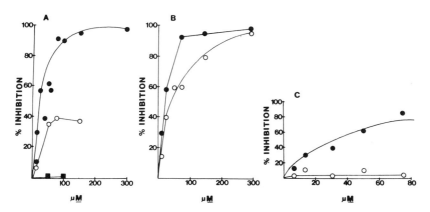

FIGURE 8. Inhibition of virus production (A) HSV-1 (F)-infected Vero cells were exposed to d-Tp*CCTCCTG* at 0 hpi (●) or 1 hpi (O) or to d-Tp*TTTTT* at 0 hpi (■). (B) HSV-1 (F)-infected Vero cells were exposed to d-Tp*CCTCCTG* 24 hr before infection (●). HSV-1 (G)-infected Vero cells were exposed to d-Tp*CCTCCTG* at 0 hpi (O). (C) HSV-1 (F)-infected Vero cells were exposed to d-Tp*CCTCCTG* (●) or d-Tp*CCCTCTG* (O) at 0 hpi. (From Smith *et al.*[14] With permission from the publisher.)

Inhibition of SV40 Large T-antigen RNA

We have synthesized Matagens with sequences complementary to the donor splice junction of SV40 large T-antigen and to the 5'-terminal sequence of U_1 RNA (FIGURE 6). U_1 RNA has been shown to be involved in the splicing of mammalian and viral pre-mRNAs. The effects of these Matagens on large T-antigen synthesis in SV40-infected African green monkey kidney cells (BSC40) were determined by an immuno-precipitation technique. As shown in the table accompanying FIGURE 6, the splice junction-complementary oligomer, d-*AATACCTCA*, and the two U_1 RNA-complementary oligomers each reduce the level of large T-antigen in the cells, while the non-specific oligomer, d-*TTTTTT*, had no effect. None of these oligomers reduced overall protein synthesis by the BSC40 cells.

Inhibition of Herpes Simplex Virus Type 1

We have synthesized the Matagen d-Tp*CCTCCTG*, whose sequence is comple-mentary to the acceptor splice junctions of HSV-1 immediate early mRNA 4 and 5.[14] The targeted binding site of this Matagen on the HSV-1 pre-mRNA is shown in FIGURE 7. To test the specificity of the Matagen, we have also synthesized a control Matagen, d-Tp*CCCTCTG*, in which positions 4 and 5 are —C T— instead of —T C—. The effects of these Matagens on virus replication are shown in FIGURE 8. Treatment of HSV-1–infected cells with d-Tp*CCTCCTG* before (1–24 hr) or at the time of infection caused a dose-dependent inhibition of virus replication. Virus titers were decreased 50% and 90% in cells treated with 25 μM and 75 μM oligomer, respectively;

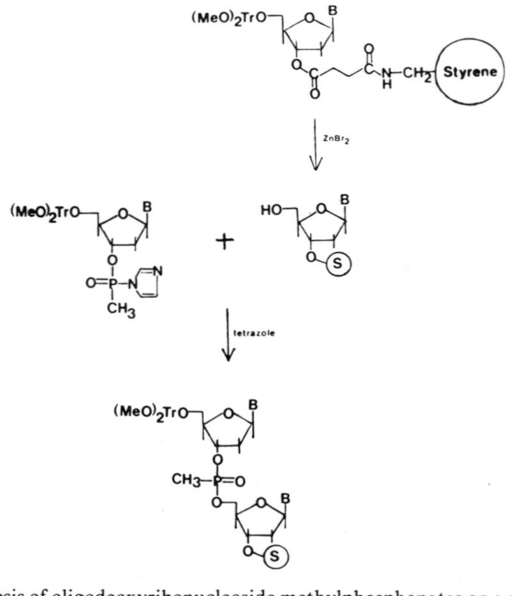

FIGURE 9. Synthesis of oligodeoxyribonucleoside methylphosphonates on a polystyrene support. (From Miller *et al.*[9] With permission from *Biochemistry*.)

TABLE 7. Reaction Cycle for Preparation of Oligodeoxyribonucleoside Methylphosphonates[a]

Step	Reagent		Time (min)
Detritylation	1 M ZnBr$_2$ in methylene chloride/iso-propanol[b]	4 × 1 ml	2 each (C, T)
		2 × 2 ml	2 each (G, A)
Wash	methylene chloride/isopropanol[b]	3 × 1 ml	5 last wash
Wash	0.5 M TEAA in dimethylformamide	3 × 1 ml	
Wash	acetonitrile	6 × 1 ml	
Dry	vacuum pump		30
Condensation	coupling mixture	400 μl[c]	60
Wash	tetrahydrofuran	5 × 1 ml	
Acetylation	capping solution [d]	2 × 1 ml	5 last wash
Wash	methylene chloride/isopropanol[b]	6 × 1 ml	

[a]Reactions were carried out on 100 mg or 200 mg of polystyrene support at room temperature.
[b]85:15 vol/vol.
[c]Use 800 μl for 200 mg of support.
[d]Capping solution: 1 ml acetic anhydride, 1 ml anhydrous pyridine, and 10 mg dimethylamino-pyridine.
Data from Miller *et al.*[9]

at 300 μM, a 99% reduction in virus production was observed. Under the same conditions the control Matagen d-Tp*CCCTCTG* had little inhibitory effect. These data clearly demonstrate the sequence specificity of the Matagen. In addition, the Matagen is more effective against HSV-1 than HSV-2, indicating a strain specificity in the action of Matagen. Finally, the timing of the addition of Matagen is important. As shown in FIGURE 8a, addition of the Matagen at the time of infection is most effective.

The Matagen specifically reduced viral DNA synthesis 70–75%.[14] A 90% reduction in the synthesis of viral proteins, including other immediate early species and viral functional and structural proteins, was also observed. The specificity of the Matagen is demonstrated by the observation that Matagen caused minimal reduction in cellular protein synthesis and minimal effects on the growth rate of uninfected cells.[14]

SYNTHESIS OF MATAGEN ON POLYMER SUPPORTS

A polymer support method was developed to prepare Matagens of defined sequence.[9] The synthetic scheme is shown in FIGURE 9. 5'-(Dimethyoxytrityl)-deoxyribonucleoside 3'-(methylphosphonic imidazolides) are condensed with polymer support-bound oligonucleotide in tetrazole, which appears to act as an acid catalyst. The half-life for dimer formation on the polystyrene support is 5 min and the reaction is 95% complete after 60 min. The reaction cycle for the preparation of Matagen is described by TABLE 7.

The yields and the HPLC retention times of six Matagens prepared by this procedure are shown in TABLE 8. In order to simplify purification and sequence analysis of the oligomer, the 5'-terminal nucleoside unit is linked via a phosphodiester bond. The singly charged oligomers are easily purified by affinity chromatography on DEAE cellulose. The chain lengths of the oligomers were confirmed after 5'-end labeling with polynucleotide kinase by partial hydrolysis of the methylphosphonate linkages with 1 M aqueous piperidine followed by polyacrylamide gel electrophoresis of the hydrolysate.[10] The positions of purine and pyrimidine bases were confirmed by treatment of 5'-end labeled oligomers with acid and hydrazine, respectively. The characterization of Cp*ATTTTTGGTTTCCA*, a 15-mer, is shown in FIGURE 10. These results show that Matagens (up to 15 nucleotides in length) can be synthesized on a polymer support and can be purified, sequenced, and characterized in a manner similar to that used for normal oligodeoxyribonucleotides.

FUTURE CHALLENGES

While our experiments show a great deal of promise that Matagen may be used to control gene expression and may also be useful as a chemotherapeutic agent, there are still problems that require further investigation.

TABLE 8. Syntheses of Oligodeoxyribonucleoside Methylphosphonates on a Polystyrene Support[a]

Oligomer	Average Yield/Phosphonate Condensation Step[b]	Isolated Yield	HPLC[c] Retention Time (min)
d-Tp*CCTCCTG*	89%	15%	13.8
d-Gp*AATCCTG*	90%	21%	14.1
	92%[d]	24%	14.1
d-Tp*GTTGGTC*	91%	25%	14.2
		18%[e]	14.2
d-Ap*ACAGACAT*	88%	12%	15.8
d-Tp*AAATAAAAAAAATT*	91%	4%[e]	16.5
d-Cp*ATTTTTGGTTTCCA*	91%	4%	15.6

[a]The reactions were carried out on 100 mg of support and the last nucleotide was added using the phosphotriester method unless otherwise noted.
[b]Determined by analysis of the dimethoxytrityl group after each coupling step.
[c]ODS-3 reversed-phase HPLC using a 50 ml gradient of 0.5% to 30% acetonitrile (8 and 9 mers) or a 0.5% to 35% acetonitrile (15 mers) in 0.1 M ammonium acetate (pH 5.8) at a flow rate of 2.5 ml/min.
[d]Reaction run on 200 mg of polystyrene support.
[e]5'-Terminal nucleotide added by phosphoramidite method.
Data from Miller *et al.*[9]

(1) Thermodynamic considerations indicate that at low binding levels, the association process predominates and binding is efficient, while at high binding levels the dissociation process predominates and binding becomes inefficient. Thus, physical binding above the 50% level is much less efficient and the efficiency approaches zero as the binding level approaches 100%.

(2) Efficient physical binding of Matagen requires high Matagen concentrations and the extent of binding depends on the binding constant. However at high concentrations the specificity of Matagen may be reduced because the Matagen may partially bind to other sequences.

(3) The specificity of Matagen binding depends upon base pairing selectivity and the uniqueness of the sequence. It will be demonstrated in a subsequent section of this chapter that a sequence of 15 nucleotides would be unique in a mammalian genome. However, Matagen of that chain length could participate in partial binding involving 5

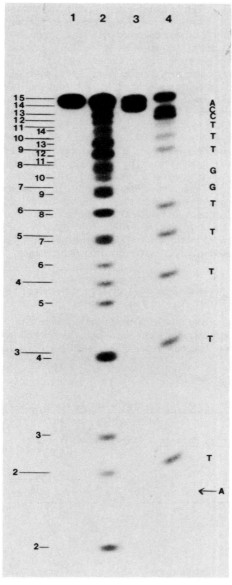

FIGURE 10. Characterization of d-^{32}pCp*ATTTTTGGTTCCA*. The autoradiogram shows: lane 1, 15-mer; lane 2, 15-mer treated with 1 M aqueous piperidine at 37°C; lane 3, 15-mer treated with 2 M hydrochloric acid at 37°C; and lane 4, 15-mer treated with 90% hydrazine at 37°C. The numbers at the far left show the chain length of oligomers terminating with a 3'-hydroxyl group while the next set of numbers show the chain length of oligomers terminating with a 3'-methylphosphonate group. The positions of purine and pyrimidine residues are shown at the right. The arrow indicates the position of the band that is observed in longer exposures of the gel. This band corresponds to the monomer formed by cleavage of the first A residue in the oligomer. (From Miller *et al.*[10] With permission from *Biochemistry*.)

to 10 contiguous bases. Under equilibrium conditions, complete binding by the oligomer is most stable and would lead to high specificity. Under transient conditions, however, partial binding to other sites could occur that would lower the specificity.

(4) A discussion on the statistical basis of the chain length of Matagen versus its sequence specificity would be instructive. The average size of the mammalian haploid genome is about 3×10^9 base pairs and the average gene expression in any given cell is only 1–3% of the total genome or 3×10^7–1×10^8 base pairs. It is estimated that only 10% of the mRNA sequences or 3×10^6–1×10^7 nucleotides have fully exposed regions of 8–12 nucleotides in length. The number of unique sequences is a combination of 4 bases, equivalent to 4^n, where n is the chain length of the sequence. Thus, 4^{10} equals 1.05×10^6, 4^{12} equals 1.68×10^7, 4^{14} equals 2.68×10^8 and 4^{16} equals 4.16×10^9. According to these considerations, a 12-mer could be a unique sequence in a genome size of approximately 1.5×10^7 base pairs. Thus, on a statistical basis, a 12-mer is sufficiently long to mask a specific mRNA species. In order to mask a specific gene in DNA, a 14-mer, which would give 3×10^8 sequence specificity, may be more appropriate. Since approximately 50% of the DNA is in the form of repetitive or mid-repetitive sequences, a chain length of 14 may be sufficient to uniquely define the sequence specificity (1.5×10^9 b.p. in a single copy sequence). In any event, a chain length of 16 is sufficiently unique on a statistical basis for the entire mammalian genome and may be used in solution hybridization experiments.

CURRENT PROGRESS AND FUTURE DIRECTIONS

To overcome some of the problems cited above, two new types of oligonucleoside methylphosphonate derivatives are currently being developed and tested. The schematic concepts of these two new types of Matagen are illustrated schematically in FIGURE 11.

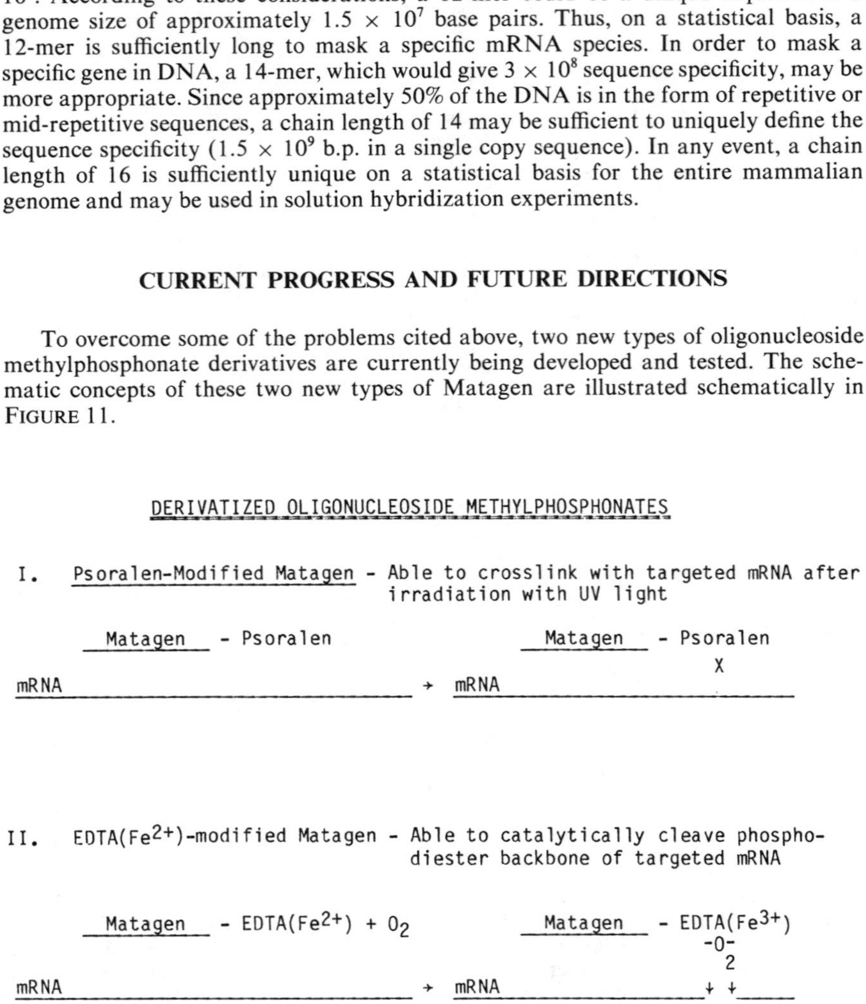
DERIVATIZED OLIGONUCLEOSIDE METHYLPHOSPHONATES
I. Psoralen-Modified Matagen - Able to crosslink with targeted mRNA after irradiation with UV light
Matagen - Psoralen
mRNA
Matagen - Psoralen
X
mRNA
II. EDTA(Fe2+)-modified Matagen - Able to catalytically cleave phosphodiester backbone of targeted mRNA
Matagen - EDTA(Fe2+) + O2
mRNA
Matagen - EDTA(Fe3+)
-O-
2
mRNA

FIGURE 11. Derivatized Matagens.

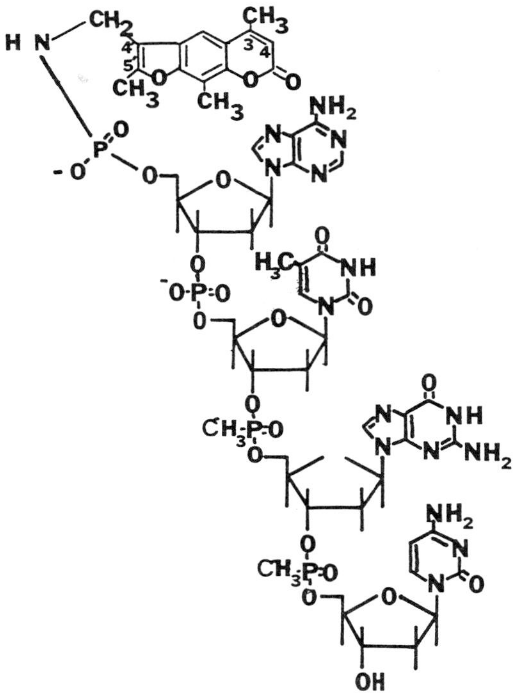

FIGURE 12. Oligodeoxyribonucleoside methylphosphonate derivatized with aminomethyltrimethylpsoralen (AMT)—Matagen-C.

Crosslinking-Matagen (Matagen-C)

The structure of one type of Matagen-C with psoralen as the photoinducible crosslinking group, is shown in FIGURE 12 and the structure of the crosslink between Matagen-C and a complementary target strand is shown in FIGURE 13. The formation of a crosslink between the target nucleic acid and the Matagen could not only irreversibly inactivate the target RNA but also provide unambiguous information about the exact binding site of the Matagen. Because the Matagen-C crosslinks only upon photoirradiation at 365 nm wavelength, it should be possible to specifically control gene expression at selected times during the cell cycle or virus replication cycle. The results of a preliminary experiment with psoralen-Matagen against VSV protein synthesis in VSV-infected cells is shown in TABLE 9. The data clearly indicate that even at low concentrations of psoralen-Matagen, the inhibition of viral yield can take place, particularly as induced by 365 nm irradiation.

Restriction-Matagen (Matagen-R)

This type of Matagen is designed to degrade the sugar-phosphate backbone of targeted complementary nucleic acids. A promising candidate is EDTA-linked Matagen, whose structure is shown in FIGURE 14. The EDTA portion of Matagen, when complexed with FeII and in the presence of molecular oxygen and a reducing agent, is capable of generating hydroxyl radicals that can cleave the complementary strand of the target nucleic acid. Dr. Peter Dervan's group as well as Dr. Leslie Orgel's group have investigated EDTA-linked conventional oligodeoxynucleotides. However, one serious problem with this family of compounds is autodegradation, a problem that appears to be less serious in oligomers without a phosphodiester backbone.

Animal Studies

Preliminary studies with Matagen anti-HSV-1 have shown that when Matagen is prepared in cream form and applied daily post-infection to the ear of a mouse, it is capable of preventing the expression of the herpetic lesions in the mouse and reducing the yield of virus in the skin region and in the ganglion region of the mouse versus the

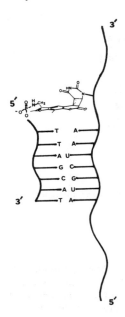

FIGURE 13. Psoralen-derivatized oligonucleoside methylphosphonate (left strand) and mRNA (right strand). A cyclobutane bridge is formed between the pyrone ring of the psoralen and the A uracil residue of the mRNA.

untreated, infected mouse. This experimental observation suggests that Matagen is able to penetrate the mouse skin.

Preliminary data with tritium-labeled Matagen (M. Colvin, unpublished results) indicate that Matagen can penetrate all organs and tissues in the mouse upon intravenous injection, with the exception of the brain. These data provide the encouraging notion that in spite of the brain barrier, there are no other internal barriers for the distribution of Matagen inside the mouse, once it has been introduced into the circulatory system. Matagen is not absorbed by serum protein and has been found to be widely distributed in all tissues.

PROSPECTS OF MATAGEN AS AN ANTIVIRAL THERAPEUTIC AGENT

The processes of viral replication and gene expression, which form a target for attack by chemotherapeutic agents, are shown in FIGURE 15. In this diagram, the

TABLE 9. Effects of a Psoralen-Derivatized Oligonucleoside Methylphosphonate on Vesicular Stomatitis Virus (VSV) Protein Synthesis in VSV-Infected Mouse L-929 Cells. The Oligomer is Complementary to the Initiation Codon Region of VSV-N Protein mRNA.

Cells Protein	$5 \mu M$	% Inhibition		
		$5 \mu M$ Oligomer Only	365 nm Light Only	$5 \mu M$ Oligomer and 365 nm Light
Uninfected L 929 cells	Cellular	-4	16	4
VSV-infected cells	L	26	41	89
	G	21	31	84
	NS	12	39	82
	N	18	38	84
	M	17	37	83

The cells were treated with oligomer at the time of infection. Six hours post infection, the cells were irradiated at 365 nm for 15 min and then labeled with [^{35}S]methionine for 30 min. The cells were then lysed and the proteins separated by polyacrylamide gel electrophoresis.

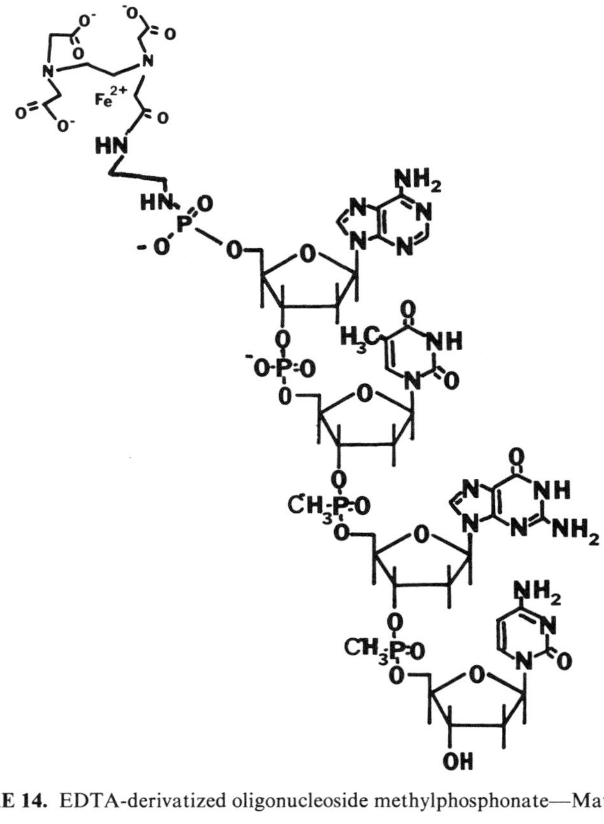

FIGURE 14. EDTA-derivatized oligonucleoside methylphosphonate—Matagen-R.

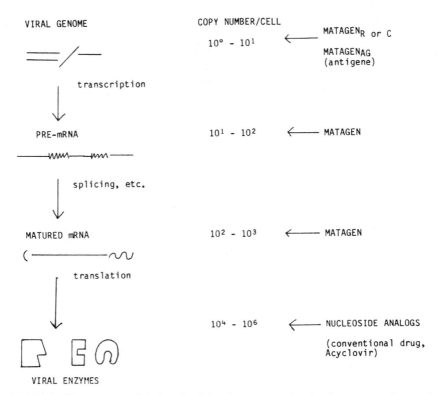

FIGURE 15. The processes of viral replication and gene expression that form a target for attack by chemotherapeutic agents.

TABLE 10. Comparison between Matagen and Nucleoside Analogs (Acyclovir) as Antiviral Agents

	Nucleoside	Matagen
1. Complexity/molecular weight	300–500	5,000–8,000
2. Information basis for design	Differences between host enzymes and viral enzymes	Differences between base sequences of viral gene and host gene
	By trial and error	By sequence information/secondary structure information
3. Development of resistant mutants	Point mutation to change the viral protein	Change of crucial viral sequence
	Entire program has to start all over again	Very easy to design a new Matagen
4. Cost of synthesis	Relatively cheap but large quantity required	Relatively more expensive but possibly very small quantities needed, particularly in Matagen-R, Matagen-AG series
5. Scientific basis	Contributes relatively little to viral biology and viral pathology	Provides unique tool to study viral biology and viral pathology

conventional point of attack of the nucleoside analog, such as acyclovir, is to inhibit viral enzymes without inhibiting the host enzymes of a similar function. Unfortunately, in terms of the number of copies of viral gene products, the number is largest at the enzyme level and smallest at the viral genome level, with the pre-mRNA level and the mature mRNA level lying in between. That is, the number of pre-mRNA or mature mRNA as gene products will certainly be much smaller than the viral enzymes but larger than the number of viral genes itself. Therefore, the quantities of Matagen needed to interrupt the viral replication process would be smaller than the nucleoside analogs needed to interrupt the viral process at the viral enzyme level.

The comparison between the approaches of Matagen and nucleoside analogs as antiviral agents is shown in TABLE 10. Currently, there is only one disadvantage of Matagen, i.e. the question of cost as compared to nucleoside analogs. It is hoped, however, that the necessary quantities of Matagen will be much smaller than those of nucleoside analogs, because of the binding affinity of Matagen and because of the number of targeted molecules in the cells. Currently, we hope to reach the level of 1 μmole concentration as an effective inhibition of viral gene function.

The most important characteristic of the Matagen concept is the development of chemotherapeutics based on information about the nucleotide sequence and secondary structure of vital target genes. The science of nucleic acid chemistry is used to design and develop new chemotherapeutic agents on a rational basis, rather than relying on a random search for effective compounds. Thus, nucleic acid chemistry and chemotherapy come together to form a common basis for drug development, as well as to provide fundamental knowledge about organisms and humans.

REFERENCES

1. RATNER, L., W. HASELTINE, R. PATARCA, K. R. LIVAK, B. STARCICH, S. F. JOSEPHS, E. R. DORAN, J. A. RAFALSKI, E. A. WHITEHORN, K. BOWMEISTER, L. IVANOV, S. R. PETTEWAY, JR., M. R. PEARSON, J. A. LAUTENBERGER, T. S. PAPAS, J. GHRAYEB, N. T. CHANG, R. C. GALLO & F. WONG-STAAL. 1985. Nature **313:** 277–284.
2. PULCIANI, S., E. SANTOS, A. V. LAUVER, L. K. LONG, S. A. AARONSON & M. BARBACID. 1982. Nature **300:** 539–542.
3. RAMSAY, G., G. E. EVAN & J. M. BISHOP. 1984. Proc. Natl. Acad. Sci. USA **81:** 7742–7746.
4. KNUDSON, JR., A. G. 1985. Cancer Res. **45:** 1437–1443.
5. CHACKO, K. K., K. LINDNER, W. SAENGER & P. S. MILLER. 1983. Nucleic Acids Res. **11:** 2801–2814.
6. KAN, L.-S., D. M. CHENG, P. S. MILLER, J. YANO & P. O. P. TS'O. 1980. Biochemistry **19:** 2122–2132.
7. MILLER, P. S., K. B. MCPARLAND, K. JAYARAMAN & P. O. P. TS'O. 1981. Biochemistry **20:** 1874–1880.
8. MILLER, P. S., J. YANO, E. YANO, C. CARROLL, K. JAYARAMAN & P. O. P. TS'O. 1979. Biochemistry **18:** 5134–5143.
9. MILLER, P. S., M. P. REDDY, A. MURAKAMI, K. R. BLAKE, S.-B. LIN & C. H. AGRIS. 1986. Biochemistry **25:** 5092–5097.
10. MURAKAMI, A., K. R. BLAKE & P. S. MILLER. 1985. Biochemistry **24:** 4041–4046.
11. JAYARAMAN, K., K. MCPARLAND, P. MILLER & P. O. P. TS'O. 1981. Proc. Natl. Acad. Sci. USA **78:** 1537–1541.
12. BLAKE, K. R., A. MURAKAMI, S. A. SPITZ, S. A. GLAVE, M. P. REDDY, P. O. P. TS'O & P. S. MILLER. 1985. Biochemistry **24:** 6139–6145.
13. AGRIS, C. H., K. R. BLAKE, P. S. MILLER, M. P. REDDY & P. O. P. TS'O. 1986. Biochemistry **25:** 6268–6275.
14. SMITH, C. C., L. AURELIAN, M. P. REDDY, P. S. MILLER & P. O. P. TS'O. 1986. Proc. Natl. Acad. Sci. USA **83:** 2787–2791.

Retrovirus-Mediated Gene Transfer into Hematopoietic Stem Cells[a]

JOHN E. DICK

Department of Genetics
Research Institute
Hospital for Sick Children
Toronto, Ontario M5G 1X8, Canada

INTRODUCTION

The ability to transfer new genetic information into hematopoietic cells offers a novel approach for understanding the genetic events governing stem cell development. Moreover, the ability to introduce cloned genes into human hematopoietic cells opens up the possibility of correcting certain human diseases by gene therapy. It has only been with the development of high efficiency gene transfer methods, based on highly infectious retroviruses, that this novel approach has become feasible. In this review, I will briefly discuss some key features of retrovirus vector life cycle and structure and describe several examples of how this technology has been applied to transfer genes into hematopoietic cells from both mice and humans.

RETROVIRUSES

Retrovirus vectors are engineered derivatives of the RNA tumor viruses.[1] The structure of a typical retrovirus is shown in FIGURE 1. The open boxes represent those sequences required in *cis* for viral gene expression and replication. The long terminal repeats or LTRs located at each end of the molecule include sequences required for RNA synthesis, such as the promoter, enhancer, poly A addition sites, and stop signals. In addition, they include sequences required for integration of the virus into the host DNA. Immediately downstream of the 5'LTR is the ψ, or packaging region required for encapsidation of the viral RNA into mature virions.

In contrast to these sequences required in *cis* are the sequences shown in the shaded areas, which contain coding sequences for *gag, pol,* and *env* proteins. These genes code for proteins involved in virion assembly and structure, reverse transcription, and virus absorption/penetration, respectively. These proteins can be supplied in *trans* for the retrovirus to complete its life cycle. Virus absorption and penetration occurs via a poorly understood process following recognition of the *env* protein by specific receptors on the cell surface. Following infection, the retrovirus RNA molecules are reverse transcribed into circular double-stranded DNA, which then integrates into the host chromosome by non-homologous recombination. The integrated provirus structure is shown in FIGURE 1. It appears retroviruses can integrate at many possible sites, although some recent evidence suggests that there may be some bias in favor of integration into transcriptionally active regions.[2]

[a]Supported by a grant from the National Cancer Institute of Canada.

242

RETROVIRUS VECTORS

It is readily apparent that the natural life cycle of retroviruses offers a number of important advantages[1] that make them particularly useful as gene transfer vectors: (1) stable insertion of a DNA copy of their genome into the host genome; (2) infection and transmission of their genetic information into a high proportion of recipient cells; (3) a broad, modifiable host range making it possible to infect cells from a variety of species and cell types; (4) stable, predictable proviral structure at low copy number in the host genome; (5) retrovirus infection is not toxic to the cell; and (6) approximately 10 kb of heterologous sequences can be packaged within a single virion.

Generation of retrovirus vectors involves removal of either part or all of the *gag, pol,* and *env* sequences, and their replacement by the foreign gene of interest, thereby generating a defective retrovirus. Since the *cis* acting sequences remain intact, infectious particles can be generated provided the deleted functions are supplied in *trans* in order to assemble the defective vector RNA. This can be achieved in two ways.

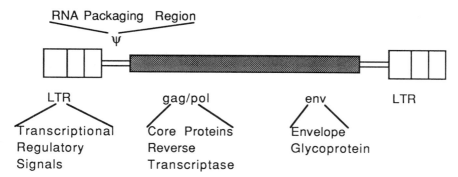

FIGURE 1. Model of a typical retrovirus. The shaded areas represent those genes whose function, if provided in *trans,* can be deleted from the virus. The open boxes indicate those sequences required in *cis* for virus gene expression and replication.

Firstly, cell lines containing a defective engineered provirus can be superinfected with a replication competent helper virus. The *gag, pol,* and *env* protein products generated from the wild type provirus can function to package both the defective RNA genome as well as the wild type RNA genome, thereby producing both replication-defective as well as replication-competent viruses.[3] For many applications, however, it is very useful to have virus preparations that contain only replication-defective virus particles with no replication-competent virus. Replication-defective viruses are only able to undergo one round of infection since the defective virus will not produce any further infectious particles. This is especially important for any *in vivo* studies where one does not want the spread of replication-competent virus throughout the animal, making it viremic. To achieve this, a second way of generating replication-defective viruses involves the use of helper cells.[4,5] Helper cells contain a defective provirus that has a deletion in the ψ or packaging region; the coding sequences of the provirus remain intact and the RNA transcript can be translated into viral proteins. However, deletion of the ψ region prevents these RNA molecules from being packaged into mature virions. A defective retrovirus vector plasmid now can be transfected into these helper cells, and since the subsequent RNA transcript from this structure contains a normal functioning packaging region, it would be recognized by the *gag, pol,* and *env* protein products produced by the packaging plasmid. In this way, infectious viral particles free of replication competent helper virus will be produced.

Many different designs of retrovirus vectors have been developed over the past several years using a variety of different strategies.[1] Unfortunately, at present, the success of a particular design of vector is still largely the result of empirical methods. Some of the choices available include whether to use a heterologous or natural promoter or the LTR promoter to activate transcription of the foreign gene, the transcriptional orientation of the foreign gene, or the inclusion of a dominant selectable gene if the foreign gene of interest is not selectable. Each of these choices may have ramifications upon the resulting virus titer because each can affect viral RNA expression causing low titer, rearranged genomes, or low expression of the newly inserted sequences in the recipient cells. For many applications, it is very useful to include a dominant selectable gene in addition to the gene of interest, and in several cases the designs shown in FIGURE 2 have been successful in obtaining expression of both the selectable gene and the non-selectable gene, as well as maintaining high virus titer. In this design the selectable gene is transcribed using the LTR promoter while the non-selectable gene is transcribed using a heterologous promoter, such as herpes simplex virus *tk, β*-actin, or the immunoglobulin promoters. It does appear, however, that the choice of promoter can be especially significant since some promoters are apparently not expressed in all cell types or tissues. For example, we have found that the SV40 early region promoter is not expressed at high levels in murine hematopoietic cells.[6]

HEMATOPOIETIC SYSTEM

A detailed understanding of the molecular events governing differentiation and development remains as a major challenge in biology. The hematopoietic system serves as an important model of differentiation.[7] It is composed of a hierarchy of cell types ranging from rare primitive stem cells, capable of extensive proliferation and differentiation, to mature differentiated cells. FIGURE 3 shows a model of the hematopoietic system that is generally consistent with the current data. Because the hematopoietic system is arranged as a hierarchy, the relationships of the cells at the right of the diagram are better understood than those at the left. Mature differentiated cells make up the bulk of the system while stem cells are found at a frequency of approximately 10^{-4} to 10^{-6}.

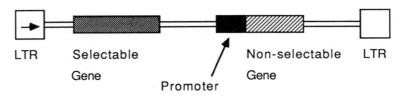

FIGURE 2. Diagram of retrovirus vector designed to transfer a selectable and non-selectable gene.

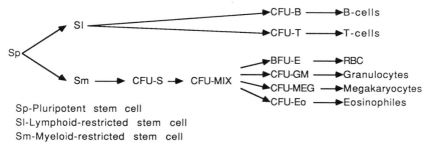

FIGURE 3. Model of murine hematopoietic stem cell organization.

The advantages of the hematopoietic system as a model of differentiation are numerous.[7,10] There is a rich diversity of differentiated cell types with all the various cell types available in readily accessible tissues (bone marrow, blood, thymus, spleen, etc.). A wide variety of growth factors that act on specific cell types have also been identified, thus making it possible to analyze the signals involved in stimulating proliferation and/or differentiation.[9] Most important, has been the development of a wide variety of *in vitro* and *in vivo* colony assays that detect individual progenitor cells.[8] The *in vitro* assays involve plating bone marrow cells in semi-solid media in the presence of appropriate growth factors; the progenitor cells will form colonies composed of mature differentiated cells. For example, the progenitor CFU-GM will produce colonies composed of granulocytes and macrophages, BFU-E colonies of erythroid cells, CFU-MEG colonies of megakaryocytes, and CFU-Eo colonies of eosinophils. In addition to these committed progenitors, a multipotential cell type called CFU-MIX produces colonies that contain both erythroid and myeloid cells and, in contrast to the more mature cell types, it is capable of limited self-renewal. Conditions have been established for the growth of these progenitors from both rodent and human bone marrow.[8] *In vivo* assays have also been established that permit detection of more primitive murine stem cells. The CFU-S assay involves short-term reconstitution of lethally irradiated mice with donor bone marrow.[11] After 10 to 14 days, the CFU-S progenitor produces a large colony on the spleen of the recipient mice. These colonies contain all the progenitors and mature cells found in the erythroid and myeloid lineages. While no colony assays exist for more primitive cells, they can nevertheless be detected in long-term reconstitution assays.[10] Briefly, these assays involve bone marrow transplantation into animals with defective hematopoietic systems. After long periods of time (greater than 3 months) the recipient mice are analyzed for the presence of donor cell types indicating successful engraftment of donor stem cells. By waiting this length of time, all the more committed cells are lost because they have a limited life span and it is the progeny of long-lived stem cells that now repopulate the recipient mice.

The nature of stem cells shown at the left in FIGURE 3 and their relationship to each other are not well understood. It is only through the use of clonal markers that identify individual stem cells that a clearer view of their organization is finally at hand. Furthermore, the regulation of stem cell proliferation and differentiation is very complex, involving growth factors as well as short-range, cell-cell interactions. It is with the advent of novel gene transfer technologies that new approaches to identifying the controlling elements in stem cell development can be approached.

GENE TRANSFER INTO MURINE HEMATOPOIETIC CELLS

The low frequency of hematopoietic progenitor and stem cells generally precludes most physical methods of DNA transfer that yield gene transfer efficiencies in the order of $<10^{-3}$. However, highly infectious retrovirus vectors developed over the past several years have proved to be efficient enough to introduce heterologous genes into even very rare pluripotent stem cells.[12,13]

The first demonstration that genes could be transferred into murine bone marrow progenitors was made by Joyner et al.[14] Bone marrow was infected with a Moloney murine leukemia virus vector containing the dominant selectable neo gene. Progenitor cells containing the neo gene were resistant to the antibiotic G418 and were able to form colonies in the presence of this antibiotic. The proportion of CFU-GM containing the neo gene was determined by plating the infected bone marrow in the presence and absence of G418. Approximately 0.3% of the CFU-GM became G418 resistant and expressed neo specific RNA transcripts.

Subsequently, Williams et al.[15] and Eglitis et al.[16] extended these studies to demonstrate gene transfer into CFU-S progenitor cells at frequencies of greater than 20%. Because spleen colonies derived from CFU-S are large (greater than 10^6 cells), gene transfer was established by detection of neo DNA sequences using Southern blotting techniques.

As described in FIGURE 3, cells more primitive than CFU-S are probably responsible for long-term reconstitution. Recently we,[17] Keller et al.,[18] and Lemischka et al.[19] have used a protocol generally similar to that outlined in FIGURE 4 to transfer the neo gene into primitive pluripotent cells. Bone marrow cells, in medium containing growth factors that support stem cells, were infected by co-cultivation for 24 hours over a monolayer of irradiated fibroblasts that release neo virus. Following infection, the infected bone marrow cells were exposed to high concentrations of G418 for a further 48 hours to enrich for those bone marrow cells that express high levels of the neo gene. The proportion of the various kinds of G418 resistant progenitor cells that express the neo gene was then determined by in vitro colony formation in the presence and absence of G418. Using this protocol, high efficiency gene transfer (ca. 60–100%) into hematopoietic progenitor was obtained with a variety of different retroviral constructs. This figure also shows that a portion of the infected bone marrow could be injected into a recipient mouse and allowed to reconstitute that animal for greater than 3 months after which Southern analysis was performed on various tissues to determine the presence of the neo gene. This reconstitution assay is a measure of gene transfer into primitive repopulating stem cells. As noted earlier, primitive stem cells can best be assayed by their ability to repopulate mice with a deficient hematopoietic system. Using this protocol, genes have been transferred into hematopoietic stem cells capable of reconstituting both W/W^v recipients or lethally irradiated mice. Mice with a mutation at the W locus are particularly good recipients for reconstitution assays. These mice carry dominant mutations that affect not only coat color, but also hematopoiesis and gametogenesis.[20] They are ideal recipients for long-term reconstitution because they contain genetically defective stem cells. Thus, the transplanted stem cells have a selective and permanent advantage in W/W^v hosts and repopulation can occur with even a single donor stem cell. A representative experiment demonstrating gene transfer into a pluripotent stem cell is shown in FIGURE 5. Bone marrow, which had been infected with a neo virus and preselected, was injected into W/W^v recipients. Mice were analyzed after more than 12 weeks to determine whether they had been reconstituted by stem cells infected with the neo vector. Southern blot analysis was carried out on DNA extracted from the bone marrow, thymus, spleen, peritoneal wash macrophages, and Peyer's patch lymphocytes probing for the presence of the neo gene.

It is clear from this analysis that (1) each of these three tissues has been reconstituted with progeny that contain the *neo* gene and (2) since the DNA was digested with restriction enzymes that do not cut within the *neo* gene, the size of the fragment is a reflection of the integration site of the *neo* provirus. Since the same size fragment is present in all three tissues, it is clear that these tissues have been reconstituted by cells derived from a common progenitor, providing conclusive evidence for the existence of a stem cell capable of producing both lymphoid and myeloid progeny (i.e. S_p in FIGURE 3). Using this approach, preliminary evidence has also been obtained for stem cells with extensive capacity to proliferate but restricted to either the lymphoid or the myeloid lineage. Keller *et al.*[18] have demonstrated that these *neo*-containing stem cells have extensive self-renewal capability as they were able to serially transfer bone

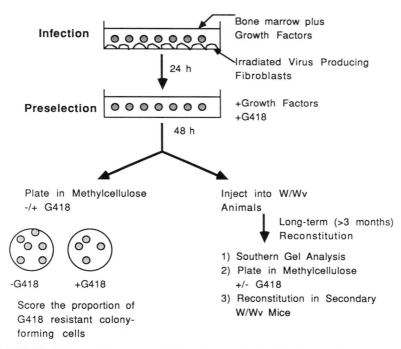

FIGURE 4. Protocol for gene transfer into hematopoietic cells using retrovirus vectors.

marrow from a primary recipient to a secondary recipient and finally to a tertiary recipient. Clonal analysis demonstrated that the same clone persisted in each serial transplant. These studies demonstrate the power of this technology at carrying out very detailed lineage analysis to determine the nature and relationship of various stem cells in the hematopoietic hierarchy. Furthermore, not only is the *neo* gene present in these cells after periods of reconstitution (up to one year), but these genes continue to be expressed in the progenitors derived from the single pluripotent stem cell clone, which reconstituted those animals.[17,18] It is, however, clear that expression from some retrovirus vectors is down regulated over long periods of time in that only a fraction of the cells that contain the gene are actually expressing it. Nevertheless, these studies

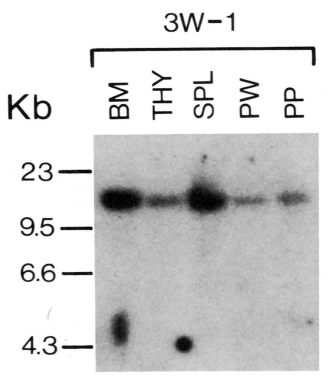

FIGURE 5. Southern blot analysis of DNA from the bone marrow, thymus, spleen, peritoneal wash macrophages, and Peyer's patch of a reconstituted W/W^v mouse. High molecular weight DNA was extracted from these tissues 15 weeks after reconstitution with bone marrow infected with a NEO vector and preselected in G418. The DNA was digested with the restriction enzyme *Bam*HI, which cuts once in the provirus, generating cell-virus junction fragments whose size reflects a particular viral integration site. The blots were probed with a *neo* fragment.

demonstrate that it should be possible to use gene transfer into hematopoietic stem cells as a means of identifying genes that play an important regulatory role in governing the developmental decisions the stem cells must make. Such genes include oncogenes, which affect the hematopoietic system and/or proliferation, and a wide variety of growth factor genes, which also affect the regulation of hematopoietic progenitor and stem cells. Furthermore, these murine experiments are also important models for any future gene therapy experiments where clinically relevant genes such as adenosine deaminase (ADA) or betaglobin are transferred into hematopoietic stem cells, to determine whether these genes continue to be expressed following long periods of reconstitution.[21-23]

GENE TRANSFER INTO HUMAN HEMATOPOIETIC CELLS

The introduction of developmentally regulated genes, lineage specific genes, growth factor genes, or oncogenes into various hematopoietic cells will provide new insights into gene expression and regulation during hematopoietic differentiation. Furthermore, the correction of certain human genetic defects may be possible by the insertion of a functional gene into the primitive bone marrow stem cells of the human hematopoietic system.[21-23] Recently, using a protocol similar to that described in FIGURE 4, gene transfer has been reported into human hematopoietic progenitor cells.[24-26] Gene transfer frequencies were in the order of 5 to 10% into human hematopoietic progenitor cells. In an attempt to devise conditions of higher efficiencies of gene transfer, we made some modifications to earlier protocols. These modifications included exposing the infected bone marrow cells to high concentrations of G418 for short periods of time *in vitro* prior to plating methyl cellulose cultures to enrich for those cells expressing high levels of the *neo* gene. The second modification was to include growth factors that support hematopoietic stem cells during liquid culture of the human bone marrow cells. The addition of these growth factors should permit the stimulation of non-cycling stem cells and make them susceptible to retrovirus infection. As shown in TABLE 1, inclusion of the pre-selection step appeared to increase the frequency of gene transfer by a factor of 3 or 4. Furthermore, recent experiments using detailed survival curves have shown that following pre-selection with the inclusion of growth factors, 100% of the population of cells can become G418-resistant following pre-selection (in preparation).

In the mouse, there is considerable heterogeneity in expression of the *neo* gene in committed hematopoietic progenitor cells derived from more primitive stem cells infected with retrovirus vectors.[6] In an attempt to determine the ability of various promoters to be expressed in human cells, a variety of constructs were analyzed for their ability to express the *neo* gene in human hematopoietic progenitor cells. Our data demonstrate that *neo* vectors containing either the viral LTR promotor or the herpes virus TK promoter to transcribe the *neo* gene can be transferred into human hematopoietic progenitor cells and continue to be expressed for at least 14 days, during which a colony is formed in the presence of G418 (in preparation). In contrast, I have investigated *neo* gene expression in human hematopoietic cell lines and primary bone marrow progenitor cells infected with a vector that uses the SV40 promoter since this is a strong promoter in a wide variety of cell types. No G418-resistant colonies were found after infection of bone marrow cells with this vector. This reduction in gene expression appears to be restricted to some hematopoietic cell types including normal progenitor cells since infection of several T cell lines did produce high numbers of G418-resistant colonies. These results suggest that the SV40 promoter appears to be

TABLE 1. Gene Transfer into Normal Human Bone Marrow with Retrovirus Vectors

		CFU-GM/2×10^5 Cells G418 μg/ml		
Pre Selection	Vectors	0	800	% Resistance
−	uninfected	77	0	0
+	uninfected	31	0	0
−	PAN2	150	20	13
+	PAN2	60	29	48

Percoll fractionated normal human bone marrow cells were cocultivated with the virus producing fibroblast cell line PAN2[18] according to the protocol outlined in FIGURE 4. Controls were performed using cell lines not producing virus. The cells were exposed to 2 mg/ml G418 for 48 hr prior to plating in methylcellulose according to the method described by Fauser and Messner.[27] Colonies were scored after 14 days.

down-regulated in human hematopoietic cell lines and progenitor cells and therefore may not be a good promotor for experiments aimed at gene therapy in humans. An understanding of the mechanisms whereby gene expression from some vectors are down-regulated is essential if vectors are to be used to study gene expression during differentiation or for gene therapy of human disease.

SUMMARY

The ability to transfer new genetic information into murine and human hematopoietic cells with retrovirus vectors offers a powerful approach to identifying the molecular mechanisms governing stem cell development. The newly integrated provirus also serves as a clonal marker for elucidating the lineage relationships of the cells in the stem cell hierarchy. High efficiency gene transfer into human cells opens the way to developing new therapy for treating genetic diseases by introducing functional genes into deficient cells. Present transplantation technology would only permit gene therapy with bone marrow cells. However, as gene transfer and transplantation technologies improve it may be possible to consider treating diseases that affect other organs and tissues.

I would like to acknowledge the support of Alan Bernstein and R. Phillips in whose labs the murine work was carried out during a post-doctoral fellowship. I also thank Sharon Kerbel for excellent assistance in the preparation of this manuscript.

REFERENCES

1. BERNSTEIN, A., S. BERGER, D. HUSZAR & J. DICK. 1985. Gene transfer with retrovirus vectors. *In* Genetic Engineering: Principles and Methods. J. K. Setlow & A. Hollaender, Eds. 7:235. Plenum.
2. ROHDEWOLD, H., H. WEIHER, W. REIK, R. JAENISCH & M. BREWOL. 1987. J. Virol. **61:** 336.
3. TEICH, N. 1984. *In* RNA Tumor Viruses. R. Wein, N. Teich, H. Varmus & J. Coffin, Eds.: 25. Cold Spring Harbor Laboratory. Cold Spring Harbor, NY.
4. MANN, R., R. MULLIGAN & D. BALTIMORE. 1983. Construction of a retrovirus packaging mutant and its use to produce helper free defective retrovirus. Cell **38:** 153.
5. MILLER, A., M. D. LAW & I. VERMA. 1985. Generation of helper free amphotropic retroviruses that transduce a dominant-acting methotrexate-resistant DHFR gene. Mol. Cell Biol. **5:**431.
6. MAGLI, M.-C., J. DICK, A. BERNSTEIN & R. PHILLIPS. 1987. Modulation of gene expression in multiple hematopoietic cell lineages following retroviral vector gene transfer. Proc. Natl. Acad. Sci. USA **84:** 789–793.
7. TILL, J. E. & E. A. McCULLOCH. 1980. Hemopoietic stem cell differentiation. Biochim. Biophys. Acta **605:** 431.
8. OGAWA, M., P. N. PORTER & T. NOHOHOTA. 1983. Renewal and commitment to differentiation of hemopoietic stem cells: an interpretative review. Blood **61:** 823.
9. STANLEY, E. & P. JUBINSKY. 1984. Clin. Haematol. **13:** 329–347.
10. PHILLIPS, R. 1985. Comparison of different assays for multipotent hematopoietic stem cells. *In* Mediators in Cell Growth and Differentiation. R. J. Ford & A. L. Maizel, Eds.: 135. Raven Press. New York.
11. TILL, J. & E. McCULLOCH. 1961. A direct measurement of the radiation sensitivity of normal mouse bone marrow cells. Rad. Res. **14:** 213–222.
12. DICK, J. E., M. -C. MAGLI, R. A. PHILLIPS & A. BERNSTEIN. 1986. Genetic manipulation of hematopoietic stem cells with retrovirus vectors. Trends in Genet. **2:** 165.
13. BERNSTEIN, A., J. DICK, D. HUSZAR, I. ROBSON, J. ROSSANT, M. -C. MAGLI, Z. ESTROV,

M. Freedman & R. Phillips. 1987. Genetic engineering of mouse and human stem cells. Cold Spring Harbor Symp. Quant. Biol. **51:**1083–1091.

14. Joyner, A., G. Keller, R. A. Phillips & A. Bernstein. 1983. Retrovirus mediated transfer of a bacterial gene into mouse hematopoietic progenitor cells. Nature **305:** 206.

15. Williams, D. A., I. R. Lemischka, D. G. Nathans & R. C. Mulligan. 1984. Introduction of new genetic material into pluripotent haemopoietic stem cells of the mouse. Nature **310:** 476.

16. Eglitis, M., P. Kantoff, E. Gilboa & W. F. Anderson. 1985. Gene expression in mice after high efficiency retroviral-mediated gene transfer. Science **230:** 1395.

17. Dick, J. E., M. -C. Magli, D. H. Huszar, R. A. Phillips & A. Bernstein. 1985. Introduction of a selectable gene into primitive stem cells capable of long term reconstitution of the hemopoietic system of W/W^v mice. Cell **42:** 71.

18. Keller, G., C. Paige, E. Gilboa & E. F. Wagner. 1985. Expression of a foreign gene in myeloid and lymphoid cells derived from multipotent haematopoietic precursors. Nature **318:**149.

19. Lemischka, I., D. Raulet & R. Mulligan. 1986. Developmental potential and dynamic behavior of hematopoietic stem cells. Cell **45:** 917.

20. Russell, E. 1979. Hereditary anemia of the mouse: a review for geneticists. Adv. Genet. **20:** 357–459.

21. Anderson, W. F. 1984. Prospects for human gene therapy. Science **226:** 401.

22. Friedman, T. 1987. Gene therapy: Fact and fiction. Biology's New Approaches to Disease. Cold Spring Harbor.

23. Belmont, J. W. & C. T. Caskey. 1987. Developments leading to human gene therapy. *In* Gene Transfer. R. Kucherlapati, Ed. Plenum. New York.

24. Hock, R. A. & A. D. Miller. 1986. Retrovirus-mediated transfer and expression of drug resistance genes in human haematopoietic progenitor cells. Nature **320:** 275.

25. Hogge, D. & R. K. Humphries. 1987. Gene transfer to primary and malignant human hemopoietic progenitors using recombinant retroviruses. Blood **69:** 611.

26. Dick, J., M. -C. Magli, Z. Estrov, M. Freedman, R. Phillips & A. Bernstein. 1987. Retrovirus-mediated gene transfer and expression in murine and human stem cells. *In* Recent Advances in Bone Marrow Transplantation. UCLA Symposium on Molecular and Cellular Biology. New Series. R. P. Gale & R. Champlin, eds. Alan R. Liss. New York.

27. Fauser, A. A. & H. A. Messner. 1978. Granuloerythropoietic colonies in human bone marrow, peripheral blood, and cord blood. Blood **52:** 1243.

Delivery of Lipophilic Drugs Using Lipoproteins[a]

J. MICHAEL SHAW

Alcon Laboratories, Inc.
Fort Worth, Texas 76134-2099

KALA V. SHAW, SAUL YANOVICH, MICHAEL IWANIK,
AND WILLIAM S. FUTCH

Medical College of Virginia
Richmond, Virginia 23298

ANDRÉ ROSOWSKY

Dana-Farber Cancer Institute
Boston, Massachusetts 02115

LAWRENCE B. SCHOOK

University of Illinois
Urbana, Illinois 61801

INTRODUCTION

Low density lipoproteins (LDLs) and high density lipoproteins (HDLs), are spherical classes of particles 7 to 25 nm in diameter with oily, nonaqueous cores (FIGURE 1). Extensive studies have been performed throughout the years with respect to the structure, metabolism, and molecular biology of lipoproteins.[1,2] Recently lipoproteins, most notably LDL, have been examined experimentally as drug-delivery vehicles.[3-15] Advantages of lipoproteins as drug carriers include: (1) their being natural components able to survive in plasma and tissue fluids for significant time periods, (2) the small particle size, which allows diffusion from vascular to extravascular compartments, (3) their interaction via receptor-mediated endocytosis enabling intracellular uptake of drug, and (4) the oily core, which provides a domain for lipophilic drugs and prodrugs. Disadvantages of lipoproteins as drug carriers include their complex and unstable nature, a general lack of targeting since receptors for some lipoproteins reside on numerous tissues, and potential drug cytotoxicity to normal tissues.

In the present studies, the preparation, composition, and stability of lipoprotein-drug complexes are described. Interactions of these complexes with cells *in vitro* were performed to establish how the modified lipoprotein particles and drugs became cell associated and what biological effects occurred on the target cells.

[a]Supported by grants from the National Institutes of Health, National Cancer Institute, and the National Science Foundation.

RESULTS

Preparation, Composition, and Stability of Lipoprotein-Drug Complexes

Four methods are available for preparing lipoprotein-drug complexes. In method 1, solvent extraction, LDL is first mixed with starch then freeze dried. The lipophilic core is extracted with solvent, such as heptane, diethyl ether, or benzene, followed by replacement of the lipid with lipophilic drug.[16,17] We found the procedure to be time consuming with poor reproducibility when using the lipophilic anthracycline, N-

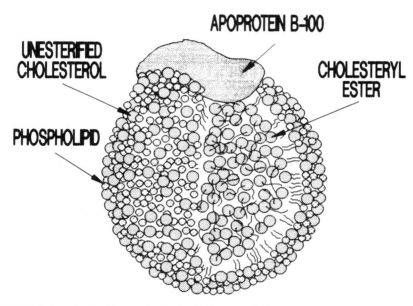

FIGURE 1. Low density lipoprotein. A spherical water-soluble particle, 20 to 25 nm in diameter with a molecular mass of ~2.5 × 10⁶ daltons. The oily core of the particle is composed of mainly cholesteryl ester (81 mol%) with lesser amounts of triglyceride (19 mol%), whereas the surface monolayer is composed of phospholipid (58 mol%) and unesterified cholesterol (42 mol%) and contains one major glycoprotein, apoprotein B-100 (350 to 550 K daltons).[1,32] The sequence of a complimentary DNA originally screened using an apoprotein B carboxy-terminal oligonucleotide probe has led to the identification of (1) an eleven amino acid region enriched in arginine and lysine residues as an LDL receptor binding site and (2) potential lipid binding regions which contain proline-enriched beta-sheets.[43] (After Brown & Goldstein.[44])

trifluoroacetyl-adriamycin-14-valerate (AD-32). Recovery of apoprotein B-100 was usually less than 40% and the reconstituted LDL–AD-32 complex was larger than native LDL and passed through 0.8 μm filters but not 0.45 μm filters. Method 2, detergent dialysis, was accomplished by solubilizing the lipophilic drug using the nonionic detergent, octylglucoside at 20 mM. The LDL was added to the mixture of octylglucoside and AD-32, followed by stirring at 25°C, then extensive dialysis. The complexes were further fractionated using Sephadex G15-120 and filtration through 0.45 μm filters. The complexes prepared by detergent dialysis were less than

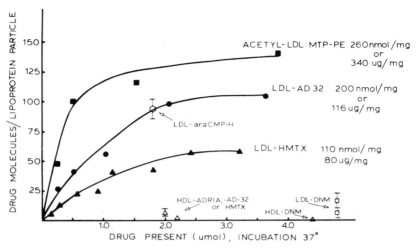

FIGURE 2. Stoichiometry of lipoprotein-drug complexes. Lipoprotein-drug complexes were prepared using drug and constant amounts of lipoprotein by a dry-film stir technique at 37°C. HDL-adria and LDL-dnm (upper point, □) were prepared by the aqueous addition and detergent dialysis methods, respectively. HDL-HMTX and HDL-AD32 were prepared by the solvent extraction method. The drug levels were determined following fractionation of each complex using Sephadex G15-120 chromatography and 0.45 μm filtration. The number of drug molecules/particle were estimated assuming molecular weights of 2.5×10^6 for LDL and acetyl-LDL and 2.5×10^5 for HDL species, with protein representing 25 wt% for LDL and acetyl-LDL, and 50 wt% for HDL.

satisfactory since upon ageing at 4°C the turbidity of the preparations slowly increased. Complete detergent removal was not successful. Method 3, aqueous addition of drug, was useful for complexing water-soluble drugs with lipoproteins and was carried out with a total human HDL fraction, purified free of apoprotein B and E lipoproteins using heparin-Sepharose chromatography. Adriamycin (adr) and dauno-mycin (dnm) have been the only drugs tested by this procedure. Adriamycin (2–3 mM) in buffer was added dropwise to HDL while stirring at 37°C for 2 hr. The resulting complex was fractionated from unbound drug by gel chromatography and then 0.45 μm filtration. The HDL-adr complex contained on the average 3 to 5 drug molecules/ particle (FIGURE 2). HDL particles are approximately 7 to 9 nm in diameter with a much smaller lipid environment than LDL and one third the mass of LDL cholesterol. Method 4, dry-film stir, was the preferred method of choice for all LDL-drug complexes. Each of the widely structured drugs illustrated in FIGURE 3 could be partitioned into the LDL or chemically modified LDL by the dry-film stir method. The method consisted of using a dry film or powdered drug and stirring with LDL at 37–40°C for 2 hr.[9] Fractionation was accomplished by gel chromatography using Sephadex G15–120 then 0.45 μm filtration.

FIGURE 2 illustrates that different drugs formed complexes with LDL or acety-lated-LDL at characteristic saturating levels. Seven dnm molecules/LDL particle, 55 hexadecyl-methotrexate (HMTX) molecules/LDL particle, 100 AD-32 molecules/ LDL particle and 140 muramyltripeptide phosphatidylethanolamine (MTP-PE) mole-cules/acetylated LDL particle. Acetylated LDL is a chemically modified LDL, prepared by the acetylation of lysine residues on apoprotein B-100 of LDL.[18]

LDL-arabinofuranosylcytosine-5'-(n-hexadecyl phosphate) (ara-CMPH) was prepared at only one drug concentration (1.8 mM) and gave 90 ara-CMPH molecules/ LDL particle. It was not possible to associate adr with LDL, since immediate aggregation and flocculation occurred at several adr concentrations. All complexes successfully prepared by dry-film stir could be passed through 0.45 μm filters with negligible losses of apoprotein B-100. In all cases, stoichiometry of LDL drug levels were confirmed after reflotation at a density of 1.063 g/ml. LDL-dnm and LDL-AD-32 showed precipitation of greater than 70% drug when treated with antibody to apoprotein B-100. Fluorescence quenching studies of LDL-dnm with iodide and calf thymus deoxyribonucleic acid (DNA) have been previously reported to locate 60% dnm in the core of the LDL and 40% dnm at surface domains.[9] HDL-adr was a surprisingly stable complex and when incubated with human plasma at 37°C for 0.5 hr, greater than 80% adr could be refloated at the density of HDL, 1.215 g/ml (FIGURE 4A). Free adr incubated with plasma refloated in the lipoprotein free fraction of the plasma at a density greater than 1.215 g/ml (FIGURE 4A). HDL-lipophilic drug complexes prepared using the solvent extraction technique with AD-32 or HMTX also contained on the average only 5 molecules/particle.

The LDL-lipophilic drug complexes prepared using MTP-PE, ara-CMPH, HMTX, and AD-32 were all examined for drug stability at 4°C (FIGURE 5). All drugs showed good stability with the exception of HMTX, which was steadily hydrolyzed to free methotrexate (MTX) at the gamma ester-linked hexadecyl group. The hydrolysis of HMTX was observed with LDL preparations purified by density flotation and

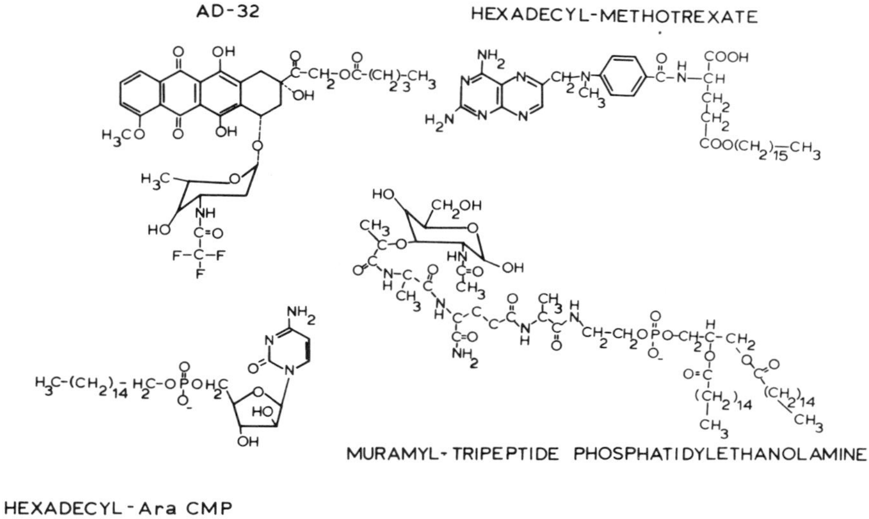

FIGURE 3. Lipophilic drugs for complexing to lipoprotein. N-trifluoroacetyl-adriamycin-14-valerate (AD-32) is an experimental fluorescent anthracycline tested in the treatment of acute myelogenous leukemia. Hexadecyl-methotrexate (HMTX) and arabinofuranosylcytosine-5'-(n-hexadecyl phosphate) (Ara-CMPH) are derivatives of methotrexate, a dihydrofolate reductase inhibitor and Ara-C, a DNA synthesis inhibitor, respectively. Both methotrexate and Ara-C are widely used in cancer chemotherapy. N-acetyl-muramyl-L-alanyl-D-isoglutamine-L-alanyl-1,2 dipalmitoyl phosphatidylethanolamine (MTP-PE), is an activator for macrophage-mediated tumoricidal activity.

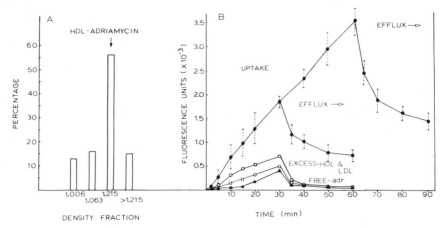

FIGURE 4. High density lipoprotein-adriamycin stability in plasma and uptake by P388 murine leukemia cells. (A) HDL-adr, prepared by the aqueous addition technique was incubated with human plasma at 37°C for 30 min, followed by density flotation at four different densities. Adr levels were determined after solvent extraction or detergent treatment, and percentages of adr calculated. (B) Uptake of HDL-adr or free adr was examined in defined media maintained, drug sensitive P388 leukemia cells using a digitized video fluorescence microscopy technique in a flow cell at 37°C. Uptake was performed during perfusion with HDL-adr (0.4 μg/ml, 70 μg protein/ml) (●) or free adr (0.4 μg/ml) (▲) in Hanks' BSS for up to 1 hr. At 30 min or 1 hr, efflux was performed for 30 min with Hanks' BSS. Uptake of HDL-adr was also performed in the presence of a 10 times excess of HDL (○) or LDL (□). The experiments represent the average of two separate experiments.

flotation followed by fractionation on Sepharose CL-4B. A half-time for HMTX hydrolysis of approximately 51 hr at 4°C was found with each of the two LDL purification procedures (FIGURE 5). The prodrug hydrolysis was a function of HMTX association with LDL since no HMTX to MTX conversion was observed over similar ageing periods with liposome-HMTX complex. The release of water-soluble MTX from LDL-HMTX could be monitored in separate studies by following an enhancement in the activity of a purified dihydrofolate reductase (J. Shaw, A. Rosowsky, R. Baichwal and V. Schirch, unpublished observations).

LDL-DNM Interaction via the LDL-Receptor Pathway

Studies performed with the LDL-dnm complex and freshly isolated P388 leukemia cells were consistent with LDL-receptor mediated uptake of dnm bound to LDL.[10] LDL-cell interactions were monitored by following the fluorescence of the anthracycline bound to LDL. Flow cell fluorescence video microscopy with digital image analysis of drug fluorescence was used for quantitation in all experiments. FIGURE 6 illustrates the uptake of LDL-dnm and free dnm in P388 leukemia cells, which were either sensitive or resistant to free dnm. The LDL-dnm uptake was rapid, saturable, and remained associated with cells during efflux experiments with buffer alone. FIGURE 7 illustrates LDL-bound dnm experiments in which a ten-fold excess of native LDL or HDL was included in the assay with sensitive cells. Marked competition by LDL, but not HDL, for LDL-bound dnm was strongly supportive of uptake predominantly by receptor-mediated endocytosis through the LDL-receptor, a 160,000 dalton glycoprotein found on numerous cell types (FIGURES 7 and 8).[19-21] FIGURE 9 demonstrates the marked retention of LDL-bound dnm relative to free dnm in P388-resistant cells. The LDL-dnm, cell efflux experiments were performed after a 30 min uptake of LDL-bound dnm at 0.1 μg dnm/ml, whereas the free dnm-cell experiments were carried out at 1 μg dnm/ml (FIGURE 9). In published studies, LDL-bound dnm after cell fractionation resided largely in cell membrane fractions, whereas free dnm was almost exclusively found in an insoluble nuclear fraction.[9] The results presented in TABLE 1 show that both sensitive and resistant P388 leukemia cells could be growth-inhibited by treatment with LDL-dnm, however the resistant cells still maintained higher growth capabilities than sensitive cells.

Acetylated-LDL Interaction via the Acetyl-LDL Receptor

The acetyl-LDL receptor-mediated endocytosis pathway, known to occur in macrophages and certain endothelial cells[22-25] has been studied using an acetyl-LDL-drug complex and thioglycolate-elicited peritoneal macrophages from mice

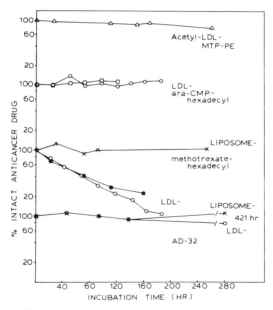

FIGURE 5. Ageing of lipoprotein and liposome-drug complexes for drug stability. Lipoprotein and liposome-drug complexes were prepared by the dry-film stir technique at 37°C, fractionated, filtered, and stored at 4°C under sterile conditions. Aliquots were taken as a function of time and drug integrity determined after solvent extraction by amino acid analysis for MTP-PE, spectrophotometry for Ara-CMP-H, HPLC for HMTX and MTX, and thin layer chromatography followed by fluorescence analysis for AD-32. The liposomes used in the study were prepared by sonication and were composed of dioleoyl phosphatidylcholine (80 mol%) and cholesterol (20 mol%). LDL preparations isolated from 3 different individuals and prepared by either density flotation (O) or density flotation followed by Sepharose CL-4B chromatography (●) gave similar results when complexed with HMTX.

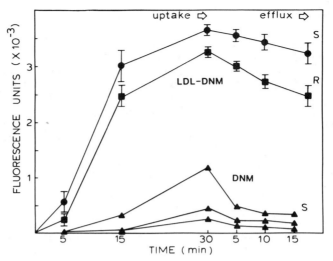

FIGURE 6. Uptake and efflux studies with sensitive (S) and resistant (R) P388 cells and LDL-dnm (●, ■) or free dnm (▲). A digitized video fluorescence microscopy technique in a flow cell at 37°C was used for determining intracellular drug levels. Uptake was performed during perfusion with LDL-dnm (0.1 μg/ml, 15 μg protein) or free dnm (0.1, 0.2, and 0.4 μg/ml) in Hanks' BSS between zero and 30 min. At 30 min, efflux was performed for 15 min with Hanks' BSS. The sensitive cell LDL-dnm experiments and the resistant cell LDL-dnm experiments represent the means for five and three separate experiments, respectively. The sensitive cell free dnm experiments (▲) represent the average of two experiments with increasing concentrations of dnm (0.1, 0.2, and 0.4 μg/ml). The same instrumental gain for the fluorescence measurements was utilized in all cases. (From Yanovich et al.[10] With permission of the publisher.)

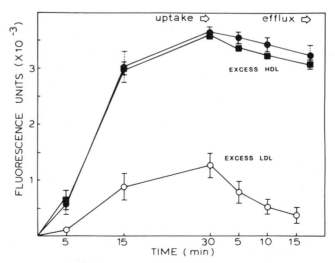

FIGURE 7. Competition of LDL or HDL for LDL-dnm uptake by sensitive P388 cells. LDL-dnm (0.1 μg dnm/ml, 11 to 15 μg protein/ml) plus excess LDL (110 to 150 μg protein/ml) were perfused for 30 min with sensitive cells followed by efflux with Hanks' BSS for 15 min. Values for LDL-dnm (●) were performed five times, values for LDL competition (○) were performed three times, and values for HDL competition (■) were performed twice. (From Yanovich et al.[10] With permission of the publisher.)

(FIGURE 8). The drug examined was MTP-PE, an immunomodulator that has been documented to activate macrophages for tumoricidal and antiviral activity.[26–28] Three independent procedures were used for examining the interactions of acetyl-LDL:MTP-PE complex with thioglycolate-elicited macrophages, (1) uptake of ^{125}I-labeled apoprotein B 100 complex, (2) uptake of dioctadecyl-tetramethylindocarbo-cyanine (DiI) fluorescent-labeled complex and (3) the MTP-PE effects on macrophage activation.

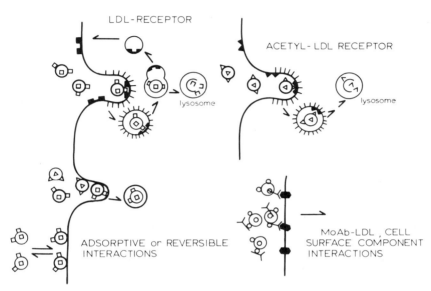

FIGURE 8. Cellular interactions of lipoproteins and modified lipoproteins. The LDL-receptor pathway is a classic model for receptor-mediated endocytosis.[19] The receptor is a 160,000 dalton glycoprotein with isoelectric point of ~4.8 and found on a variety of cell types. The K_d for LDL is 1×10^{-9} M. Following endocytosis of LDL in clathrin-coated vesicles ($t_{1/2} \sim 5$ min) and endosome formation, LDL is processed by lysosomal enzymes and the receptor is recycled to the cell surface.[19–21] The acetyl-LDL receptor pathway is found on a more restricted number of cell types, macrophages, monocytes, sinusoidal endothelial cells, and to a lesser extent aortic and microvascular endothelial cells.[22–24,37,38] The receptor is a 260,000 dalton glycoprotein with isoelectric point of ~6.0 and has no calcium requirement. The K_d for acetyl-LDL is 3×10^{-8} M. Endocytosis and lysosomal processing of acetyl-LDL is accompanied by rapid re-esterification of liberated cholesterol and a general lack of control over receptor synthesis.[23,25] Adsorptive, receptor-independent LDL transport and reversible binding of LDL at the cell surface are established pathways.[29,31,45] Receptor-independent LDL transport cannot be accounted for by bulk fluid pinocytosis and uptake does not occur in clathrin-coated vesicles.[45] HDL species lacking apoprotein E do not appear to interact with cells via a protein receptor.[30] Monoclonal antibody modified LDL has the potential for interacting with cell surfaces by (1) antibody/cell surface antigen interaction and (2) adsorptive interactions due to the LDL. The cell surface component for the MoAb, anti-H2K^k, is the k haplotype region of H2 complex, a 45,000 dalton glycoprotein associated with beta$_2$microglobulin. Adsorptive endocytosis is presumed to be the dominant pathway for uptake of LDL-anti-H2K^{k}.[34]

At 4 and 37°C, thioglycolate-elicited macrophages interacted with ^{125}I]acetyl-LDL and showed approximately 90% competition with a thirty-fold excess of unlabeled acetyl-LDL. In addition, association of MTP-PE with ^{125}I]acetyl-LDL did not alter the lipoprotein intereaction with macrophages (J. Shaw, W. Futch, and L.

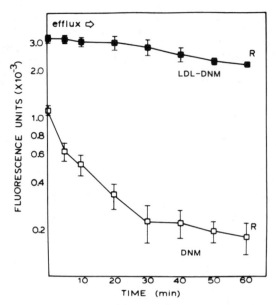

FIGURE 9. Logarithmic plot of Hanks' BSS efflux of resistant (R) P388 leukemia cells after a 30-min incubation with LDL-dnm (■, 0.1, μg dnm/ml, 21 μg protein/ml) or free dnm (□, 1.0 μg dnm/ml). The digitized video fluorescent microscopy technique was utilized with the same instrumental gain for each curve. Points, means of two separate experiments. (From Yanovich *et al.*[10] With permission of the publisher.)

TABLE 1. P388 Colony Growth Inhibition

		% of Colony Growth			
	Incubation with Daunomycin	LDL	Control	Free Daunomycin	LDL-Daunomycin
Daunomycin-sensitive cells (0.2 μg/ml)	2 hr	100	100	5	5
Daunomycin-sensitive cells (0.4 μg/ml)	10 min	ND	100	60	20
Daunomycin-resistant cells (0.4 μg/ml)	2 hr	100	100	100	12
Daunomycin-resistant cells (0.4 μg/ml)	10 min	ND	100	100	55

Sensitive or resistant cells (1.25 to 1.5 × 10⁶) were incubated with LDL-dnm (0.2 to 0.4 μg dnm/ml, 26 to 68 μg protein), free dnm (0.2 to 0.4 μg/ml), LDL (26 to 68 μg protein), or buffer alone for 10 min or 2 hr at 37°C. The cells were washed, resuspended in complete medium containing semisoft agar, and seeded in plastic multiwell dishes (5,000 cell/well). The cells were counted for colony formation after 10 days in a 5% CO_2 incubator. Each experiment was performed in triplicate, and the number of colonies was expressed as a percentage of the control. (After Yarovich *et al.*[10])

Schook, unpublished results). The lipophilic immunomodulator, MTP-PE and the lipophilic fluorescent dye, DiI, were complexed with acetylated-LDL. FIGURE 10 shows the uptake of acetyl-LDL:MTP-PE-DiI complex by thioglycolate-elicited macrophages, with the DiI being monitored by fluorescence spectrofluorometry. The inset in FIGURE 10 illustrates the specificity of the interaction with excess acetyl-LDL showing excellent competition. Excess LDL or excess liposomes were poorly competing nonparticles. When the same experiment was performed with liposome-MTP-PE-DiI, virtually no specificity was observed since competition was found with excesses of liposomes, acetyl-LDL, or LDL (J. Shaw, W. Futch and L. Schook, unpublished

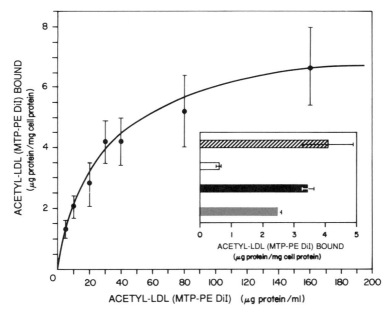

FIGURE 10. Binding and uptake of acetyl-LDL:MTP-PE-DiI by thioglycolate elicited macrophages. The binding and uptake of acetyl-LDL:MTP-PE-DiI was carried out at 37°C and the fluorescence intensity of cell-associated DiI recorded. The μg acetyl-LDL:MTP-PE-DiI bound was determined by knowing the quantity of DiI associated with the complex (1.34 ± 0.76 nmol DiI/mg acetyl-LDL protein). The data points represent an average of three separate experiments. *Insert:* Uptake of 30 μg of acetyl-LDL:MTP-PE-DiI (▨) and in the presence of a 30-fold excess of acetyl-LDL (▢), a 30-fold excess of LDL (■), or a 30-fold excess of liposomes (▦).

results). In addition, the uptake of liposome-MTP-PE-DiI was not easily saturable and showed continued uptake by cells well beyond 2 hr. TABLES 2 and 3 show the effects of acetyl-LDL bound MTP-PE on activation of macrophages for cytostatic or cytotoxic effects on tumor cells. In TABLE 2, concentrations up to 5 μg/ml of acetyl-LDL bound MTP-PE were observed to increase the cytostasis (inhibition of [³H]thymidine uptake) of B16F10 melanoma cells. The addition of excess liposome bilayers during the incubation of macrophages with acetyl-LDL:MTP-PE were important in showing the negligible effects by excess endocytic vesicles on macrophage activation by acetyl-LDL:MTP-PE. TABLE 3 shows the effects of acetyl-LDL:MTP-PE, free MTP-PE, or

TABLE 2. *In Vitro* Activation of Murine Peritoneal Macrophages for Cytostatic Activity by the Acetyl-LDL:MTP-PE Complex (B16F10 Melanoma Tumor Target Cells)

		% Cytostasis	
Acetyl-LDL (μg Protein/ml)	MTP-PE (μg/ml)	Acetyl-LDL:MTP-PE (Complex)	Acetyl-LDL:MTP-PE[a] (Complext + Excess) Liposomes
100	0.0	$\leq$5	$\leq$5
100	9.9	30 $\pm$ 11	44 $\pm$ 5
50	0.0	$\leq$5	$\leq$5
50	5.0	59 $\pm$ 19	45 $\pm$ 5
25	0.0	25 $\pm$ 12	$\leq$5
25	2.5	31 $\pm$ 3	21 $\pm$ 6
12.5	0.0	$\leq$5	$\leq$5
12.5	1.3	15 $\pm$ 8	$\leq$5
6.25	0.0	$\leq$5	$\leq$5
6.25	0.62	$\leq$5	$\leq$5

Thioglycolate-elicited macrophages (1×10^5 cells) were treated with different concentrations of the acetyl-LDL:MTP-PE complex (97.2 μg MTP-PE/mg protein) for 24 hr, unbound complex was washed away, and B16F10 melanoma cells (1×10^4) were added. After 24 hr the cultures were pulsed with [³H]thymidine and harvested after 24 hr (effector:target ratio, 10:1). The results were expressed as a percent inhibition (cytostasis) of [³H]thymidine incorporation into the B16F10 target cells.

$$\% \text{ cytostasis} = 1 - \frac{(\text{CPM B16F10} + \text{CPM macrophages})}{(\text{CPM B16F10 alone})} \times 100$$

[a]Addition of acetyl-LDL:MTP-PE complex in the presence of excess liposomes (300 μg lipid/mL) to thioglycolate-elicited macrophages. Liposomes alone induced a cytostatic activity of $\leq$5%.

TABLE 3. *In Vitro* Activation of Murine Peritoneal Macrophages for Cytotoxic Activity by the Acetyl-LDL:MTP-PE Complex (P815 Mastocytoma Target Cells)

Effector to Target Cell Ratio	% Cytotoxicity			
	None	Acetyl-LDL:MTP-PE	MTP-PE	Acetyl-LDL
40:1	5 $\pm$ 2	20 $\pm$ 8	7.5 $\pm$ 7	3 $\pm$ 2
20:1	1.2 $\pm$ 2.5	12 $\pm$ 2.2	4.3 $\pm$ 1.2	6 $\pm$ 2
10:1	0.8 $\pm$ 2.5	14 $\pm$ 3	8.6 $\pm$ 4	4 $\pm$ 2
5:1	0.5 $\pm$ 1	3.5 $\pm$ 2	6 $\pm$ 4	4.5 $\pm$ 4
1:1	0.0 $\pm$ 0.6	3 $\pm$ 3	3 $\pm$ 4	0.5 $\pm$ 1

Thioglycolate-elicited macrophages plated at varying numbers of cells/well were incubated with acetyl-LDL:MTP-PE (18 μg protein, 3.6 μg MTP-PE), free MTP-PE (3.6 μg), acetyl-LDL (18 μg protein) or buffer for 24 hr at 37°C. Following washing, [³H]thymidine labeled P815 mastocytoma cells (1×10^4) were added and after 24 hr the percent specific release (cytotoxicity) calculated. The addition of 10 ng lipopolysaccharide had no effect on the macrophage cytotoxicity activity (data not shown). The results represent the mean $\pm$ S.D. of two separate experiments performed in triplicate.

$$\% \text{ cytotoxicity} = \frac{\text{CPM experimental} - \text{CPM spontaneous release}}{\text{total CPM in cells}} \times 100.$$

acetyl-LDL alone on the activation of macrophages for cytotoxicity (release of [^{3}H]thymidine) against P815 mastocytoma tumor cells. Acetyl-LDL bound MTP-PE was more effective than free MTP-PE alone at 10:1, 20:1, and 40:1 effector-target cell ratios. Acetyl-LDL alone showed only slight macrophage-activating effects above no additions, and no enhancement in cytotoxicity was observed with increased effector/ target cell ratios.

Adsorptive and Reversible Interactions of Lipoprotein-Drug Complexes

A variety of studies have examined the interactions of reductive-methylated-LDL-dnm with P388 leukemia cells (J. Shaw and S. Yanovich, unpublished results) and the dose response cytotoxicity of LDL-HMTX, acetyl-LDL-HMTX and liposome-HMTX, and in L1210 leukemia cells (J. Shaw, C. Barlow and L. Matherly, unpublished results). These studies support other non-receptor adsorptive or reversible interactions of the lipoprotein-drug complexes with cells *in vitro* (FIGURE 8). Exchange of drug at the lipoprotein particle–plasma membrane interface was also consistent with results from these studies. Receptor-independent lipoprotein transport and reversible interactions of lipoproteins at cell surfaces are additional pathways for lipoprotein metabolism.[29–31]

Experiments with HDL-bound adr are illustrated in FIGURE 4B and demonstrate a different adsorptive interaction at the P388 leukemia cell surface as compared to lipoprotein-mediated receptor pathways. Uptake of HDL-bound adr at 30 min was approximately four times greater than free adr at the same drug concentration. The uptake appeared to be adsorptive but not specific since excess HDL and LDL showed competition. The addition of Ca^{2+} or heparin during the influx experiments with HDL-adr complex and P388 cells had no significant effects on adr uptake. Fluorescence video microscopy pictures suggested the drug to be internalized by the P388 cells (data not shown). HDL-bound adr did not appear saturable for up to 1 hr and showed an almost linear pattern of uptake in P388 cells (FIGURE 4B). The cellular fluorescence from adr in contrast to LDL-bound dnm either was rapidly quenched or lost from the cell during efflux (FIGURE 4B, efflux pattern).

Monoclonal Antibody Directed Interactions of LDL

Anti-H2K^k, an IgG2a monoclonal antibody, has been covalently bound to the oligosaccharide group of apoprotein B-100, a glycoprotein having 5–10% carbohydrate (FIGURE 11).[32] The LDL-antibody conjugate was prepared as described in the flow chart of FIGURE 11 and represents an adaptation of a procedure by Heath and Papahadjopoulos for coupling monoclonal antibody (MoAb) to ganglioside-enriched liposomes.[33] Following periodate oxidation of LDL, coupling of oxidized LDL to anti-H2K^{kl}, and lastly borohydride reduction, the LDL-anti-H2K^k complex was fractionated from free anti-H2K^k by flotation at density 1.150 g/ml or preferably Sepharose CL-4B chromatography.[34] The complex was larger in size than LDL-drug complexes and was filterable through 0.8 μm but not 0.45 μm filters. The anti-H2K^k complex was dry-film stirred with AD-32 and the composition of the resulting complex is given in TABLE 4. The lipid composition of LDL-anti-H2K^k and LDL-anti-H2K^k-AD-32 complexes agreed closely with native LDL.

The LDL-MoAb complexes were predicted to interact with cells via antibody-cell surface antigen interactions provided LDL receptor activity was lost during the chemical coupling (FIGURE 8).[34] The interaction of the LDL[^{125}I]anti-H2K^k has been

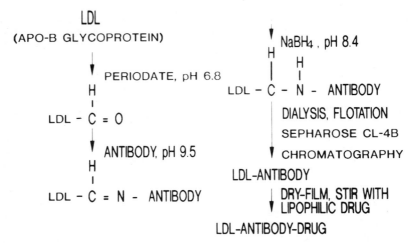

FIGURE 11. Procedure for coupling monoclonal antibody to ganglioside-enriched liposomes.

examined in H-2K^k haplotype-positive L-929 cells and haplotype-negative Vero kidney or HeLa cells *in vitro* (FIGURE 12). As illustrated in the figure, LDL[^{125}I]anti-H2K^k and free H-2K^k bound poorly to antigen-negative cells, but strongly to antigen-positive L-929 cells at two concentrations. In general, LDL-anti-H2K^k bound to cells about 60% as well as free anti-H2K^k, at similar anti-H2K^k concentrations. FIGURE 13 shows the interaction of haplotype-positive L-929 cells with the LDL-anti-H2K^k complex in the presence or absence of excess LDL or anti-H2K^k. The results indicate that LDL-anti-H2K^k interacts with L-929 positive cells by antigen/antibody interactions with little or no cellular binding through the LDL-receptor mediated pathway.

DISCUSSION

Preparation, Composition, and Stability of Lipoprotein-Drug Complexes

Lipoproteins (LDL and HDL) are a heterogeneous group of water-soluble nanoparticles whose core is composed of a water-insoluble oil, namely cholesterol ester

TABLE 4. Composition of Low Density Lipoprotein Monoclonal Anti-H-2K^k Complexes

Complex	Antibody (μg)	AD-32 (nmol)	Cholesterol (nmol)	Cholesterol Ester (nmol)	Phospholipid (nmol)
LDL-anti-H-2K^k	63 ± 12	—	1263 ± 198	2477 ± 281	834 ± 200
LDL-anti-H-2K^k-AD-32	54 ± 13	49 ± 41	1132 ± 160	2050 ± 147	740 ± 90

Values are expressed per mg apoprotein B for the LDL-anti-H2K^k complexes. N-trifluoroace-tyl-adriamycin-14-valerate (AD-32). (After Shaw *et al.*[34])

and triglyceride. Lipoproteins are uniquely designed for transporting the enclosed oil droplet in the blood, across vascular and sinusoidal endothelial linings and in the cell interiors of tissues via receptor and non-receptor–mediated pathways.[1,2,19,29]

Our studies have been directed toward procedures for partitioning and complexing lipophilic drugs into and at the interface of the water-insoluble core of lipoproteins. Of the four techniques examined, only stirring at the phase transition of LDL with a dry film or powder of excess drug resulted in an LDL-drug complex that resembled native LDL structurally and fuctionally. Even at the upper end of drug incorporation per LDL particle, there was minimal perturbation as the drug quantities represented only

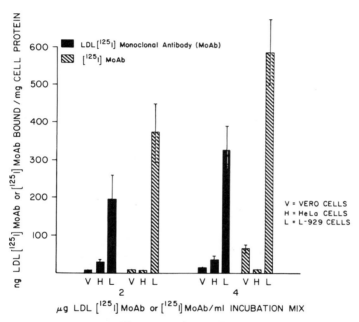

FIGURE 12. Interaction of LDL[[125I]]anti-H2K^k and [[125I]]anti-H2K^k with H-2K^k negative and positive cells. Cultured L-929 (H-2K^k positive), HeLa and Vero (H-2K^k negative) cells were incubated with complex or free antibody for 2 hr at 37°C. After three wash steps, cells were solubilized in 0.1% SDS in water, and then radioactivity and protein values were determined. The ng/ml and μg/ml values represent MoAb protein only. (From Shaw *et al.*[34] With permission of the publisher.)

5% of the lipid. The four lipophilic drugs used in the studies varied widely in structure with the only common feature being the presence of one or more alkyl chains. AD-32 contains an ester-linked valeric acid, HMTX exhibits an esterified sixteen carbon alkyl chain at the gamma carboxyl group of glutamate, ara-CMPH contains a 5'-hexadecyl phosphate ester, and MTP-PE represents a muramic acid tripeptide coupled to a phospholipid with two hexadecyl esterified chains. With drugs of higher water-solubility such as dnm or adr, it is clear that only small levels of drug can be incorporated per particle. Consequently, satisfactory pharmacological levels for *in vivo* studies would only be possible with highly active drugs. The finding that the more water-soluble drug, adr, caused aggregation of LDL may be a more common observation with intermediate solubility drugs of amphipathic character.

We have used a variety of techniques to evaluate the integrity of lipoprotein-drug complexes. These include reflotation of lipoprotein-drug complex, antibody precipitation studies, fluorescence quenching measurements to distinguish surface-core drug localization, and complete compositional analysis (drug, phospholipid, cholesterol, cholesteryl ester, apoprotein B-100 integrity on SDS gels). In one instance, the drug compositional analysis identified drug analogue/parent drug conversion of LDL-bound HMTX to water-soluble MTX.

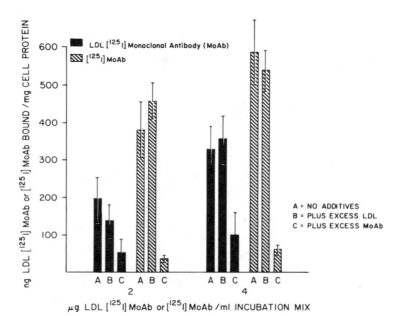

FIGURE 13. Interaction of LDL[^{125}I]anti-H2K^k and [^{125}I]anti-H2K^k with H-2K^k positive L-929 cells in the presence of excess LDL or MoAb. Cultured L-929 cells were incubated with [^{125}I] complex or free [^{125}I]anti-H-2K^k for 2 hr at 37°C in the presence or absence of a 25-fold excess of LDL or MoAb. After three wash steps, cells were solubilized in 0.1% SDS in water then radioactivity and protein determined. The ng/ml and µg/ml values represent MoAb protein only. (From Shaw et al.[34] With permission of the publisher.)

LDL-DNM Interaction via the LDL-Receptor Pathway

At least four distinct classes of interaction and cellular uptake for the lipoprotein-drug complexes are supported by our studies (FIGURE 8). The first class represented interaction via the LDL-receptor mediated pathway. The studies were performed with LDL-dnm complex and freshly isolated sensitive and resistant P388 leukemia cells. Image analysis of flow-cell fluorescence microscopy video pictures showed a marked retention of LDL-dnm within the cells. These results were consistent with endocytosis of LDL-dnm within coated vesicles with a slow processing of the lipoprotein and drug within lysosomes. Clearly, intracellular uptake of lipoprotein-bound dnm was more efficient than free dnm. Resistant cells were susceptible to the cytotoxic effects of only lipoprotein-bound dnm. Other workers have also demonstrated the uptake of LDL-bound anthracyclines, namely AD-32 and N-(N-retinoyl)-L-leucyldoxorubicin-14-linoleate, by the LDL receptor mediated pathway in human mononuclear, leukemia, and cultured fibroblast cells.[12,17]

In the *in vivo* situation, the actual targeting of an LDL-drug complex does not seem feasible due to receptors residing on a variety of tissues. At the present time, two approaches may be possible for circumventing the "targeting problem" in the *in vivo* experiment. First, investigation is underway in some laboratories for maintaining a degree of targeting by understanding and taking advantage of down regulation of LDL-receptor synthesis at the gene level, which occurs on normal tissues, but is lost or uncontrolled in certain diseased tissues like cancerous tumors.[35] Secondly, direct perfusion into diseased areas or compartmental delivery (i.e. peritoneal cavity, lymphatic system, etc.) of lipoprotein-drug complexes may help avoid the need for targeting yet take advantage of the rapid cellular uptake of lipoprotein-lipophilic drug complexes.

Acetylated-LDL Interaction via the Acetyl-LDL Receptor

Uptake of acetyl-LDL bound MTP-PE by thioglycolate-elicited peritoneal macrophages from mice was demonstrated to occur through the acetyl-LDL receptor. This endocytic receptor pathway, also known as the scavenger pathway, utilizes a large surface glycoprotein not normally subject to feedback regulation.[23,25] Consequently, acetyl-LDL uptake can lead to high levels of accumulation of the lipoprotein in macrophages and blood monocytes.[23] The present studies were monitored using a fluorescent dye, DiI, which contains as part of its chemical structure two ester-linked acyl chains, analogous to MTP-PE. Both cytostasis and cytotoxicity assays with B16F10 melanoma and P815 mastocytoma tumor cells confirmed the tumoricidal activation of thioglycolate-elicited macrophages. Murine macrophages, such as those elicited by thioglycolate, are characterized as "responsive" for antitumor activation but are normally more difficult to activate by lymphokine (i.e. MTP-PE) alone.[36] "Responsive" peritoneal macrophages are thought to require a primary signal, e.g., gamma interferon, to reach the "primed state" followed by a second "triggering" signal, such as endotoxin or bacterial lipopolysaccharide, to become fully "activated."[36]

The acetyl-LDL:MTP-PE complex appears to have excellent potential for *in vivo* testing for the following reasons. (1) A targeting advantage can be gained with the acetyl-LDL receptor as it resides on a more restricted number of cell types, i.e. macrophages, blood monocytes, sinusoidal endothelial cells, and to a lesser extent microvascular endothelial cells.[22–25,37,38] (2) The immunomodulator, MTP-PE exerts its major actions largely on macrophage/blood monocyte cell types.[26,27,39] A question of concern, however, is the identity of the natural lipoprotein ligand, *in vivo* for the receptor.[40] If the concentration of this "modified lipoprotein" is substantially high, it will provide a competing lipoprotein particle for the acetyl-LDL-immunomodulator complex and lower its effectiveness. This competition by plasma lipoproteins is also a major problem in the use of any lipoprotein delivery system, *in vivo*.

Adsorptive and Reversible Interactions of Lipoprotein-Drug Complexes

The third class of lipoprotein-drug–cellular interactions that we have observed represented nonspecific adsorptive interactions and possibly reversible interactions of lipoprotein-bound drug at the particle–plasma membrane interface (FIGURE 8). The best example of these interactions were illustrated using an HDL-adr complex and

P388 leukemia cells maintained in defined media. The HDL-bound adr/cell interactions exhibited three characteristics, nonsaturable uptake, a lack of specificity, and an enhanced uptake relative to free adr. In addition, no cell surface receptors have been conclusively identified for apoproteins AI and AII-HDL lipoproteins. Nonreceptor-mediated uptake of lipoproteins is also a well established finding, *in vivo*,[29,45] and reversible interactions have been reported for LDL at the fibroblast cell surface.[31] Drug-cell interactions not mediated via the LDL receptor have been previously described for LDL-dnm, LDL-benzopyrene, LDL-AD-32, and certain LDL-cytotoxic drug complexes.[4,10,11,17,41] It must be stressed, however, that a stable lipoprotein-drug complex must be established before a description of cellular interactions can be made when using the complex. Lastly, it should be realized that lipoprotein–cell interactions have been monitored in the vast majority of cases using ^{125}I-labeled apoproteins with far fewer studies being performed with radiolabeled lipids, fluorescent probes, or drugs.

Monoclonal Antibody Directed Interactions of LDL

In an effort to learn how to direct LDL to any specified site, the MoAb, anti-H2K^k was covalently coupled to the particle (FIGURE 11). The LDL–anti-H2K^k complex could still be complexed with a lipophilic drug by the dry-film stir technique (FIGURE 11). The anti-H2K^k–LDL–AD-32 complex was larger than the other lipoprotein-drug complexes and tended to aggregate if concentrated. The LDL–anti-H2K^k expressed a lower affinity than free anti-H2K^k for binding to cells. This finding likely reflects the one MoAb/LDL particle stoichiometry and the inability of designating the Fc end of the anti-H2K^k for covalent attachment to LDL. In addition, the native anti-H2K^k (MW 150,000) and the LDL-anti-H2K^k (MW greater than 2.5×10^6), must encounter different stereochemical and thermodynamic factors during cell surface antigen binding. LDL–anti-H2K^k interacted with H-2K^k haplotype-positive but not haplotype-negative cells. The apparent loss of interaction via the LDL-receptor was not surprising since periodate oxidation/borohydride treatments were harsh conditions for a particle such as LDL. The characteristic yellow, carotene color of LDL was largely lost during the chemical coupling of the anti-H2K^k. The H2K^k is a cell surface glycoprotein of approximately 45,000 daltons and the LDL–anti-H2K^k interaction with the L-929 cells presumably represented adsorptive endocytosis.[34,42] Further studies are required to determine the comparative and contrasting interactions of LDL-drug and MoAb-LDL-drug complexes with cells.

CONCLUSION

Lipoproteins are naturally occurring colloidal particles found in mammalian blood and tissue fluids. These lipid-protein emulsions have been well characterized structurally and serve as transport carriers for lipids. LDLs and HDLs have been examined as model vehicles for carrying lipophilic drugs. Drug delivery and targeting studies with lipoprotein-drug complexes can be effectively explored for receptor-mediated endocytosis and metabolism in tissues and cell culture.

ACKNOWLEDGMENTS

We wish to express our thanks to Drs. R. Scartazzine and D. G. Braun (CIBA-GEIGY, Basle) for the gift of MTP-PE, Dr. Merwyn Israel (Department of

Pharmacology, University of Tennessee) for AD-32 and Drs. Narayanan and Kedda (Drug Synthesis and Chemistry Branch, NCI) for a variety of anthracyclines. Ms. Ellen Smith and Shelly Delgado (Alcon Laboratories) provided excellent typing of the manuscript and slide preparation. J.M.S. thanks Drs. Laverne Schirch and Larry Matherly and students Roopa Baichwal and Charles Barlow (Medical College of Virginia, Richmond, VA) for collaborative work with MTX and HMTX not reported here.

REFERENCES

1. SEGREST, J. P. & J. J. ALBERS, Eds. 1986. Plasma lipoproteins, Part A, preparation, structure, and molecular biology. *In* Methods in Enzymology. Vol. 128. Academic Press. New York.
2. ALBERS, J. J. & J. P. SEGREST, Eds. 1986. Plasma lipoproteins, Part B, characterization, cell biology, and metabolism. *In* Methods in Enzymology. Vol. 129. Academic Press. New York.
3. KREIGER, M., L. SMITH, R. ANDERSON, J. GOLDSTEIN, Y. KOA, H. POWNALL, A. GOTTO & M. BROWN. 1979. Reconstituted low-density lipoprotein: A vehicle for the delivery of hydrophobic fluorescent probes in cells. J. Supramol. Struct. **10**: 467–478.
4. REMSEN, J. & R. SHIREMAN. 1981. Effect of low-density lipoprotein on the incorporation of benzo(a)pyrene by cultured cells. Cancer Res. **41**: 3179–3185.
5. GAL, D., M. OHASHI, P. C. MCDONALD, H. J. BUCHSBAUM & E. R. SIMPSON. 1981. Low-density lipoprotein as a potential vehicle for chemotherapeutic agents and radionucleotides in the management of gynecologic neoplasms. Am J. Obstet. Gynecol. **139**: 877–885.
6. MOSLEY, S. T., J. L. GOLDSTEIN, M. S. BROWN, J. R. FALCK & R. G. ANDERSON. 1981. Targeted killing of cultured cells by receptor dependent photosensitization. Proc. Natl. Acad. Sci. USA **78**: 5717–5721.
7. COUNSELL, R. & R. POHLAND. 1982. Lipoproteins as potential site-specific delivery systems for diagnostic and therapeutic agents. J. Med. Chem. **25**: 1115–1120.
8. RUDLING, M. J., V. P. COLLINS & C. O. PETERSON. 1983. Delivery of aclacinomycin A to human glioma cell *in vitro* by the low-density lipoprotein pathway. Cancer Res. **43**: 4600–4605.
9. IWANIK, M., K. V. SHAW, B. LEDWITH, S. YANOVICH & J. M. SHAW. 1984. Preparation and interaction of a low-density lipoprotein: daunomycin complex with P388 leukemic cells. Cancer Res. **44**: 1206–1215.
10. YANOVICH, S., L. PRESTON & J. M. SHAW. 1984. Characteristics of uptake and cytotoxicity of a low-density lipoprotein: daunomycin complex in P388 leukemia cells. Cancer Res. **44**: 3377–3382.
11. FIRESTONE, R. A., J. M. PISANO, J. R. FALCK, M. M. MCPHAUL & M. KRIEGER. 1984. Selective delivery of cytotoxic compounds to cells by the LDL pathway. J. Med. Chem. **27**: 1037–1043.
12. VITOLS, S. G., M. MASQUELIER & C. O. PETERSON. 1985. Selective uptake of a toxic lipophilic anthracycline derative by the low-density lipoprotein receptor pathway in cultured fibroblasts. J. Med. Chem. **28**: 451–454.
13. HALBERT, G. W., J. F. STUART & A. T. FLORENCE. 1985. A low density lipoprotein-methotrexate covalent complex and its activity against L1210 cells *in vitro*. Cancer Chemother. Pharmacol. **15**: 223–227.
14. SEKI, J., A. OKITA, M. WATANABE, T. NAKAGAWA, K. HONDA, N. TATEWAKI & M. SUGIYAMA. 1985. Plasma lipoproteins as drug carriers: Pharmacological activity and disposition of β-sitosteryl-β-D-glucopyranoside with plasma lipoproteins. J. Pharm. Sci. **74**: 1259–1264.
15. MASQUELIER, M., S. VITOLS & C. PETERSON. 1986. Low-density lipoprotein as a carrier of antitumor drugs: *In vitro* fate of drug-human low-density lipoprotein complexes in mice. Cancer Res. **46**: 3842–3847.
16. KRIEGER, M., M. J. MCPHAUL, J. L. GOLDSTEIN & M. S. BROWN. 1979. Replacement of

neutral lipids of low-density lipoprotein with esters of long-chain unsaturated fatty acids. J. Biol. Chem. **254:** 3845–3853.

17. VITOLS, S. G., G. GAHRTON & C. PETERSON. 1984. Significance of low-density lipoprotein (LDL) receptor pathway for the *in vitro* accumulation of AD-32 incorporated into LDL in normal and leukemic white blood cells. Cancer Treat. Rep. **68:** 515–520.

18. BASU, S. K., J. L. GOLDSTEIN, R. G. ANDERSON & M. S. BROWN. 1976. Degradation of cationized low-density lipoprotein and regulation of cholesterol metabolism in homozygous familial hypercholesterolemia fibroblasts. Proc. Natl. Acad. Sci. USA **73:** 3178–3182.

19. GOLDSTEIN, J. L. & M. S. BROWN. 1977. The low-density lipoprotein pathway and its relation to atherosclerosis. Ann. Rev. Biochem. **46:** 897–930.

20. MAHLEY, R. W. & T. L. INNERARITY. 1983. Lipoprotein receptors and cholesterol homeostasis. Biochim. Biophys. Acta **737:** 197–222.

21. SCHNEIDER, W. J., U. BEISIEGEL, J. L. GOLDSTEIN & M. S. BROWN. 1982. Purification of the low-density lipoprotein receptor, an acidic glycoprotein of 164,000 molecular weight. J. Biol. Chem **257:** 2664–2673.

22. GOLDSTEIN, J. T., Y. K. HO, S. K. BASU & M. S. BROWN. 1979. Binding site on macrophages that mediates uptake and degradation of acetylated low-density lipoprotein producing massive cholesterol deposition. Proc. Natl. Acad. Sci. USA **76:** 333–337.

23. BROWN, M. S. & J. L. GOLDSTEIN. 1983. Lipoprotein metabolism in the macrophage; implications for cholesterol deposition in atherosclerosis. Ann. Rev. Biochem. **52:** 223–261.

24. NAGELKERKE, J. F., K. P. BARTO & T. J. VAN BERKEL. 1983. *In vivo* and *in vitro* uptake and degradation of acetylated low-density lipoprotein by rat liver endothelial, Kupffer and Parenchymal cells. J. Biol. Chem. **258:** 12,221–12,227.

25. VIA, D. P., H. A. DRESEL, S. L. CHENG & A. M. GOTTO. 1985. Murine macrophage tumors are a source of a 260,000-dalton acetyl-low-density lipoprotein receptor. J. Biol. Chem. **260:** 7379–7386.

26. KEY, M., J. TALMADGE, W. FOGLER, C. BUCANA & I. FIDLER. 1982. Isolation of tumoricidal macrophages from lung melanoma metastases of mice treated systemically with liposomes containing a lipophilic derivative of muramyl dipeptide. J. Natl. Cancer Inst. **69:** 1189–1198.

27. KLEINERMAN, E., K. ERICKSON, A. SCHROIT, W. FOGLER & I. FIDLER. 1983. Activation of tumoricidal properties in human blood monocytes by liposomes containing lipophilic muramyl tripeptide. Cancer Res. **43:** 2010–2014.

28. KOFF, W., S. SHOWALTER, B. HAMPAR & I. FIDLER. 1985. Protection of mice against fatal herpes simplex Type 2 infection by liposomes containing muramyl tripeptide. Science **228:** 495–497.

29. SPADY, D. K., S. D. TURLEY & J. M. DIETSCHY. 1985. Receptor-independent low-density lipoprotein transport in the rat *in vivo*. J. Clin. Invest. **76:** 1113–1122.

30. TABAS, I. & A. R. TALL. 1984. Mechanism of the association of HDL_3 with endothelial cells, smooth muscle cells, and fibroblasts. J. Biol. Chem. **259:** 13897–13905.

31. HOEG, J. M., J. C. OSBORNE & H. B. BREWER. 1982. Analysis of reversible lipoprotein-cell interactions. J. Biol. Chem. **257:** 2125–2128.

32. CHAPMAN, M. J. 1986. Comparative analysis of mammalian plasma lipoproteins. *In* Methods of Enzymology. Segrest, J. P. & J. J. Albers, Eds. **128:** 70–143. Academic Press. New York.

33. HEATH, T., B. MACHER & D. PAPAHADJOPOULOS. 1981. Covalent attachment of immunoglobulins to liposomes via glycosphingolipids. Biochim. Biophys. Acta **640:** 66–81.

34. SHAW, J. M., K. V. SHAW & L. B. SCHOOK. 1987. Drug delivery particles and monoclonal antibodies. *In* Monoclonal Antibodies: Production, Techniques and Applications. L. B. Schook, Ed. **15:** 285–310. Marcel Dekker, Inc. New York.

35. HYNDS, S. A., J. WELSH, J. M. STEWART, A. JACK, M. SOUKOP, C. S. MCARDLE, K. C. CALMAN, C. J. PACKARD & J. SHEPERD. 1983. Low-density lipoprotein metabolism in mice with soft tissue tumors. Biochim. Biophys. Acta **795:** 589–595.

36. ADAMS, D. O. & T. A. HAMILTON. 1984. The cell biology of macrophage activation. Ann. Rev. Immunol. **2:** 283–318.

37. VOYTA, J. C., D. P. VIA, C. E. BUTTERFIELD & B. R. ZETTER. 1984. Identification and

isolation of endothelial cells based on their increased uptake of acetylated-low-density lipoprotein. J. Cell Biol. **99:** 2034–2040.

38. PITAS, R. E., J. BOYLES, R. W. MAHLEY & D. M. BISSELL. 1985. Uptake of chemically modified low-density lipoproteins *in vivo* is mediated by specific endothelial cells. J. Cell Biol. **100:** 103–117.

39. OLDHAM, R. K. 1985. Biologicals and biological response modifiers: New approaches to cancer treatment. Cancer Invest. **3:** 53–70.

40. PARTHOSARATHY, S., U. P. STEINBRECKER, J. BARNETT, J. L. WITZTUM & D. STEINBERG. 1985. Essential role of phospholipase A2 activity in endothelial cell-induced modification of low-density lipoprotein. Proc. Natl. Acad. Sci. USA **82:** 3000–3004.

41. PLANT, A. L., D. M. BENSON & L. C. SMITH. 1985. Cellular uptake and intracellular localization of Benzo(a)pyrene by digital fluorescence imaging microscopy. J. Cell Biol. **100:** 1295–1308.

42. STEINMAN, R., I. MELLMAN, W. MULLER & Z. COHN. 1983. Endocytosis and the recycling of plasma membrane. J. Cell Biol. **96:** 1–27.

43. KNOTT, T. J., S. C. RALL, T. L. INNERARITY, S. F. JACOBSON, M. S. URDEA, B. L. WILSON, L. M. POWELL, R. J. PEASE, R. EDDY, H. NAKAI, M. BYERS, L. M. PRIESTLY, E. ROBERTSON, L. B. RALL, C. BETSHOLTZ, T. B. SHOWS, R. W. MAHLEY & J. SCOTT. 1985. Human apolipoprotein B: Structure of carboxyl-terminal domains, sites of gene expression, and chromosomal localization. Science **230:** 37–43.

44. BROWN, M. S. & J. L. GOLDSTEIN. 1984. How LDL receptors influence cholesterol and atherosclerosis. Sci. Am. **251:** 58–66.

45. SHEPHERD, J. & C. J. PACKARD. 1986. Receptor-independent low-density lipoprotein catabolism. *In* Methods of Enzymology. J. J. Albers & J. P. Segrest, Eds. **129:** 566–590. Academic Press. New York.

Saccharide Determinants in Selective Drug Delivery

T. Y. SHEN

Department of Chemistry
University of Virginia
Charlottesville, Virginia 22901

INTRODUCTION

The possible use of saccharide determinants in selective drug delivery has been explored in the past few years in several laboratories with limited success.[1-3] The potential of this approach is being enhanced by recent biochemical studies of the structure and characteristics of various saccharide binding proteins, which facilitate the molecular design of novel carriers or drug conjugates for greater target cell selectivity and *in vivo* efficacy.

Carbohydrate determinants of many glycoproteins and glycolipids play key roles in numerous biological recognition processes.[4] Cellular interactions, the infection of mycoplasma and viruses, the formation of antibody complexes of blood group–related substances and tumor-associated antigens,[5] the receptor binding of epidermal growth factor, and the translocation of enzymes[6] and toxins[7] via saccharide receptor-mediated endocytosis are well known examples. Saccharide determinants are not limited to common carbohydrate molecules. Endogenous enzymatic transformation of saccharide may also be involved in the production of unique carbohydrate determinant as in the transport and uptake of lysosomal enzymes.[6] The targeting of lysosomal enzymes to lysosomes and the intercellular exchange of these enzymes in many cases depend upon the phosphorylation of the terminal mannose groups of their complex oligosaccharide side-chains.[8] The newly formed mannose-6-phosphate ligand displays a high affinity for the membrane mannose-6-phosphate receptors, with K_D values in the nanomolar range, comparable to those of many receptor ligands. Chemically synthesized carbohydrate derivatives[9,10] with high affinity for saccharide binding proteins further expand the scope of potentially useful saccharide ligands.

SACCHARIDE BINDING PROTEINS (RECEPTORS)

Following the initial observation by Ashwell and Morell that hepatocytes possess saccharide binding proteins on their surface,[11] which showed high affinity for D-galactose and N-acetyl D-galactosamine but not other carbohydrates, several other cell surface binding proteins have been identified. In addition to the fibroblasts receptor for D-mannose-6-phosphate mentioned above,[8] Kupffer cells and alveolar macrophages have binding proteins in the coated pit region with specificity for D-mannose and to a lesser extent N-acetyl D-glucosamine. A D-galactose recognizing protein was recently suggested to be involved in the lysis of murine tumor cells by activated mouse macrophages.[12] The saccharide binding proteins in general recognized a short oligosaccharide sequence. Their affinity for glycoprotein ligands is greatly enhanced by multivalency binding of a cluster of determinants with a preferred configuration.[10]

Considerable efforts have been devoted to the isolation and characterization of plant lectins and mammalian saccharide binding proteins.[13] Analytical techniques, such as X-ray crystallography, nuclear magnetic resonance, and gene cloning, have brought forth many critical details at the molecular level. For example, the primary sequence of two distinct but homologous mannose binding proteins from rat liver were recently determined by Drickamer et al.[14] by sequencing peptides from the proteins, isolation and sequencing of cDNAs for both proteins, and partial characterization for one of the genes (FIGURE 1). Each of the two 29,000 molecular weight subunits consists of three structural regions, an amino terminal segment rich in disulfide linkages, a collagen-like sequence, and a binding domain of approximately 150 amino acids near the carboxyl end. Interestingly, the sequence of the binding domain shows a clear homology with binding domains of glycoprotein receptors for N-acetyl D-glucosamine and several asialoproteins from different species. Indeed, saccharide binding appears to be one of the nature's early recognition mechanisms.[14] The rabbit alveolar macrophage mannan receptor was identified by Stahl et al.[15] as a 175 Kd membrane protein. The binding site was radioiodinated with mannosyl lactoperoxidase. The protein binds mannosyl BSA and GlcNAc-agarose with K_D in the 10^{-8} molar range.

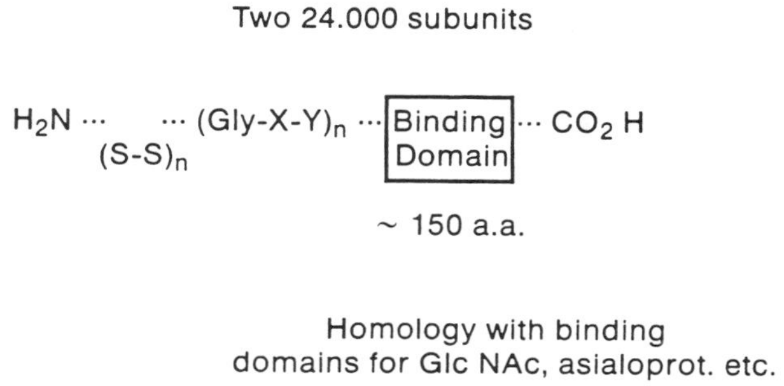

Two 24.000 subunits

$$H_2N \cdots \quad \cdots (Gly\text{-}X\text{-}Y)_n \cdots \boxed{\begin{array}{c} \text{Binding} \\ \text{Domain} \end{array}} \cdots CO_2 H$$
$$(S\text{-}S)_n$$

~ 150 a.a.

Homology with binding
domains for Glc NAc, asialoprot. etc.

FIGURE 1. Structural features of rat liver mannose binding proteins. (Adapted from Drickamer et al.[14])

The very high degree of specificity of hepatic lectins were well illustrated by Lee et al.[16] The Gal/GalNAc lectin binds N-acetyl lactosamine-type oligosaccharides over a million fold affinity range (K_D = 1 nM–1 mM). It binds a bovine fetuin glycopeptide, which has a triantenary Gal-β-(1,4)-GlcNAc structure, with a K_D of 4.4 nM. Replacement of one terminal disaccharide with its position isomer Gal-β(1,3)-GlcNAc decreased affinity almost 100 fold. The interaction of saccharides with their binding proteins is clearly determined by their composition as well as configuration.

The apparent number and the affinity of Gal/GalNAc binding sites on the surface of rabbit hepatocytes vary according to the ligand used in the determination. Both high and low affinity binding sites were found for asialo-orosomucoid, an asialoglycopeptide from $\alpha1$ protease inhibitor and a synthetic ligand di-tri-lac.[17] Considerable variations both in K_D values and in number of sites per cell for these ligands were observed. The synthetic ligand, possibly because of its smaller size, has significantly more binding sites than the other two macromolecular ligands.

Regarding the nature of bonding, a survey of X-ray crystallographic data[13] indicated that charged groups in the binding domain contribute to approximately 40% of the important hydrogen bonds of ca. 2.8 Å in length. Van der Waals interactions at ca. 3.2–4 Å often involve nonpolar atoms in Trp, Tyr, and His residues. Hydrophobic interactions between the nonpolar side of saccharides and lipophilic peptide regions contribute to a lesser degree. The hydroxyl groups in saccharide ligands simulaneously serve both as hydrogen donors and hydrogen acceptors in the formation of a multivalent hydrogen bond network. Most planar hydrogen bonds are tetrahedral but some arrangements have also been observed in the X-ray structures. A remarkable ligand-receptor complex of L-arabinose and its binding protein was elucidated by Quiocho et al. recently (FIGURE 2).[13] An inner shell of amino acid residues forms an intricate network of hydrogen bonds with the oxygen functions of the carbohydrate ligand, which is supported by an outer shell of water molecules and polar functional groups. Similar analysis of oligosaccharide binding proteins should greatly facilitate the design and synthesis of more effective targeting saccharide ligands for drug delivery.

LIPOSOMES WITH CARBOHYDRATE DETERMINANTS

To use carbohydrate determinants in targeted delivery, a variety of naturally occurring and synthetic carbohydrate derivatives have been incorporated into liposomes or conjugated to bioactive substances (FIGURE 3).[1-3] As liposome components, ceramide-β-lactoside and asialo-ganglioside are most commonly used to anchor carbohydrate chains into the bilayer vesicles.[18] Phospholipid derivatives of asialo-orosomucoid and amylopectin have also been used. We have synthesized a series of carbohydrate cholestrol conjugates that effectively place mono- or disaccharide determinants on the surface of lipid vesicles, and which form liposomes more stable

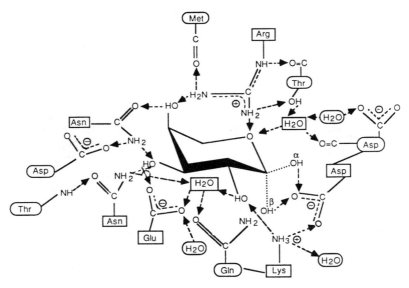

FIGURE 2. The complex hydrogen-bonding network of L-arabinose and its binding protein. (Adapted from Quiocho.[13])

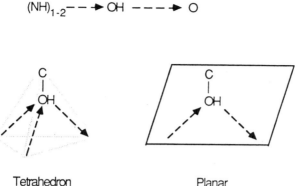

$(NH)_{1-2} - - - \rightarrow OH - - - - \rightarrow O$

Tetrahedron   Planar

Multivalency

FIGURE 3. Carbohydrate ligands used in preparing glycosylated liposomes and conjugates of bioactive substances.

than those prepared from glycosylated ceramides (FIGURE 4). The cholestrol conjugate of a modified saccharide, 6-amino-6-deoxy-D-mannose, turned out to be particularly interesting, it increased the *in vivo* stability and reduced membrane permeability of liposomes very significantly.[19] More recently, saccharide derivatives of other lipophilic anchoring groups, such as phosphatidyl ethanolamine, diacyl glycerol, and sterols were also employed.

A number of laboratories have investigated the *in vivo* distribution or targeting of these glycosylated liposomes. Earlier, Scherphof *et al.*[20] showed that incorporation of lactosylceramide into small unilamellar vesicles increased the clearance rate three fold and the hepatic uptake two fold, presumably via the galactose receptor on the surface of hepatocytes. In contrast, only a slight increase of uptake by nonparenchymal cells, which possess mannose receptors, was observed in the same experiment. Similarly, Bachhawat *et al.*[21] showed a differential uptake of liposomes carrying asialo-GM1 by liver cells. The enhanced uptake by hepatocytes was partially blocked by a competitive ligand asialofetuin. In using liposomes for gene transfer and expression *in vivo,* most of plasmid DNA of preproinsulin gene 1 was found to be taken up by Kupffer cells and not by the secretory hepatocytes as desired. This was remedied by incorporation of lactosylceramide in the liposome, which delivered 19% of the exogenous plasmid to hepatocytes.[22,23]

Glycosylated lectin-specific liposomes were also used to target the delivery of a genetically missing enzyme to different liver cells for possible application in enzyme replacement therapy. Gaucher's disease is an inherited metabolic disorder caused by a deficiency of β-glucocerebrosidase and the consequent accumulation of the glycolipid glucocerebroside in Kupffer cells. Infusion of the native enzyme, which has galactose terminals, delivers the enzyme mostly to hepatocytes via their Gal receptor and not to the Kupffer cells. This undesirable distribution pattern would be reversed by entrapping ^{125}I-labeled β-glucocerebrosidase in liposomes, which are readily phagocytosed by rat nonparenchymal cells. Interestingly, another five-fold increase in radioactivity in the nonparenchymal cells was achieved by using mannosylated liposomes (TABLE 1).

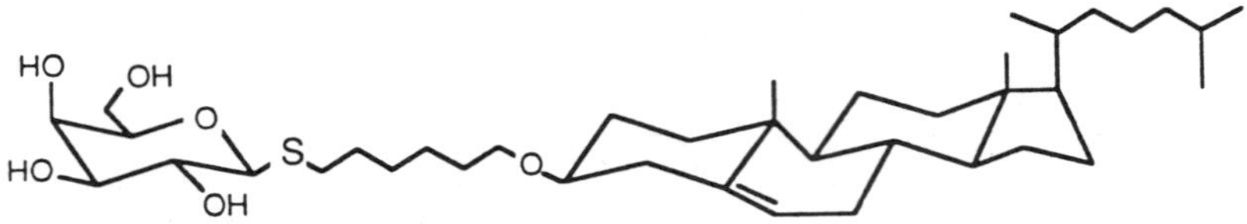

GalChol

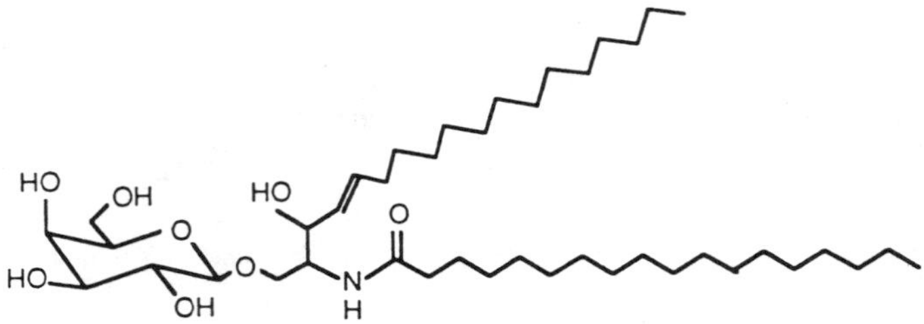

GalCer

FIGURE 4. Chemical structure of galactose derivative of cholesterol and ceramide.

The involvement of Man receptor in this case was demonstrated by the reversal of increased clearance rate and uptake by a competing ligand, hydrolyzed mannan, and not by the Gal ligand asialo-orosomucoid.

In addition to the placement of saccharide determinants on the surface of liposomes, the incorporation of glycolipid and glycopeptide derivatives into the bilayer structure also modify other properties of liposomes, sometimes very significantly. The lipophilic anchor and the hydrophilic carbohydrate head group may affect both the stability and permeability of the vesicle.[25,26] While the saccharide moiety is designed to alter the clearance rate, tissue distribution, and liver uptake, its immunogenicity may also be enhanced by the adjuvanticity of the liposome carrier (TABLE 2).[27]

Earlier, inclusion of 6-amino-6-deoxy-D-mannose on the surface of liposomes was

TABLE 1. Uptake of ^{125}I-Labeled β-Glucocerebrosidase Entrapped in Liposomes of Glycosylated Liposomes by Rat Liver Cells after Infusion

Carbohydrate Ligands
Liposome components
Ceramide-β-lactoside
Asialo ganglioside
Lipid derivative of orosomucoid, amylopectin
Saccharide derivatives of PE, DAG, sterols
Oligosaccharide conjugates

(Data from Das et al.[24])

TABLE 2. Modification of the Physical and Biological Properties of Liposomes by Incorporation of Saccharide Ligands into the Bilayer Membrane

Surface Polar Groups, Lipid Composition, Size
• Stability • Permeability • Clearance rate/Liver uptake • Tissue distribution • Immunological responses

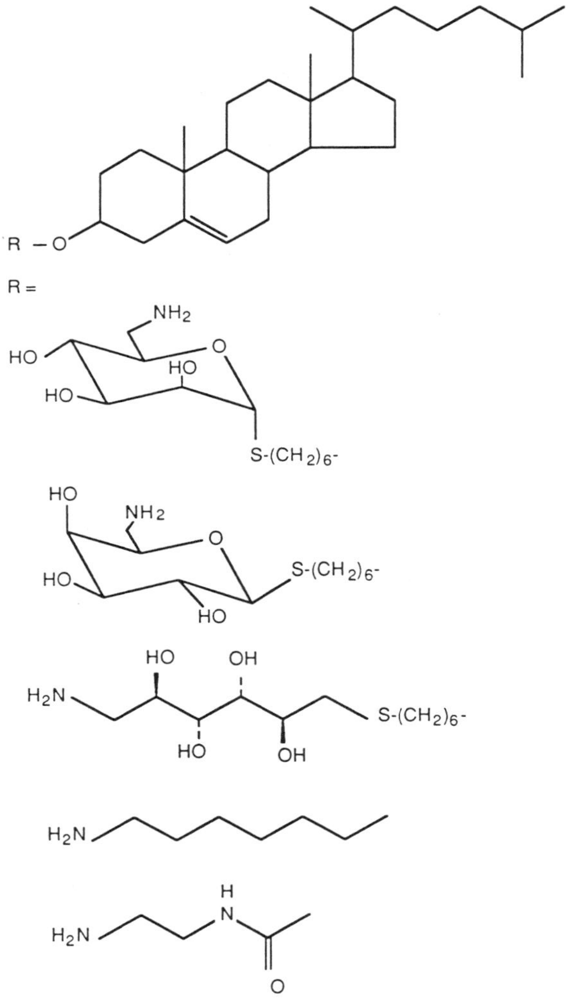

FIGURE 5. Chemical structure of cholesterol derivative of (from the top) 6-amino-6-deoxy-mannose, 6-amino-6-deoxy-galactose, 6-amino-6-deoxy-D-mannitol, and two aliphatic amines.

reported to increase the rate of phagocytosis by macrophages.[28] Several modified phospholipid vesicles containing cholesterol derivatives of polyhydroxyamines (e.g., 6-amino-6-deoxy-D-mannose, 6-amino-6-deoxy-D-galactose, and the acyclic 6-amino-6-deoxy-D-mannitol) synthesized in our laboratory (FIGURE 5) were found by Baldeschwieler et al.[29] to be endocytosed by mouse peritoneal macrophage at a greater rate than those vesicles containing the cholesterol conjugate of hexylamine, acetylethylenediamine, or various pentoses and hexoses. Cationic groups in a hydrated environment appear to be helpful, but the exact nature of their stimulation of macrophage uptake is not yet clear.

SACCHARIDE DERIVATIVES FOR SELECTIVE DELIVERY

Instead of glycosylated liposomes, soluble synthetic saccharide derivatives may also be used as carriers for selective delivery with certain advantages. With increasing knowledge of the molecular basis of receptor specificity (e.g., terminal determinants, neighboring sequence, and anomeric linkage, etc.), oligosaccharide clusters or novel structures may be designed, as illustrated by Lee et al. in the case of di-tri-lac,[17] with higher affinity and more binding sites than natural macromolecules (TABLE 3). From the pharmacokinetic point of view, having relatively low molecular weight ($\leq 5,000$) synthetic ligands should encounter lower in vivo distribution barriers and suffer less nonspecific uptake by the reticuloendothelial system. With these considerations in mind, we synthesized a group of glycopeptide analogs simply by attaching three saccharide molecules to the free amino groups in the dipeptide lysyl-lysine as potential carriers.[9] The carboxyl terminal conveniently provides a site for attachment of various drug molecules, polysaccharide vaccine, or polypeptides. The Bolton-Hunter derivative of a mannosyl ligand, Man_3Lys_2BH has a K_D value of 2.7 μM in binding to the macrophage mannan receptor and a maximal binding of 5.2×10^5 molecules per cell at $0°C$.[30] Kinetic data showed that the ligand of this ligand conjugate is recognized and pinocytosed by macrophage with a K_m of uptake to be 5.6 μM and a maximal velocity V_{max} of 1.7×10^5 molecules per minute per cell. In other words, the rate of entry is approximately 1 conjugate molecule/receptor/3 min, similar to the rate of other receptor-mediated endocytosis. The in vivo targeting of the ligand was demonstrated by the uptake of ^{125}I-labeled Man_3Lys_2-Bolton Hunter derivative by the liver in rats. The enhanced clearance and uptake are both inhibited by coinjection with unlabeled Man_3Lys_2 but not with the isomeric Gal_3Lys_2.

The potential application of this soluble macrophage ligand in enzyme replacement was explored in collaboration with Brady's laboratory.[31] Purified human β-glucocerebrosidase was chemically coupled to 8–9 molecules of Man_3Lys_2 per each subunit of

TABLE 3. Possible Advantages of using Soluble Saccharide Derivatives as Carriers for Selective Delivery

Saccharide Derivatives for Selective Delivery
Δ Receptor specificity
Terminal, anomeric linkage, sequence
Δ High affinity, more sites
Clusters, oligosaccharides
Δ Low molecular weight $\leq 5,000$
Lower distribution barriers
Less nonspecific RE uptake

TABLE 4. Distribution of Human β-Glucocerebrosidase (G), (Man$_3$Lys$_2$) Derivatized Enzyme (Man$_3$Lys$_2$-G), and Partially Deglycosylated Enzyme (AHEXO-G) in Rat Liver Cells after Infusion

| | Distribution of Modified Glucocerebrosidase (G) (Enzyme Activity/mg Cell Protein) | |
	Hepatocytes	Nonparenchymal
Control	66 ± 12	44 ± 17
G	87 ± 7	251 ± 116
Man$_3$Lys$_2$-G	102 ± 5	766 ± 346
AHEXO-G	113 ± 14	2532 ± 655

Data from Murray et al.[32]

67,000 molecular weight. The reaction product retained 60% of the original enzymatic activity without any loss of specificity. The K_m and V_{max} values of the derivative enzyme were improved slightly. Its clearance rate *in vivo* was twice that of the native enzyme, and which could be reduced by coinfusion with a competing ligand yeast mannan *in vivo*, the addition of Man$_3$Lys$_2$ groups to the enzyme increased the uptake into rat alveolar macrophage from 23 to 68 U/10^6 cells/hr. Using a second preparation,[32] infusion of modified enzyme in rats resulted in an 18-fold increase in specific activity in nonparenchymal cells and only 1.5-fold in hepatocytes compared to uninjected animals. The former increase is greater than the 6-fold increase seen for native enzyme, but is lower than the 50-fold increase seen after injection of partially deglycosylated glucocerebrosidase. Nevertheless, it is encouraging to see that the active enzyme can be selectively delivered to target cells by covalent attachment of a synthetic carbohydrate ligand (TABLE 4). Further optimization of the ligand structure and enzyme modification procedure for possible therapeutic experiments would seem warranted.

In perspective, synthetic saccharide derivatives have been shown to be effective ligands for receptor-mediated selective delivery of bioactive substances in some cases. However, several practical limitations remain to be resolved. The preparation of multivalent oligosaccharide ligands requires dedicated and extensive synthetic effort to handle their chemical complexity. To obtain these ligands by partial degradation of polysaccharides, glycopeptides, or other natural products is often complicated by heterogeneity and low yields. Additional analytical data on the sequence and stereochemical specificity of binding proteins are still needed. Finally, to broaden the application of this approach to many therapeutic conditions, the discovery of new saccharide binding proteins on more target cells of clinical importance is eagerly awaited.

REFERENCES

1. PONPIPOM, M.M. & T.Y. SHEN. 1985. *In* Receptor-Mediated Targeting of Drugs. G. Gregoriadis, G. Poste, J. Senior & A. Trouet, Eds.: 373–392. Plenum Publishing Corp. New York.
2. PONPIPOM, M.M., R.L. BUGIANESI, J.C. ROBBINS, T.W. DOEBBER & T.Y. SHEN. 1985. *In* Receptor-Mediated Targeting of Drugs. G. Gregoriadis, G. Poste, J. Senior & A. Trouet, Eds.: 53–71. Plenum Publishing Corp. New York.
3. POZNANSKY, M.J. & R.L. JULIANO. 1984. Pharmacol. Rev. **36**:277–336.
4. NEUFELD, E.F. & G. ASHWELL. 1980. Carbohydrate recognition systems for receptor-

mediated pinocytosis. *In* The Biochemistry of Glycoproteins and Proteoglycans. W.J. Lennarz, Ed.: 241–261. Plenum Press. New York

5. FEIZI, T. & R.A. CHILDS. 1985. Trends Biochem. Sci. 24–29.
6. VON FIGURA, K. & A. HASILIK. 1986. Ann. Rev. Biochem. **55:**167–193.
7. NEVILLE, D.M. JR. & T.H. HUDSON. 1986. Ann. Rev. Biochem. **55:**195–224.
8. HICKMAN, S. & E.F. NEUFELD. 1972. Biophys. Biochem. Res. Commun. **48:**992–999.
9. PONPIPOM, M.M., R.L. BUGIANESI, J.C. ROBBINS, T.W. DOEBBER & T.Y. SHEN. 1981. J. Med. Chem. **24:**1388-1395.
10. LEE, R.T., P. LIN & Y.C. LEE. 1984. Biochem **23:**4255–4261.
11. ASHWELL, G. & A.G. MORELL. 1974. Adv. Enzym. 99–128.
12. MERCURIO, A.M. 1986. Proc. Natl. Acad. Sci. USA **83:**2609–2613.
13. QUIOCHO, F.A. 1986. Ann. Rev. Biochem. **55:**287–315.
14. DRICKAMER, K., M.S. DORDAL & L. REYNOLDS. 1986. J. Biol. Chem. **162:**6878–6884.
15. WILEMANN, T.E., M.R. LENNARTZ & P.D. STAHL. 1986. Proc. Natl. Adad. Sci. USA **83:**2501–2505.
16. TOWNSEND, R.R., M.R. HARDY, T.C. WONG & Y.C. LEE. 1986. Biochem. **25:**5716–5725.
17. HARDY, M.R., R.R. TOWNSEND, S.M. PARKHURST & Y.C. LEE. 1985. Biochem. **24:**22–28.
18. PONPIPOM, M.M., R.L. BUGIANESI & T.Y. SHEN. 1980. Can. J. Chem. **58:**214–220.
19. WU, P.S., H.M. WU, G.W. TIN, J.R. SCHUH, W.R. GROASMUN, J.D. BALDESCHWIELER, T.Y. SHEN & M.M. PONPIPOM. 1982. Proc. Natl. Acad. Sci. USA **79:**5490–5493.
20. ROERDINK, F.H., J. DIJKSTRA, H.H. SPANJER & G.L. SCHERPHOF. 1984. Biochem. Soc. Trans. **12:**335–336.
21. DASGUPTA, P. & B.K. BACHHAWAT. 1985. Biochem. Int. **10:**327–336.
22. SOVIANO, P., J. DIJKSTRA, A. LEGRAND, H. SPANJER, D. LONDONS-GAGLIANDI, F. ROERDINK, G. SCHERPOS & C. NICOLAU. 1983. Proc Natl. Acad. Sci. USA **80:**7128–7131.
23. NICOLAU, C. 1984. Biochem. Soc. Trans. **12:**349–350.
24. DAS, P.K., G.J. MURRAY, G.C. ZIRZOW, R.O. BRADY & J.A. BARRANGER. 1985. Biochem. Med **33:**124–131.
25. PATEL, K.R., M.P. LI, J.R. SCHUH & J.D. BALDES-CHWIELER. 1985. Biochim. Biophy. Acta **814:**256–264.
26. MOELLERFELD, J., W. PRASS, H. RINGSDORF, H. HAMAZAKI & J. SUNAMOTO. 1986. Biochim. Biophy. Acta. **857:**265–270.
27. LATIF, N. & B.K. BACHHAWAT. 1984. Immunol. Lett. **8:**75–78.
28. WU, P.S., G.W. TIM & J.D. BALDESCHWIELER. 1981. Proc. Natl. Acad. Sci. USA **78:**2033.
29. BALDESCHWIELER, J.D. 1985. Ann. N.Y. Acad. Sci. **446:**349–367.
30. ROBBINS, J.C., M.H. LAM, C.S. TRIPP, R.L. BUGIANESI, M.M. PONPIPOM & T.Y. SHEN. 1981. Proc. Natl. Acad. Sci. USA **78:**7294–7298.
31. DOEBBER, T.W., M.S. WU, R.L. BUGIANESI, M.M. PONPIPOM, F.S. FURBISH, J.A. BARRANGER, R.O. BRADY & T.Y. SHEN. 1982. J. Biol. Chem. **257:**2193–2199.
32. MURRAY, G.J., T.W. DOEBBER, T.Y. SHEN, M.S. WU, M.M. PONPIPOM, R.L. BUGIANESI, R.O. BRADY & J.A. BARRANGER. 1985. Biochem. Med. **34:**241–246.

Some Perspectives on Targeted Delivery with Prodrugs

ANTHONY A. SINKULA

Research Laboratories
The Upjohn Company
Kalamazoo, Michigan 49001

INTRODUCTION

Historically, research in the area of targeted delivery by the use of prodrugs has been undertaken primarily by intuition and empiricism. The fault lies not with the biologist or chemist but rather with the paucity of definitive information that might be used for the design of experiments based on rational drug delivery theory.

The concept of targeted or site-directed prodrug delivery can be separated into two processes: (1) *Site direction,* in which the prodrug is transported and distributed preferentially to specific tissues or cells according to the physicochemical properties of the prodrug, as well as the nature of the barriers encountered in the transport process within the organism and (2) *Site activation,* in which the prodrug is taken up by the cell and transformed into the active drug species.

TRADITIONAL PRODRUG APPROACHES

The rationale for the synthesis of site-directed prodrugs evolved in the area of cancer chemotherapy but can be summarized by certain principles that apply to the chemical treatment of any localized disease state. (1) Certain disease conditions and symptomatology are localized in specific tissue. (2) Drugs utilized in certain disease states are affected by both normal and diseased tissue and are subjected to degradation and elimination prior to bioactivation. (3) Diseased tissue possesses enzyme systems differing in their nature and abundance from normal tissue. (4) Such enzyme systems are capable of promoting bioactivation of the prodrug. Several reviews have expanded on these principles in more detail.[1-5]

The ideal site-specific prodrug might possess the following characteristics: (1) Exclusive and complete transport to the target cell with subsequent uptake. (2) Absence of binding of the prodrug to normal protein or tissue and with no biochemical intervention prior to contact with diseased bioenviroment; lack of toxicity toward normal tissue during the transport and distribution phases. (3) Complete elimination of drug from the organism once disease symptomatology is eliminated or controlled. The ideal prodrug, then, consists of a bioactive parent molecule containing a suitable transport group sufficiently stable to deliver the molecule to the site of activity (site-direction) and responsive to the necessary enzyme systems and/or chemical bioenvironment to regenerate the parent molecule at the cellular or subcellular site (site-activation).

While the ideal prodrug is yet to be made, several approaches have been utilized to provide optimal therapeutic response and site-specificity. They can be categorized as (1) utilization of the enhanced or ligand specific enzymatic activity present in diseased cells or subcellular components but not present in normal cells, (2) utilization of the

TABLE 1. Promoieties Used as Transport Modifiers and Enhancers of Drugs to Site-Specific Tissue

Parent Drug Molecule	Promoiety	Route of Administration	Target Tissue/Cell	Reference
Cytosine arabinoside (cytarabine)	5'-acylate	Intraperitoneal	L-1210 leukemia	6
	5'-sulfonate	Subcutaneous		
Nitrogen mustard	Peptide (glycine, phenylalanine)	Intraperitoneal	Hepatoma	7
			Walker carcinoma	8
Dichlorodiamine, dichlorodialkylamine	Platinum coordination complex	Intraperitoneal	Solid sarcoma 180	9
		Intravenous	Dunning leukemia	10
			Primary Lewis lung carcinoma	
Morphine, phenazocine	Ether	Subcutaneous	CNS	11
Dopamine	Diacyl esters		Brain	12
L-Dopa	L-γ-glutamyl-D-Val-Leu-Lys			13, 14
Melphalan	N-(2-hydroxypropyl) methacrylamide (HPMA) copolymers	Intraperitoneal	B16 melanoma	2
Daunomycin, puromycin, adriamycin, bleomycin, bestatin		Intraperitoneal	L-1210 leukemia	15
Methotrexate	poly (L-lysine)	Intraperitoneal	L-1210 leukemia	16

lower pH of neoplastic tissue relative to that of most normal cells, which is especially important for prodrugs with acid-labile promoieties, and (3) manipulation of physico-chemical parameters (lipophilic/hydrophilic balance, pK_a, molecular size, and geometry, etc.) to enhance transport and distribution to site-specific tissue. TABLE 1 summarizes attempts to use a variety of promoieties designed to deliver drugs, by several routes of administration, to specific organs, tissues, and cells within the living organism. While none have been particularly successful in achieving the objective, the list does illustrate the variety of carrier groups attempted. Most were used in cancer chemotherapy.

NEWER APPROACHES TO TARGETED DELIVERY

Present and future targeted prodrug delivery should focus on and involve a blend of current theory and practice in molecular and cell biology, as well as physical and organic chemistry. The recent advances in disciplines such as biochemistry, biophysics, immunology, and cellular physiology, provide a rich source of interdisciplinary research that will lead to an understanding of the underlying physiological, biochemical, and physicochemical processes governing the delivery of drugs. It is known, for example, that prodrugs require the intervention of enzymes to regenerate the parent drug *in vivo* and the design of most prodrugs take this into consideration. Preliminary experiments usually validate this premise by *in vitro* studies. Extrapolation of these laboratory results to ultimate biochemical or enzymatic behavior in the host organism, however, remains a fertile area for investigation. The assumption usually is made that bioactivation will occur immediately prior to or at the actual subcellular site where the active drug species is needed to exert its therapeutic response. Rarely considered is the potential for biochemical intervention during the early stages of the transport process and metabolism/deactivation of the prodrug or drug prior to receptor interaction is disregarded or assumed to be of minor importance. A high enough dose is usually administered in the hope that the receptor will be swamped with drug to elicit a response. Understanding morphological and subtle physiological differences in cells as they affect drug transport should enable investigators to tailor prodrug molecules that participate in cellular transport processes in a manner that enhances efficacy.

The great strides made in understanding the molecular basis of immunoreactivity as it pertains to immunotherapy suggest approaches to other challenges encountered in targeted prodrug delivery. An understanding of antigen/antibody interactions, for example, provides a method for a targeted delivery by the use of immunoreagents or with monoclonal antibodies as surface recognition agents on liposomal carriers containing prodrugs. Design, synthesis, and physicochemical characterization complete the expertise necessary to approach the complex problems associated with prodrug delivery from an interdisciplinary perspective.

While it is acknowledged that most challenges pertaining to targeted prodrug delivery involve transport phenomena and processes, little is known how these processes operate *in vivo*. From the moment that the prodrug is administered until the therapeutic effect is achieved, forces are operative within the organism to maintain homeostasis against any foreign substances. FIGURE 1 presents in schematic form the main phases of drug transport and action. The pharmaceutical phase represents the traditional approach to drug delivery and is concerned with performance characteristics of the dosage form (disintegration and solubility). Modeling of pharmacokinetic processes (phase 2) has extended knowledge in terms of describing kinetic processes involved in drug delivery but does not provide insight into the biochemical mechanisms driving these processes. Little is presently known about the biochemical, physiological,

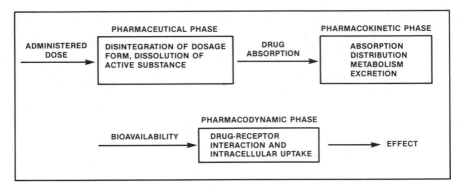

FIGURE 1. Main phases of drug transport and bioactivity.

and immunological implications of the pharmacokinetic phase (both animal and human) of prodrug transport and research in this area is needed. Finally, a most important area being intensively studied is the pharmacodynamic phase of drug transport, which involves attempts to describe events at the cellular and subcellular level. The sequence of events that lead to engulfment and subsequent disposition of a prodrug at the cellular level is shown in FIGURE 2. The interactions and processes that determine the ultimate fate of the drug, resulting in a response, occur intracellularly. Most of these processes are presently poorly understood. After receptor interaction occurs, the ligand/receptor complex collects in coated pits and is internalized to form vesicles, which fuse to form endosomes. The endosomes undergo differentiation and uncouple receptor and drug by mechanisms that are vaguely understood but are probably controlled by a pH drop from 7 to ~5. The tubular portion of the endosome separates, with receptor material, and returns to the cell surface membrane. Subsequent fusion of the remaining vesicles fuses with a lysosome where degradation (prodrug hydrolysis and metabolism?) occurs. Since endosomes contain some hydrolytic activity, perhaps prodrug metabolism can also possibly occur at this stage. Other types of cell processing besides receptor-mediated endocytosis might also occur with prodrugs especially if the prodrug contains large molecular weight polymeric backbones. Examples are phagocytosis and fluid-phase pinocytosis. Most studies carried out to date have involved understanding the transport of naturally occurring biochemicals, e.g. lipids and peptides/proteins. Thus, investigation of the cell processing of synthetically derived drugs and biochemicals remains a fertile research area.

Attempts have been made to design prodrugs that will be effectively delivered to site-specific tissue. Polymer backbones have been utilized as "hitching-posts" for a variety of chemical components intended to serve unique functions for targeting the drug molecule. Several synthetic or naturally derived biopolymers with varying degrees of solubility and containing functional groups and spacers for attaching drug molecules are being studied that can be actively or passively transported to specific organs, tissue, and cells. In general, the pharmacokinetic properties of the polymer can be altered to reflect desirable traits in the prodrug. Addition of solubilizing moieties, for example, to one region of the polymer can render the entire macromolecule nontoxic and soluble at physiological pH. A second area of the backbone can serve as the locus for drug attachment in which the parent drug molecule is covalently linked with or without spacer groups. A third part of the macromolecule can function as the targeting transport system for the entire prodrug polymer. Technology is already available to design such prodrugs using block copolymerization and cross-linking agents. A generic example of such a prodrug is illustrated in FIGURE 3. Certain assumptions must be made when fabricating such complex prodrug delivery systems. First, the polymer backbone should possess no intrinsic activity but should act only as the delivery system for the active drug molecule. Second, the backbone serves as the regulator of those pharmacokinetic properties that direct the entire molecule to site-specific tissue. Finally, regeneration of the parent drug molecule is essential since the covalent linkage of the pharmacophore almost always, without exception, renders the drug biologically inactive, i.e. the polymeric prodrug must be hydrolyzed to afford parent bioactive drug.

An early example of this approach is provided by Rowland et al.[19] The delivery of the alkylating drug p-phenylenediamine mustard (PDM) was covalently attached to a

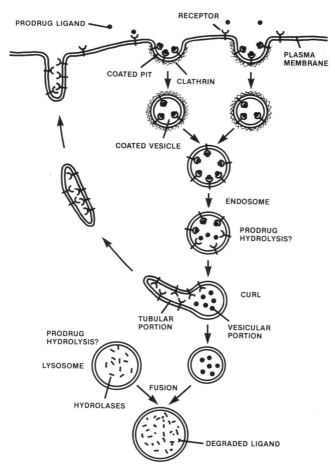

FIGURE 2. Prodrug-receptor interaction and the endocytotic process. (Adapted from Dautry-Varsat & Lodish.[17])

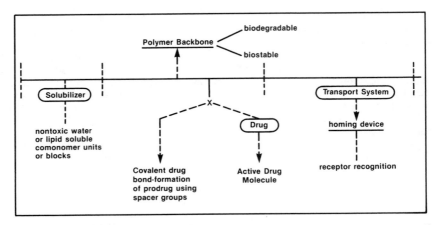

FIGURE 3. Generic example of a site-directed polymeric prodrug. (Adapted from Ringsdorf.[18])

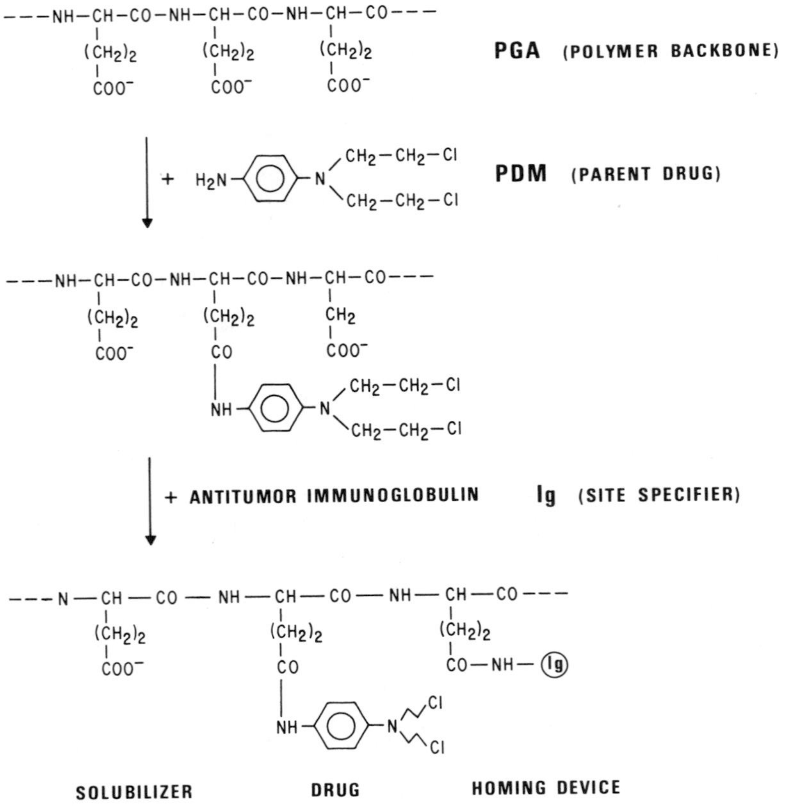

```
---NH-CH-CO-NH-CH-CO-NH-CH-CO---          PGA   (POLYMER BACKBONE)
      |           |           |
    (CH2)2      (CH2)2      (CH2)2
      |           |           |
     COO⁻        COO⁻        COO⁻
```

$$\downarrow \quad + \quad H_2N-\bigcirc-N\Big\langle {}^{CH_2-CH_2-Cl}_{CH_2-CH_2-Cl} \qquad \textbf{PDM} \quad \text{(PARENT DRUG)}$$

```
---NH-CH-CO-NH-CH-CO-NH-CH-CO---
      |           |           |
    (CH2)2      (CH2)2       CH2
      |           |           |
     COO⁻         CO         COO⁻
                  |
                  NH-◯-N⟨ CH2-CH2-Cl
                              CH2-CH2-Cl
```

$$\downarrow \quad + \text{ ANTITUMOR IMMUNOGLOBULIN} \qquad \textbf{Ig} \quad \text{(SITE SPECIFIER)}$$

```
---N—CH—CO—NH—CH—CO—NH—CH—CO---
     |           |           |
   (CH2)2      (CH2)2      (CH2)2
     |           |           |
    COO⁻         CO         CO—NH—(Ig)
                 |
                 NH-◯-N⟨ Cl
                            Cl

  SOLUBILIZER        DRUG        HOMING DEVICE
```

FIGURE 4. A PDM polymeric prodrug. (Adapted from Rowland et al.[19])

polyanionic polymer backbone, polyglutamic acid (PGA). This PGA-PDM conjugate resulted in a low (20%) survival rate (tumor suppression) for several groups of C57BL/6 mice inoculated intraperitoneally with 5×10^4 EL4 cells. The covalent addition of a site-specific transport moiety, rabbit antitumor immunoglobulin (Ig), enhanced the median survival time for 50% of the mice to >100 days. Further, 5/5 mice were alive and free of tumor at day 60 with treatment of the PGA-PDM-Ig conjugate whereas 1/5 of mice survived to day 60 after administration of the PGA-PDM conjugate. This polymeric prodrug delivery system is illustrated in FIGURE 4. The evidence would suggest that the conjugated PGA-PDM-Ig coplymer possesses the requisite balance of solubility, site-specificity, and biolability to make PDM an effective cytotoxic agent as a prodrug. Many more recent examples of the use of targeted prodrug chemotherapy are cited in a comprehensive review by Sezaki and Hashida.[20]

SUMMARY

Targeted delivery using prodrugs is becoming an important means for studying approaches to the efficient delivery for complex and often toxic molecules to specific sites within the body. Especially true for polymeric prodrugs containing targeting moieties, the future offers many possibilities for improvement of the therapeutic ratio by delivering drugs exclusively to diseased cellular and subcellular components within the organism. The fact that this type of research is highly interdisciplinary in nature requires the creative input of the biology disciplines as well as chemistry and pharmaceutical science.

Our perspective on what constitutes the true delivery system, as it applies to targeted delivery, needs to be redefined. The use of the prodrug to target drug molecules to specific sites is merely the chemical delivery device that has been conceived and designed after considering the implications of those biochemical, physiological, and immunological processes that ultimately affect the transport and distribution of the prodrug within the host organism.

REFERENCES

1. SINKULA, A. A. & S. H. YALKOWSKY. 1975. Rationale for design of biologically reversible drug derivatives: prodrugs. J. Pharm. Sci. **64:** 181–210.
2. CARL, P. L. 1983. Plasmin-activated prodrugs for cancer chemotherapy. *In* Development of Target-Oriented Anticancer Drugs. Y.-C. Cheng, B. Goz & M. Minkoff, Eds.: 143–155. Raven Press. New York.
3. SINKULA, A. A. 1985. Sustained drug action accomplished by the prodrug approach. *In* Design of Prodrugs. H. Bundgaard, Ed.: 157–176. Elsevier Science Publishers B.V. (Biomedical Division). Amsterdam.
4. STELLA, V. J. & K. J. HIMMELSTEIN. 1985. Site-specific drug delivery via prodrugs. *In* Design of Prodrugs. H. Bundgaard, Ed.: 177–198. Elsevier Science Publishers B.V. (Biomedical Division). Amsterdam.
5. TOMLINSON, E. 1986. (Patho) physiology and the temporal and spatial aspects of drug delivery. *In* Site-Specific Drug Delivery. E. Tomlinson & S. S. Davis, Eds.: 1–26. John Wiley and Sons Ltd. Chichester, Great Britain.
6. GRAY, G. D., F. R. NICOL, M. M. MICKELSON, G. W. CAMIENER, D. T. GISH, R. C. KELLY, W. J. WECHTER, T. E. MOXLEY & G. L. NEIL. 1972. Immunosuppressive, antiviral and antitumor activities of cytarabine derivatives. Biochem. Pharmacol. **21:** 465–475.
7. FRIEDMAN, O. M. & R. CHATTERJI. 1959. Synthesis of derivatives of glutamine as model substrates for anti-tumor agents. J. Am. Chem. Soc. **81:** 3750–3752.

8. BERGEL, F. & J. A. STOCK. 1954. Cyto-active amino acid and peptide derivatives. Part 1. Substituted phenylalanines. J. Chem. Soc.: 2409–2417.

9. ROSENBERG, B. 1973. Platinum coordination complexes in cancer chemotherapy. Naturwissenschaften 60, No. 9: 399–440.

10. CLEARE, M. J. 1973. Anti-cancer platinum compounds. Chem. Ind. (London): 921–923.

11. KUPCHAN, S. M. & A. F. CASY. 1967. Drug latentiation. II. Labile ether derivatives of phenolic analgesics. J. Med. Chem. 10: 959–960.

12. CASAGRANDE, C. & G. FERRARI. 1973. 3,4-0-Diacyl derivatives of dopamine. Farmaco, Ed. Sci. 28: 143–148.

13. WILK, S., H. MIZOGUCHI & M. ORLOWSKI. 1978. γ-Glutamyl DOPA: A kidney-specific dopamine precursor. J. Pharmacol Exp. Ther. 206: 227–232.

14. KYNCL, J. J., F. N. MINARD & P. H. JONES. 1978. L-γ-Glutamyl dopamine, an oral dopamine prodrug with renal selectivity. In Peripheral Dopaminergic Receptors. J.-L. Imbs & J. Schwartz, Eds.: 369–380. Pergamon Press. Oxford.

15. European Patent Application 85309560.2 Synthetic Polymeric Drugs. Dec. 31, 1985.

16. DUNCAN, R. & J. KOPECEK. 1984. Soluble synthetic polymers as potential drug carriers. In Polymers in Medicine. K. Dusek, Ed.: 51–101. Springer-Verlag. Berlin.

17. DAUTRY-VARSAT, A. & H. F. LODISH. 1984. How receptors bring proteins and particles into cells. Sci. Am. 250, No. 5: 52–58.

18. RINGSDORF, H. 1975. Structure and properties of pharmacologically active polymers. J. Polymer Sci.: Symposium No. 51: 135–153.

19. ROWLAND, G. F., G. J. O'NEILL & D. A. L. DAVIES. 1975. Suppression of tumour growth in mice by a drug-antibody conjugate using a novel approach to linkage. Nature 255: 487–488.

20. SEZAKI, H. & M. HASHIDA. 1984. Macromolecule-drug conjugates in targeted cancer chemotherapy. In CRC Critical Reviews in Therapeutic Drug Carrier Systems. S. D. Bruck, Ed. 1: 1–38.

Redox Drug Delivery Systems for Targeting Drugs to the Brain[a]

NICHOLAS BODOR

College of Pharmacy
J. Hillis Miller Health Center
Center for Drug Design and Delivery
University of Florida
Gainesville, Florida 32610

INTRODUCTION

Drug targeting to specific receptors or specific organs has been one of the main objectives of the medicinal and pharmaceutical chemists from the beginning of the century. However, only in the past 15 years or so have there been any promising developments in achieving this goal. The term "site-specific drug delivery" covers targeting to receptors or organs or any other specific part of the body to which we wish to deliver the drug exclusively. The site-specific delivery of drugs is indeed a very attractive goal because this provides one of the most significant potential ways to improve the therapeutic index (TI) of the drugs.[1] When a drug is delivered preferentially to the site of the action by virtue of this desired differential distribution, it will spare the rest of the body; thus, it will significantly reduce the overall toxicity while maintaining its therapeutic benefits.

At the present time, there are three basically different approaches for site-specific drug delivery. The first, the physical or mechanical approach, is based on effectively formulating a drug in a delivery device, which by virtue of its physical localization will allow differential release of the drug. The site specificity thus is due to exclusively producing higher drug concentrations wherever the device is localized, while the drug concentration in the rest of the body is very much diminished due to the simple dilution factor. The limitations of this approach are clearly due to the fact that many desired target sites are simply not available for the physical approach. In addition, often the distributional differences due to the dilution effect may not be sufficient to produce significant improvement in the TI.

The second basic approach is the biological one, according to which a drug is potentially targeted by a biological carrier that would have specific affinity for certain receptor sites, organs or other biological targets. This kind of approach, such as using monoclonal antibody–drug conjugates, erythrocyte carriers, or macromolecular product carriers (such as liposomes) has been the subject of many investigations. The limitations of this approach are primarily problems presented by stoichiometry, controlling the processes related to releasing the drugs from the biological carriers, as well as biological incompatibility of the carriers.

The third approach is the chemical approach, the use of the site-specific chemical delivery systems (CDSs),[1,2] which provide a wide variety of possibilities for site-enhanced or site-specific delivery. The CDS is produced by chemical reactions (at least

[a]Supported by National Institutes of Health Grant GM27167 and by a grant Pharmatec, Inc.

formally) from the target drug, which is then covalently coupled with one or more carrier moieties ($C_1 - C_n$) and if necessary one or more protective moieties ($F_1 - F_n$). By design, after delivery the CDS will undergo a variety of enzymatic conversions, which produce intermediates such as $CDS_1 CDS_2 \ldots CDS_n$, all having different physical properties and varying rates of formation and elimination, thus ultimately allowing a preferential and favorable distribution of a precursor [PD] at the site of action where ultimately the drug is released. The complex design process thus involves knowledge and use of the various enzymatic reactions ($1 - n$) and the rate differences between these reactions and elimination ($E_1 \ldots E_n$). One important concern is that the various forms of the CDS, including the direct precursor are inactive and nontoxic, thus allowing that the distributional processes will lead to the release of the active drug only at the site. This is summarized in Scheme 1 ("s" superscript indicates the site and superscript "r," the rest of the body).

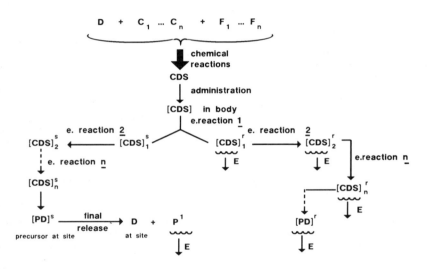

As a result of the design process, simple criteria can be represented as:

$$[CDS]_n^s \gg [CDS]_n^r; \qquad [PD]^s \gg [PD]^r$$

Thus, the concentrations of the important precursors and intermediates will be significantly higher at the site of action than in the rest of the body. This approach can allow not only the site-enhanced specific delivery, but also the sustained release of pharmacologically active concentrations at the active sites as desired. The drug released at the site will then produce the desired pharmacological activity, after which it will undergo the usual metabolism-elimination. By design, the ultimate [P'] and the intermediate moieties produced by the various enzymatic reactions should also be nontoxic and easily eliminated from the body.

Scheme 1 illustrates a general case when the CDS is based on enzymatic reactions producing preferential distribution and ultimate specific release of the drug at the site of action. The chemical approach, however, allows other types of delivery design as well. For example, a properly designed CDS can release the active drug at the site of action if the intermediate or final enzymatic reactions occur only at the site of action.

$$\text{CDS} \longrightarrow [\text{CDS}] \overset{\displaystyle \nearrow [\text{CDS}]_n^r \xrightarrow{\quad E \quad} \text{out}}{\underset{\displaystyle \searrow [\text{CDS}]_n^s \dashrightarrow [\text{PD}]^s \xrightarrow{\quad} \underset{\text{at site}}{D}}{}}$$

in body

This case is illustrated in Scheme 2. The drug is produced only at the site of action, as enzymatic reactions responsible for producing the drug do not take place at or, if they do, at a much lower rate in the rest of the body, than at the site. For example, enzymes present in the iris-ciliary body are used to produce the active drugs only at that site, which is the site of action, while the CDS distributed throughout the rest of body will not produce the active drug.[3,4]

The concept of site-specific chemical delivery systems represents a significant step forward from the original prodrug concept. While a prodrug,[5] a direct chemical precursor of a drug, can significantly alter overall delivery properties of a drug by modifying its lipophilicity, release, or metabolism, a prodrug in general cannot solve the site- and organ-specific delivery problems.

THE CONCEPT OF BRAIN-SPECIFIC DRUG DELIVERY BASED ON REDOX SYSTEMS

The brain, the major organ in the body, has a unique protective barrier, the so-called blood-brain barrier (BBB), which provides a very efficient exclusion from the brain of a wide variety of blood-borne compounds.[6–8] The basic morphologic feature of the BBB is the presence of epithelial-like, high resistance-type junctions that fuse brain capillaries and epithelia together into a continuous cellular layer separating blood and brain interstitial space. In addition, due to the lack of fenestrae and vesicular traffic in the brain capillary endothelia, the free flow between brain interstitium and the blood is restricted. What this means is that this lipid-like barrier prevents penetration into the brain of hydrophilic compounds (various neurotransmitters, amino acids, etc.) unless they are transported into the brain by an active transport system. The blood-brain barrier contains highly active enzyme systems as well, which further enhance the already very effective protective function. It is recognized that transport of molecules to the brain is not determined solely by molecular size but by the permeabilities governed by specific chemical characteristics of the permeating substance. Thus, besides the molecular size and lipophilicity, the affinity of the substances to various blood proteins, specific enzymes in the blood, or the BBB will very much influence the amount of the drug reaching the brain. While the blood-brain barrier is highly impermeable to a variety of compounds, such as neurotransmitters, when these are injected into the blood stream, this impermeability prevents their loss to blood plasma after their synthesis in the brain. This function actually confines the neurotransmitters to near their site of release and action.

The recognition that the BBB should act as a barrier against the efflux of hydrophilic molecules formed *in situ* in the brain[9] led to the idea of developing a brain-enhanced or brain-specific drug-delivery system.[10] The basic concept is a simple physical-chemical one, which fits very well into Scheme 1. That is, if by an enzymatic process, ubiquitous in nature, a lipophilic molecule that can penetrate the BBB is converted into a hydrophilic compound, then its efflux from the brain will be hindered, while at the same time its elimination from the overall system is accelerated.[10] Clearly, the most dramatic change that can occur in the physical-chemical properties of a molecule is to acquire a permanent charge. This generally will lead to about a 4-log unit change in the partition coefficient, providing a truly dramatic difference in membrane permeability of the compound. According to the CDS concept, this change in physical-chemical properties should occur on the carrier part of the molecule, that is, the enzymatic modification of the properties of the whole molecule should not affect ultimately the pharmacologically active compound to be delivered. Finally, the active drug species should be released from the newly formed hydrophilic precursor, and the carrier moiety separated should not be toxic and should also be quickly eliminated from the brain. That is, while the drug-carrier charged precursor should be locked in the brain, the charged, hydrophilic carrier, upon cleavage, should be easily eliminated from the brain.

In order to satisfy all necessary requirements, we have concentrated on a dihydropyridine-quaternary pyridinium salt-type redox system, which is analogous to the ubiquitous $NAD^+ \rightleftharpoons NADH$ coenzyme system. The idea was that if we can introduce a covalently bound but bioreversible redox moiety of this type, the ubiquitous conversion of the initial lipophilic form to the very hydrophilic charged species is assured. For this reason, the N_1-substituted nicotinic acid amides and esters were the first choice to provide the site-specific delivery. The system is summarized in a simplistic way in Scheme 3, where D represents the drug converted via various

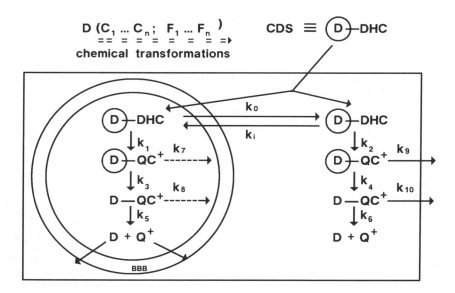

chemical transformations involving the redox carrier, and if necessary other protective moieties, into a chemical delivery system described as D-DHC. The circle around the drug D represents additional protective or modifying functions. This species is lipophilic, that is, lipophilic enough that after administration it will easily distribute throughout the body, including the brain. As with other compounds that penetrate the BBB, this lipophilic species is in continuous equilibration between the brain and the whole body, as long as it is present. The lipophilic dihydropyridine-type carrier is converted throughout the body into the charged quaternary pyridinium form represented by the ⓓ-QC$^+$. This intermediate is now already locked in the brain. At the same time its elimination from the general circulatory system is very much accelerated due to its suddenly acquired high hydrophilicity. After shedding any additional protective functions (ⓓ-QC$^+$ → D-QC$^+$), the D-QC$^+$, the direct precursor of the drug, is formed in the brain and it is still "locked in." To the extent of the same deprotection taking place in the body, some of the D-QC$^+$ is also forming there. This part is, however, eliminated even faster than the previous species (ⓓ-QC$^+$) due to the further increased hydrophilicity. If the rate of oxidative conversion of the ⓓ-DHC (corresponding rate constant k^1) is relatively slow (in general, a half-life of 20 to 50 minutes), the brain concentration of the locked-in species containing the QC$^+$ form of carrier will increase beyond the initial concentration of the ⓓ-DHC, due to the charged form being taken out of the facile distributional blood-brain equilibrium of ⓓ-DHC. What this means is that against the concentration gradient, one can increase the concentration in the brain of the locked-in species ⓓ-QC$^+$ and D-QC$^+$ until practically all the initial CDS is consumed. Generally, when this point is reached, the peripheral concentrations have substantially decreased. Thus, after a relatively short time following administration, there is a very favorable brain versus blood distributional ratio of the still inactive precursor form. Finally, the drug is released in a sustained manner from the locked-in precursor in the brain, producing the desired pharmacological activity. However, in the peripheries very little free drug will be released due to the fact that the hydrophilic charged precursors are quickly eliminated.

The use of this brain-specific redox chemical delivery system has now been successfully demonstrated for a large number of compounds. The substrates for this delivery system can be divided into two major categories. In the first class, are compounds that have difficulties in penetrating the brain, such as neurotransmitters like dopamine and GABA, which do not cross the BBB at all, antiviral agents like trifluorothymidine (TFT), or antiinfective agents like most penicillins, cephalosporins, and others. The advantage of using the delivery system approach for these compounds is quite clear. In the second class are compounds that readily penetrate the BBB. These compounds can also greatly benefit from this approach, as a substantial and effective separation of the brain from the rest of the body will allow reduction of peripheral effects and toxicity. For example, steroid hormones like estradiol, or various antiepileptic drugs like phenytoin or valproic acid, can show dramatic improvement in the brain-blood concentration ratio. Ultimately, all CNS active compounds can benefit from this approach by providing a sustained release of them in the brain and, on the other hand, by cutting off the initial peak brain concentrations. Thus, one can expect in most cases that even the central toxicity will be reduced.

CNS DELIVERY OF SOME NEUROTRANSMITTERS USING THE REDOX SYSTEM

The case of dopamine delivery illustrates very well how the concept works. As shown in Scheme 4, dopamine is converted into the CDS 2 and 3 in which the sensitive catechol is also protected by esterification, while the dihydrotrigonelline is hooked to the amine function of dopamine.[11] According to the general CDS concept, following administration of 2 or 3, sequential hydrolytic steps and oxidative conversion of the redox carrier part take place, leading ultimately to the locked-in direct precursor 5. Further cleavage of this compound leads to the release of dopamine in the brain.

Detailed studies have indicated that after i.v. dosing of the CDS 2 to rats, at 40 min following administration there is already about a 15-fold difference in the brain versus

R=COC(CH$_3$)$_3$ 2
    COCH(CH$_3$)$_2$ 3

R$_1$ or R$_2$ = R or H

blood concentration of compound **5**. Very high actual concentrations of **5** can be achieved in the brain, and the brain concentrations decrease relatively slowly allowing, thus, a very significant and prolonged central dopaminergic activity to be achieved. A 1 mg/kg dose of **2** resulted in about an 80% decrease in the serum prolactin levels, the effect of which lasted for over 12 hr.[12] Subsequent studies have clearly demonstrated that this is not due to circulating **5** (which is inactive and disappears quickly from the blood) or to the central action of **5** itself. Direct evidence was also provided for the release of dopamine in the brain.[13] In this experiment, following administration of the CDSs **2** and **3** and dopamine itself, 30 min later the aromatic amino acid decarboxylase inhibitor, m-hydroxybenzylhydrazine (NSD-1015) was given to block formation of endogenous **1** in the brain. While administration of dopamine did not alter the brain concentration of **1** or its major metabolites, dihydroxyphenylacetic acid (DOPAC, **6**) and homovanillic acid (HVA, **7**) in the striatum or hypothalamus, **2** and **3** caused about a 20% increase in striatal levels of **1** and a dramatic 4- to 5-fold increase in hypothalamic levels of **1**. As expected, concentrations of **6** were increased in both the striatum and hypothalamus after **2** and **3**, while levels of **7** were increased in the hypothalamus and decreased in the striatum. A summary of these data can be seen in TABLE 1. The observed regional differences in concentrations of **1** in response to **2** or **3** were explained in terms of the differences in nerve terminal composition of the striatum and the hypothalamus.

Another major neurotransmitter, GABA (**8**), was converted among others to the CDS **9**, where the dihydrotrigonelline carrier was put on the amine function similarly to the dopamine case, while the carboxy function was protected in the form of a benzyl ester.[14] Interestingly, this GABA delivery system showed significant CNS activity both as an anticonvulsant (ED$_{50}$ ~25 mg/kg by the bicuculline-induced convulsions) but the GABA-CDS, **9**, showed very significant anxiolytic activity.[15] The paradigm of shock-induced suppression of drinking in naive rats was used to determine the

TABLE 1. Comparison of the Concentrations of Dopamine (**1**) and Its Major Metabolites in Relevant Brain Tissues at One Hour Following Intravenous Administration of Dopamine (**1**) and Its CDSs **2** and **3a**[a]

Drug	Dose (μmol/kg)	N	DA	DOPAC(6)	HVA(7)
			Hypothalamus		
Control	1	13	2.27 ± 0.25	0.18 ± 0.04	0.25 ± 0.04
Dopamine (**1**)	17.5	7	2.27 ± 0.31	0.19 ± 0.02	0.28 ± 0.04
DA-CDS (**2**)	68	7	9.83 ± 3.71[c]	1.09 ± 0.22[c]	0.31 ± 0.04
DA-CDS (**3**)	72	7	10.40 ± 5.54[c]	0.82 ± 0.13[c]	0.33 ± 0.03
			Striatum		
Control	1	13	64.4 ± 6.78	2.39 ± 0.72	4.19 ± 0.73
Dopamine (**1**)	17.5	7	62.1 ± 3.20	1.99 ± 0.31	3.96 ± 0.42
DA-CDS (**2**)	68	7	75.5 ± 5.87[c]	12.03 ± 1.18[c]	1.87 ± 0.24[c]
DA-CDS (**3**)	72	7	81.5 ± 2.94[c]	9.15 ± 1.16[c]	1.52 ± 0.18[c]

[a]NSD 1015 (100 mg/kg i.p.) was administered 30 min after administration of the drugs, in order to block synthesis of dopamine in the brain.
[b]Dopamine could not be given at equivalent concentration with **2** and **3**, due to its toxicity.
[c]$p = 0.05$ Mann-Whitney.

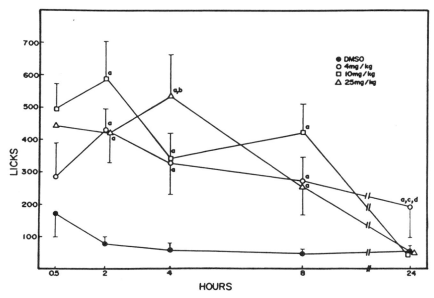

FIGURE 1. Effect of G-DH (**9**) on the anxiolytic response of naive male rats administered either 0, 4, 10, or 25 mg/kg body weight or the control vehicle (DMS). The number of animals used in each treatment group was 5–9. The number of licks were determined by multiplying the total number of sec of drinking per 3 min by a factor of 7. Each symbol represents the mean ± SEM. Analyses were performed by ANOVA and Student-Newman-Keuls statistics and level of significance chosen was $p < 0.05$. The letters indicate the following differences: (a) different from DMSO; (b) different from 4 mg/kg; (c) different from 10 mg/kg; and (d) different from 25 mg/kg.

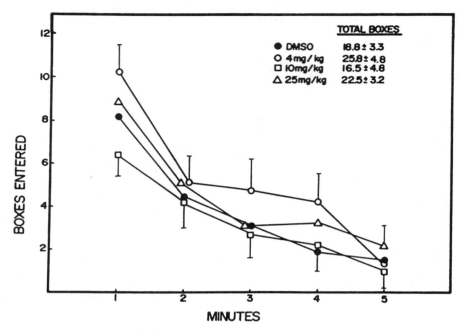

FIGURE 2. Assessment of sedation of male rats 2 hours after the administration of G-DH (**9**) dose of either 4, 10, 25 mg/kg or the control vehicle DMSO. The number of boxes entered indicates the number of squares that an animal places its feet/min for a 5 min test period. Analyses were performed by ANOVA and Student-Newman-Keuls statistics ($N = 8$; $p < 0.05$).

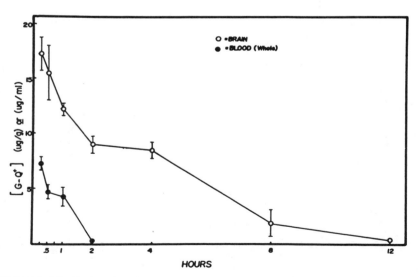

FIGURE 3. Distribution of the hydrophilic quaternary salt, G-O⁺ (**10**), in the brain and whole blood after an intravenous injection of the GABA-CDS, G-DH (**9**). After one injection, the lipophilic dihydropyridine compound rapidly enters the brain and is oxidized. The quaternary salt is found in the brain for up to 12 hr and the half-life for disappearance is 2.3 hr. The disappearance of this compound with time is attributed to ester hydrolysis and efflux from the brain. No **9** could be detected in the blood after 60 min.

anxiolytic activity. As shown in FIGURE 1, the delivery system G-DH (9) produced maximum anxiolysis at about 10 mg/kg, but interestingly at the three dose levels tested, 9 had no sedative activity (FIGURE 2). The observed CNS activity is consistent with the distribution of the locked-in form $(G-Q^+ 10)$ in the brain and whole blood (FIGURE 3). While the G-DH, 9, was very effective, neither GABA nor the $G-Q^+$ form showed any activity when injected intravenously. The delivery form G-DH did not show any analgesic activity.

BRAIN DELIVERY OF SELECTED DRUGS

In addition to neurotransmitters, various drugs have difficulty reaching the brain or producing a sustained pharmacologically active concentration level there. Most antiviral agents belong to this class. Herpes simplex virus (HSV) encephalitis is a devastating disease that is notoriously difficult to diagnose and has a mortality rate of over 70% if untreated.[16] Therapy with acyclovir reduces this mortality to the range of about 30%, but an additional 30 to 40% of survivors have significant neurologic sequelae.[17,18] Trifluorothymidine (TFT), 11, was converted to the CDS 12, which after administration to rats at 25 mg/kg dose, resulted in 16 μg/g brain concentration in rats, at 4 hr after administration.[19]

TFT   11   12   13

As a result of this, the concentration of the plaque-forming units of HSV-1 in the infected brains of mice was significantly reduced when the animals were treated with the CDS 12.[19] The more important antiviral agent, acyclovir (14), which exhibits a high potency and selectivity for HSV viruses but low toxicity, was also converted to the corresponding CDS 15. Transport of acyclovir into the brain is an important factor in treating viral infections. Under normal circumstances, only a very small amount of acyclovir is delivered into the brain by repeated intravenous administration of the drug using an infusion pump. In our laboratories, when 13 mg/kg dose of acyclovir itself was administered as an i.v. bolus, the acyclovir levels in the brain at any time interval following administration were undetectable, while appreciable levels were found, as expected, in the blood, liver, and kidney. An equimolar dose of the CDS 15 resulted in a dramatic difference in the brain delivery. As shown in FIGURE 4, significant concentrations (up to 5 μg/g) of the locked-in form 16 could be detected, and the levels of this precursor were maintained at 2 μg/g even 2 days following the administration. As a result of this and due to the hydrolytic cleavage of the locked-in 16, significant and

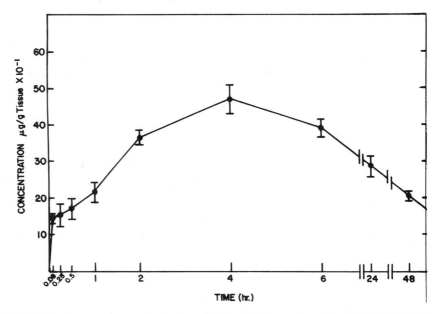

FIGURE 4. Appearance in rat brain tissue of "locked-in" form of acyclovir-CDS (**16**), following i.v. administration of the AC-CDS (**15**) at 20 mg/kg dose.

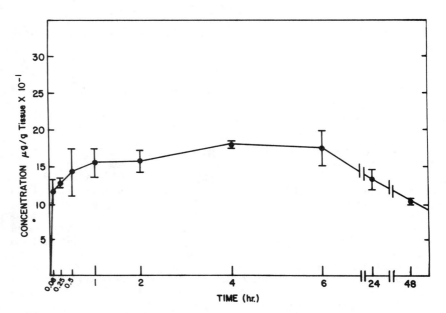

FIGURE 5. Appearance in rat brain tissue of free acyclovir (**14**) following administration of 20 mg/kg dose of **15**. The same groups of animals were studied as for **16** (FIG. 4).

sustained levels of the free acyclovir (**14**) were found in the brain of the same animals again even at 2 days following administration (FIGURE 5). The case of acyclovir demonstrates the two very important features of this redox system. On the one hand, by coupling the dihydrotrigonelline function to acyclovir, the resulting CDS **15** is more lipophilic than **14** itself (**15** is about 30 times more lipophilic than **14**). Accordingly, **15** penetrates the brain more easily. On the other hand, oxidative conversion of **15** to **16** results in an effective lock-in of this intermediate, which then provides a source for the sustained release of the active acyclovir.

The brain delivery of a very important class of antibiotics was recently demonstrated using some modified versions of the redox delivery system. The case can be illustrated by penicillin G (**17**, not shown), which was converted to the delivery system **18**, inserting a hydrolytically labile function between the carboxy group of penicillin and the carboxy group of the dihydrotrigonelline. The delivery studies were conducted on dogs, which were administered by the i.v. route 10 mg/kg penicillin G and an equimolar dose of the delivery system **18**, respectively.

As shown in FIGURE 6, there is practically no penicillin G found at any time interval in the cerebral spinal fluid (CSF) of the dogs after the penicillin G was

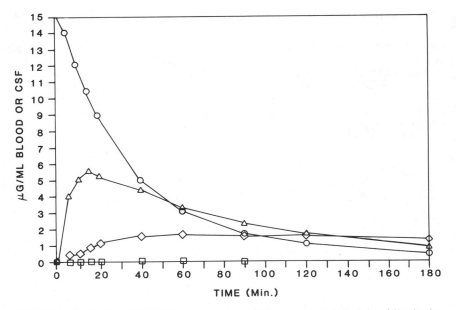

FIGURE 6. Blood (○) and CSF (□) concentrations of benzylpenicillin (**17**) in dog, following i.v. administration of a 10 mg/kg dose of benzylpenicillin (**17**), and blood (△) and CSF (◇) concentrations of **17** following i.v. administration of the P-CDS **18**, at dose equivalent to 10 mg/kg **17**. The same dogs were used in both experiments.

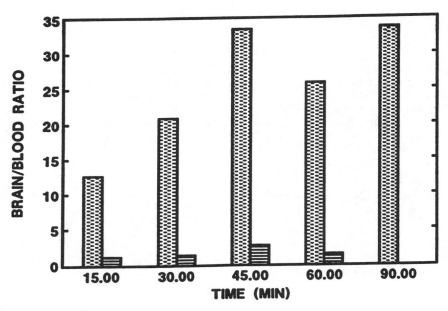

FIGURE 7. Brain/blood concentrations ratio (▤) of CCNU-OH (**19**) after its i.v. administration to rats and brain/blood concentrations ratio (▨) of the "locked-in" form **21** after administration of the CDS for CCNU-OH (**20**).

administered. On the other hand, the delivery system **18** resulted in lower blood levels but significantly higher and sustained CSF levels of the active penicillin.[21]

The use of the brain-specific drug delivery system provides a very important potential for the treatment of brain tumors. Although many systemically administered anticancer agents have been proven effective against peripheral tumors, there are very few examples of these drugs showing activity against either primary brain tumors or against metastatic tumors from cell lines that are susceptible to chemotherapy extracerebrally. The major problem associated with the treatment of tumors of the CNS is drug delivery to the tumor site. The (2-chloroethyl) nitrosoureas are among the most effective antitumor agents with demonstrated clinical activity against a variety of malignant diseases,[22] particularly brain tumors.[23] However, the high lipid solubility of nitrosoureas, which enables them to achieve a high CSF–plasma ratio, would not suffice to achieve significant levels of the drug in the tumor because of the intracellular and transcapillary exchange. The first compound in this class selected for the application of the delivery system was hydroxy cyclohexylchloroethylnitrosourea (hydroxy CCNU), **19.** The brain-to-blood ratios achieved with the basic nitrosourea **19** were compared to those obtained for the corresponding locked-in form **21,** at equimolar doses. The results (FIGURE 7) clearly demonstrate the dramatic effects obtained when this anticancer agent is hooked to the redox delivery system.[24]

SUSTAINED BRAIN-SPECIFIC DELIVERY OF ESTRADIOL CAUSES LONG-TERM EFFECTS

It is known that most steroid hormones readily pass into and out of the brain due to their lipophilicity. However, the necessary blood-brain equilibrium has limited their usefulness in treating brain-specific steroid deprivation syndromes. Also, the use of steroidal hormones to achieve reduction in gonadotropin secretion for achieving contraception or for the treatment of steroid-dependent diseases, such as endometriosis and prostatic hypertrophy, is limited by the unwanted peripheral side effects of these hormones. For this reason a variety of steroid hormones were recently studied for brain delivery using the redox delivery system. One of the most interesting cases is estradiol (22). It was converted to the CDS 23, which was found to cross readily the BBB and be converted to the corresponding hydrophilic quaternary pyridinium salt 24.[25] Kinetic studies have shown again the sustained presence of 24 in the brain while from all other organs the compound is eliminated rather easily. To evaluate the pharmacological effect of this unique system, the response of luteinizing hormone (LH) was studied. Using orchidectomized male rats, it was found that both estradiol (22) and the CDS (23) reduced serum LH concentrations equivalently by 68 to 79% from 4 to 48 hr. From 4 to 12 days after drug administration, the LH levels in estradiol-treated animals increased progressively to levels equivalent to those in the control rats. By contrast, LH concentrations in animals treated with 23 continued to be suppressed by 82, 88, and 90% when compared to control values at 4, 8, and 12 days after treatment, respectively. When estradiol was again compared to 23 in similar studies extended to 12 to 24 days after administration, it was found that while estradiol did not suppress serum LH from 12 to 24 days after a single intravenous injection, the CDS 23 reduced LH concentrations by 88, 86, and 66% relative to controls at 12, 18, and 24 days, respectively.[26]

TABLE 2 summarizes these results together with the serum concentrations of estradiol. It can be seen that estradiol blood concentrations were not different among treatment groups. Thus, a persistent elevation in circulating concentrations of estradiol subsequent to administration of compound 23 was not responsible for the observed chronic suppression of LH release. Rather, local release of estradiol in the brain, and in particular the hypothalamus, would appear to be responsible for the sustained suppression of LH release. It must be emphasized again that while the lipophilic character of the dihydropyridine derivative 23 facilitates brain delivery, this alone is not enough for the prolonged action. Thus, the "lock-in" of the positively charged form 24 is the major conceptual difference from the usual lipophilic "prodrug" approach.

The estradiol-CDS for the first time provided an insight of the central versus peripheral site of action of this gonadal steroid in behavioral and physiological processes. Thus, recent studies[27] were performed to study the effects of the estradiol-

TABLE 2. Serum Concentrations of LH and Estradiol after Intravenous Administration of DMSO, Estradiol (E_2), or Compound **23** in Orchidectomized Rats[a]

Drug	Days After Drug Administration		
	12	18	24
	Serum LH (ng/ml)		
DMSO	6.8 ± 0.08 (7)[b]	12.4 ± 2.5 (7)	8.6 ± 1.7 (7)
Estradiol (2.1 mg/kg)	12.9 ± 1.7 (6)[d,e]	12.1 ± 0.9 (6)	11.6 ± 1.4 (7)
23 (3.0 mg/kg)	0.8 ± 0.7 (7)[e]	1.7 ± 0.7 (7)[e]	2.9 ± 1.1 (7)[e]
	Serum E_2 (pg/ml)		
DMSO	27.5 ± 3.8 (4/7)[c]	<20 (7/7)	24.4 ± 3.3 (4/7)
Estradiol (2.1 mg/kg)	29.3 ± 5.9 (4/6)	<20 (6/6)	31.2 ± 8.6
23 (3.0 mg/kg)	25.9 ± 3.9 (5/7)	<20 (7/7)	24.1 ± 3.2 (5/7)

[a]Animals were killed by decapitation, and serum was assayed for LH and estradiol in duplicate.
[b]Mean ± SEM (number of animals per group).
[c]Mean ± SEM (number of samples that were below the sensitivity limits of the assay (20 pg/ml) number of animals per group.
[d]Significantly ($p < 0.05$) different from both other groups.
[e]Significantly ($p < 0.05$) different from DMSO control group.

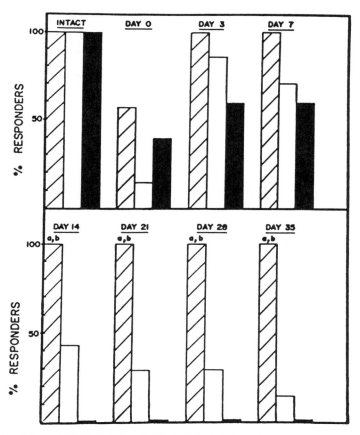

FIGURE 8. Effect of E2-CDS (**23**) (▨), E2-VAL (**25**) (□), and DMSO (■) on the mounting percentage (percent responders) in castrated male rats from day 0 to day 35 after a single i.v. injection. Groups were analyzed by the Fisher exact test and differences ($p < 0.05$) from control are depicted by (a) and from E2-VAL by (b).

CDS (E_2-CDS) versus an equimolar dose of estradiol-17-valerate (E_2-VAL, **25**) on copulatory behavior in orchidectomized rats. The data revealed that a single dose of E_2-CDS (**23**) was much more efficacious than E_2-VAL (**25**) in stimulating mounting behavior (percent responding), and the effect was 100% through 5 weeks. This is shown in FIGURE 8. The estradiol-CDS has also increased intromission behavior more than the control compound **25** through 28 days, as shown in FIGURE 9. Mount and

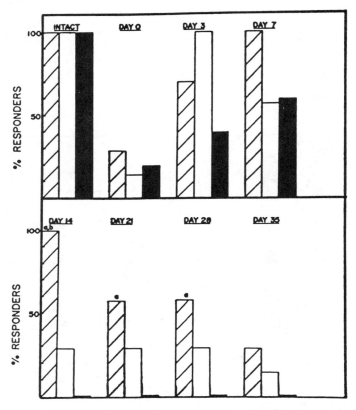

FIGURE 9. Effect of E2-CDS (**23**) (▨), E2-VAL (**25**) (□), and DMSO (■) on the intromission percentage (percent responders) in castrated male rats from day 0 to day 35 after a single i.v. injection. Groups were analyzed by the Fisher exact test and group differences are indicated by (a) (different from control) and by (b) (different from E2-VAL).

intromission latencies were also reduced by **23** for at least 28 days. These data suggest that the E_2-CDS causes a potent and long-acting stimulation of the proceptive components of male sexual behavior presumably acting through the local brain release of estradiol.

Since gonadal steroids are believed to influence a variety of actions of the CNS, this and analogous steroid delivery systems may have uses beyond those related to regulation of gonadatropin secretion.

CONCLUSIONS

The usefulness of the dihydropyridine-pyridinium salt-type redox system for brain-enhanced and brain-specific delivery of a wide variety of pharmacologically active compounds was demonstrated recently. This method provides a good example of significant improvement in therapeutic index of drugs by separating the active site from the rest of the body.

ACKNOWLEDGMENTS

Special thanks are extended to Laurie Johnston and Joan Martignago for their help in the preparation of the manuscript.

REFERENCES

1. BODOR, N. 1984. Novel approaches to the design of safer drugs: Soft drugs and site-specific chemical delivery systems. *In* Advances in Drug Research. B. Testa, Ed. **13:** 255–331. Academic Press. London.
2. BODOR, N. & H. FARAG. 1983. Improved delivery through biological membranes 11. A redox chemical drug delivery system and its use for brain specific delivery of phenylethylamine. J. Med. Chem. **26:** 313–318.
3. BODOR, N. & G. VISOR. 1984. Formation of adrenaline in the iris-ciliary body from adrenalone diesters. Exp. Eye Res. **38:** 621–626.
4. EL-KOUSSI, A. & N. BODOR. 1987. Formation of propranolol in the iris-ciliary body from its propranolol ketoxime precursor—a potential antiglaucoma drug. Exp. Eye. Res.
5. SINKULA, A. A. & S. H. YALKOWSKY. 1975. Rationale for design of biologically reversible drug derivatives prodrugs. J. Pharm. Sci. **64:** 181–210.
6. PARDRIDGE, W. M., J. D. CONNOR & I. L. CRAWFORD. 1975. Permeability changes in the blood-brain barrier: causes and consequences. CRC Crit. Rev. Toxic. **3:** 159–199.
7. RAPOPORT, S. I. 1976. The blood-brain barrier in physiology and medicine. Raven Press. New York.
8. BODOR, N. & M. BREWSTER. 1983. Problems of delivery of drugs to the brain. Pharm. Ther. **19:** 337–389.
9. BODOR, N., R. ROLLER & S. SELK. 1978. Elimination of a quaternary pyridinum salt delivered derivative from brain of mice. J. Pharm. Sci. **67:** 685–687.
10. BODOR, N., H. FARAG & M. BREWSTER. 1981. Site-specific and/or sustained release of drugs to the brain. Science **214:** 1370–1372.
11. BODOR, N. & H. FARAG. 1983. Improved delivery through biological membranes 13. Brain-specific delivery of dopamine with a dihydropyridine $\rightleftharpoons$ pyridinium salt type redox delivery system. J. Med. Chem. **26:** 528–534.
12. BODOR, N. & J. SIMPKINS. 1983. Redox delivery system for brain-specific, sustained release of dopamine. Science **221**(4605): 65–67.
13. SIMPKINS, J., N. BODOR & A. ENZ. 1985. Direct evidence for brain-specific release of dopamine from a redox delivery system. J. Pharm. Sci. 1033–1036.
14. WOODARD, P., D. WINWOOD, M. BREWSTER & N. BODOR. 1986. Improved delivery through biological membranes XXI. Design, synthesis and antiseizure activity of brain-specific anticonvulsive agents.
15. ANDERSON, W., J. SIMPKINS, P. WOODARD, D. WINWOOD, W. STERN & N. BODOR. 1987. Anxiolytic activity of a brain delivery system for GABA. Psychopharmacology **92**(2): 157–163.
16. WHITLEY, R. J., S. SOONG, R. DOLIN, G. T. GORLASSO, L. T. CHIEN & C. A. ALFORD. 1977. Adenine arabinoside therapy of biopsy-proved herpes simplex encephalitis. New Eng. J. Med. **297:** 289–294.

17. SKOLDENBERG, B. *et al.* 1984. Acyclovir versus vidarabine in herpes simplex encephalitis. Lancet **ii:** 707–712.
18. WHITLEY, R. J. *et al.* 1986. The NIAID collaborative antiviral study group. Vidarabine versus acyclovir therapy in herpes simplex encephalitis. New Eng. J. Med. **314:** 144–149.
19. RAND, K., N. BODOR, A. EL-KOUSSI, I. RAAD, A. MIYAKE, H. HOUCK & N. GILDERSLEEVE. 1986. Potential treatment of herpes simplex virus encephalitis by brain-specific delivery of trifluorothymidine using a dihydropyridine ⇌ pyridinium salt type redox delivery system. J. Med. Virology **20:** 1–8.
20. VENKATRAGHAVAN, V., M. E. BREWSTER, E. SHEK & N. BODOR. 1987. A brain-specific chemical delivery system for acyclovir.
21. WU, W., E. POP & N. BODOR. 1987. Brain delivery of penicillin G to dogs using a redox system.
22. AHMANN, D. L. 1976. Nitrosourea in the management of disseminated malignant melanoma. Cancer Treat. Rep. **60:** 747–760.
23. LEVIN, V. A. & C. B. WILSON. 1976. Nitrosourea chemotherapy for primary malignant gliomas. Cancer Treat. Rep. **60:** 719–726.
24. RAGHAVAN, K., E. SHEK & N. BODOR. 1987. Improved delivery through biological membranes XXX. Synthesis and biological aspects of 1,4-dihydropyridine based chemical delivery system for brain-sustained delivery of hydroxy CCNU. Anti-Cancer Drug Design **2:** 25–36.
25. BODOR, N., J. MCCORNACK & M. BREWSTER. 1987. Improved delivery through biological membranes XXII. Synthesis and distribution of brain-selective estrogen delivery systems. Int. J. Pharm. **1:** 275–283.
26. SIMPKINS, J., J. MCCORNACK, K. ESTES, M. BREWSTER, E. SHEK & N. BODOR. 1986. Sustained brain-specific delivery of estradiol causes long-term suppression of luteinizing hormone secretion. J. Med. Chem. 1809–1812.
27. ANDERSON, W., J. SIMPKINS, M. BREWSTER & N. BODOR. 1986. Evidence for the reestablishment of copulatory behavior in castrated male rats with a brain-enhanced estradiol-chemical delivery system. Pharmacol. Biochem. Behav. **27:** 265–271.

Bioadhesive Polymers for Controlled Drug Delivery

JOSEPH R. ROBINSON, MARK A. LONGER,
AND MICHEL VEILLARD

School of Pharmacy
University of Wisconsin
Madison, Wisconsin 53706

Bioadhesion may be defined[1] as the state in which two materials, at least one of which is of a biological nature, are held together for an extended period of time by interfacial forces. Thus, attachment of a biological object to another biological object, e.g., cell attachment, or a synthetic polymer to a biological substrate, e.g., denture fixative, are examples of bioadhesion. For drug delivery purposes the term bioadhesion infers attachment of a drug carrier system to a specific biological location. The biological surface can be epithelial tissue or it can be the mucous coat on the surface of the tissue. If adhesive attachment is to the mucin coat the phenomena is referred to as mucoadhesion. Bioadhesion can be modeled after bacterial attachment to tissue surfaces and mucoadhesion can be modeled after mucin organization on epithelial tissue.

Earlier work by Nagai[2] has shown that mucoadhesion can be used as a platform for delivery of drugs locally to the mouth or to the cervix with concomitant improvement in therapy or, alternatively, a decrease in body load of the drug. A number of workers[3–5] have been exploring both the mechanism(s) of adhesion as well as ways to utilize mucoadhesion as a platform for both local and systemic delivery of drugs. This presentation will review the concept of mucoadhesion with emphasis on attachment of polyanionic swelling hydrogels. In addition, it will review some of the recent applications of mucoadhesion with particular emphasis on buccal delivery.

MECHANISM(S) OF MUCOADHESION

Orifices of the body into which drugs are placed have a coating of mucin over the epithelial tissue. The coating varies in thickness and chemical composition in these areas but all are capable of picking up about 30–50 times their weight of water and all are highly organized on the surface of the tissue. Mucin itself consists of a protein backbone with pendant sugar groups at appropriate locations. Characteristic of mucins is that they are heavily populated with an anionic charge as a result of sialic acid or sulfonic acid residues. Hence, mucin can be viewed as a polyelectrolyte with a high charge density holding an enormous quantity of water.

Using the attachment of mucin to the epithelial surface as a model, a number of charged and neutral polymers can attach very well to the mucin through non-covalent bonds to establish an essentially irreversible attachment. Numerous polymers have been examined for such attachment[3,6] and both polycationic and polyanionic polymers show strong attachment. The polyanionic polymers, such as the lightly crosslinked polyacrylates, have been examined in some detail as to the mechanism of attachment to mucin. The following description outlines the current understanding of the mechanism of attachment of these polycarboxylic acids to mucin. (1) The polymer undergoes

TABLE 1. Relative Mucoadhesive Performance of Some Test Compounds

Substance	Mucoadhesive Force[a]	Adhesive Performance[b]
Carboxymethylcellulose	193	Excellent
Carbopol	185	Excellent
Polycarbophil	—	Excellent
Sodium alginate	126	Excellent
Gelatin	116	Fair
Pectin	100	Poor
Acacia	98	Poor
Povidone	98	Poor

[a]Percent of a standard, tested *in vitro*.[6]
[b]Assessed *in vivo*.[7]

swelling in water and this permits entanglement of the polymer chains with mucin on the surface of the tissue. (2) The unionized carboxylic acid groups on the polymer hydrogen bonds to the mucin molecule. A sufficiently high charge density on the polymer is necessary for both swelling and hydrogen bonding for firm attachment to occur.

Typically, the force of attachment of the adhesive polymer to mucin is sufficiently strong so that removal occurs primarily through mucin turnover, i.e., the weaker bond is the mucin-mucin rather than the mucin-polymer bond.

While a number of polymers will attach to mucin through both covalent and non-covalent bonds, non-covalent attachment is preferred given that the strength of attachment in many cases appears sufficiently strong to be considered essentially irreversible. In addition, while both water-soluble and water-insoluble polymers can be used it would appear that the lightly cross-linked and hence water swellable but still water-insoluble polymers are preferred as mucoadhesives given that they are not as easily removed from the site of application. Drug release from such systems should be easier to maintain and there should be less toxicity concerns for an insoluble polymer. The mucoadhesive polycarbophil (partial structure) is shown in scheme 1. Note that this is not a repeating unit since there is less than 0.2% crosslinking.

Representative mucoadhesive polymers are shown in TABLE 1. Note the correlation between mucoadhesive measurement and the subjective *in vivo* adhesive performance.

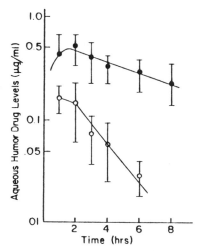

FIGURE 1. Progesterone levels in aqueous humor following topical administration of 0.3% suspension of progesterone-entrapped polymer (●) and 0.3% suspension of progesterone without polymer (○).

APPLICATION OF MUCOADHESIVES TO DRUG DELIVERY

A number of applications of mucoadhesives to drug delivery have already been reported. Nagai,[1] employing a water-soluble polymer, has shown that retention of drug delivery systems to the tongue, nasal area, and cervix leads to either an improved clinical picture for locally acting drugs or an increase in systemic absorption of drug. Other areas that have been explored are described below.

Ocular Drug Delivery

Topical delivery of drugs to the eye is significantly constrained by tear turnover, instilled solution drainage, and drug absorption into other than target tissues. Of these, drug loss through instilled solution drainage or tear turnover, i.e., clearance from the front of the eye, are the most important. Retaining the drug on the front of the eye' through the use of a mucoadhesive, which attaches to the conjunctival mucin, would substantially improve ocular drugs in terms of ocular drug bioavailability.[8]

FIGURE 1 shows progesterone levels in aqueous humor of albino rabbits in the

TABLE 2. Oral Mucosal Tissues Available for Bioadhesive Drug Delivery

Tissue	General Location
Buccal	Cheek
Sublingual	Ventral tongue; floor of mouth
Gingival	Gums surrounding teeth
Palatal	"Roof" of mouth

TABLE 3. Blood Flow in Various Regions of the Oral Mucosa of the Rhesus Monkey

Tissue	Blood Flow (ml/min/100 cm^2)
Buccal	2.40
Sublingual	
Floor of the mouth	0.97
Ventral tongue	1.17
Gingival[a]	1.47
Palatal[b]	0.89

[a]Average value of the anterior and posterior hard palatal mucosa.
[b]Average value of maxillary and mandibular attached gingival mucosa.
Data from Squier & Nanny. 1985. Archs. Oral Biol. 30:313.

presence and absence of a mucoadhesive polymer. Clearance of drug from the anterior segment of the eye is governed primarily by aqueous humor turnover and hence any prolongation of drug levels in this fluid would demonstrate a sustaining effect in the front of the eye. It is clear that the mucoadhesive substantially prolongs drug levels in the eye.

Oral Drug Delivery

The greatest practical use of mucoadhesives is for enterally administered drugs. Minimally, assuming successful retention at desired locations in the gastrointestinal tract, delaying gastrointestinal transit would lead to a decrease in dosing frequency, i.e., once daily administration. Similarly, targeting drugs locally would also be possible as would the ability to maintain a drug delivery system at a particular location for an extended period of time if it was desirable to alter tissue permeability or inhibit protease activity in a localized region.

Experiments in rats[9] showed unequivocally that mucoadhesive polymers were retained in the stomach for extended periods of time and that stomach emptying of mucoadhesive-treated particles was prolonged to more than a day. Furthermore, administering a poorly bioavailable test drug, chlorothiazide, with a mucoadhesive dosage form led to a substantial improvement in bioavailability for this drug.

TABLE 4. Some Characteristics of Human Oral Epithelia

Epithelium	Thickness (μ)	Keratinization	Membrane-Coating Granules
Buccal	767	—	+
Sublingual	168	—	+
Floor of mouth			
Ventral tongue	169	—	+
Gingival	193	+	+
Oral epithelium			
Junctional epithelium	—	—	—
Palatal	—	+	+

Data from Squier et al. 1975. Br. Med. Bull. 31:169. 1984. Arch. Oral Biol. 29:45.

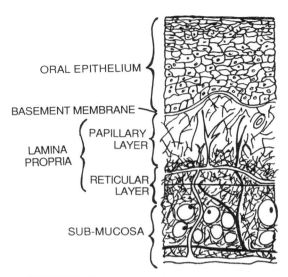

FIGURE 2. Representation of oral mucosal tissue.

When these experiments were repeated in dogs, less satisfactory results were obtained. The explanation for the difference in findings stems from the amount of soluble mucin in the stomach of the rat versus the dog. In the rat, there is very little soluble mucin so that an ingested mucoadhesive has an opportunity to adhere to the mucin-epithelial surface. In the dog, however, there is considerable soluble mucin in the stomach so that an ingested mucoadhesive would first encounter and be bound to the soluble mucin thus being unable to adhere to the mucin-epithelial surface.

Presumably, humans are between the dog and the rat in terms of the amount of stomach-soluble mucin and one expects a proportional degree of mucoadhesion. Strategies can be developed to overcome the soluble mucin issue, but to date there are no reports in the literature regarding successful approaches.

TABLE 5. Regional Differences in Permeability of Porcine Skin and Oral Mucosa to Water and Horseradish Peroxidase

	Thickness (μm)		Permeability[a] (cm/min)	
Tissue	Total Epithelium	Permeability Barrier	H_2O	Horseradish Peroxidase
Buccal	772	282	173	00
Sublingual				
Floor of mouth	192	23	1271	332
Gingival	208	35	98	79.5
Skin	69	16	21	9.4

[a]Expressed in terms of a uniform permeability barrier 100 μm thick.
Data from Squier & Hall. 1985. J. Invest. Dermatol. **84:**176.

TABLE 6. Plasma Thyrotropin and Prolactin Levels in Humans after Intravenous and Buccal Administration of TRH

	Intravenous Injection (200 μg)		Buccal Application (20 mg/10 cm² for 30 min)		
	0 min	30 min	0 min	30 min	60 min
Thyrotropin (μU/ml)	1.0–4.3	4.0–25.1	0.9–5.0	1.8–10.8	3.2–17.5
Prolactin (ng/ml)	3.0–18.2	7.6–44.0	5.2–14.8	11.7–35.7	13.1–31.4

Data from Anders & Merkle. 1983. J. Pharm. Sci. **72:**1481.

Buccal Drug Delivery

An available, but not extensively utilized area of the body for drug delivery, is the mouth. Some emergency drugs, e.g., nitroglycerin sublingual, are routinely used but it is presumably not considered a useful area for drug delivery despite its accessibility and reasonably good permeability characteristics.

TABLE 2 describes the tissues and general locations of potential drug delivery sites within the mouth. Blood flow to these regions is shown in TABLE 3 and some general characteristics of the membranes are shown in TABLE 4. As can be seen in TABLE 3, the buccal area is well perfused with blood, as are other areas of the mouth. The sublingual region, in particular, is of interest since the blood vessels are close to the surface. The general thicknesses of these membranes are averages and there is considerable difference at the low and high side of this average. Thus, for example, the buccal thickness varies from about 100 to 900 μm.

A pictorial representation of the buccal mucosa is shown in FIGURE 2. The lamina propria is well perfused with capillaries and the rate-limiting section of the membrane, the epithelium, is a non-keratinized tissue.

TABLE 5 provides some perspective on the permeability of the buccal area to water and horseradish peroxidase, as compared to skin. Note in this table that the data are normalized to a 100-μm thick barrier so that when thicknesses are taken into account, the buccal area appears to be about as permeable as skin.

From the permeability constants it would appear that the buccal area is capable of absorbing approximately 10–20 mg of a drug in a 24 hr period, assuming a 2 cm² surface is used.

To provide some additional perspective on buccal absorption of small molecules, TABLES 6 and 7 show that short exposure of buccal tissues to primitive drug delivery

TABLE 7. Plasma Isosorbide Dinitrate Levels in Humans after Buccal, Sublingual, and Palatal Administration

	Concentration (ng/ml)			
Tissue	1 min	5 min	15 min	30 min
Buccal	0.70	1.39	0.87	1.21
Sublingual	0.28	3.11	1.40	1.13
Palatal		undetected		

Data from Pimlott & Addy. 1985. Oral Surg. Oral Med. Oral Pathol. **59:**145.

systems permits relatively good systemic absorption of drugs. It is important to note that many studies exploring buccal absorption have employed drug delivery systems that are very primitive. Thus, it is common to soak a piece of filter paper with the drug and then impress this on the buccal tissue or perhaps place the drug in a dissolving system wherein the drug is released into the oral cavity and subsequently swallowed. It is assumed that a very good buccal drug delivery system, that maintains intimate contact with the absorbing surface, and permits drug to travel in only one direction, i.e., towards the tissue, would optimize the likelihood of the drug being absorbed through buccal tissue. Moreover, if it is necessary to modify buccal tissue permeability or inhibit protease activity, it is essential that the drug delivery system be localized.

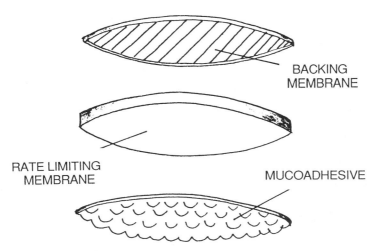

FIGURE 3. Prototype buccal mucoadhesive delivery system.

DEVELOPMENT OF A MUCOADHESIVE BUCCAL PATCH

In conjunction with scientists at 3M/Riker laboratories we have developed a buccal patch. FIGURE 3 shows a schematic of this patch. In dogs, the patch remains in place for approximately 17 hr, irrespective of food or drink consumed, and a similar finding was observed in humans. The presence of the polycarbophil permits tight attachment to the buccal mucosa. Because polycarbophil is a swelling hydrogel it imbibes water and is quite comfortable to wear for extended periods.

The rate-limiting membrane can be altered to accommodate a range of drug properties to generate a once daily delivery system. This is particularly attractive for drugs that undergo first-pass metabolism since buccal delivery bypasses first-pass metabolism and continuous delivery of such a drug would be an advantage.

Preliminary work on delivery of a small peptide is currently underway but preliminary data are not yet available.

REFERENCES

1. GOOD, R. J. 1976. Adhesion **8:** 1–9.
2. NAGAI, T. & Y. MACHIDA. 1985. Pharm. Int. **6:** 196–200.
3. PARK, K. & J. R. ROBINSON. 1984. Int. J. Pharm. **19:** 107–127.
4. PARK, H. & J. R. ROBINSON. 1985. J. Control. Release **2:** 47–57.
5. PEPPAS, N. A. & P. A. BURI. 1985. J. Control. Release **2:** 257–275.
6. SMART, J. D., I. W. KELLAWAY & E. C. WORTHINGTON. 1984. J. Pharm. Pharmacol. **36:** 295–299.
7. CHEN, J. L. & G. N. CYR. 1970. *In* Adhesion in Biological Systems. R. S. Manly, Ed. 163–181. Academic Press.
8. HUI, H.-W. & J. R. ROBINSON. 1986. J. Pharm. Sci. **75:** 280–287.
9. CH'NG, H. S., *et al.* 1985. J. Pharm. Sci. **74:** 399–411.

Utilizing Bile Acid Carrier Mechanisms to Enhance Liver and Small Intestine Absorption

N. F. H. HO

Drug Delivery Systems Research
The Upjohn Company
Kalamazoo, Michigan 49001

INTRODUCTION

Structural modifications of drug molecules aimed at delivering drugs to specific target tissues by oral or systemic administration may be accomplished by the prodrug approach, whereby the pro-moiety is an endogenous chemical structure and, therefore, is recognized as unique by the membrane carrier-mediated process of the target tissue. This research focuses on the derivatives and analogs of bile acids as novel molecular delivery system in the intestinal tract and the liver by exploiting the active transport mechanism for naturally occurring bile acids (FIGURE 1).

Small Intestinal and Liver Absorption of Bile Acids

Bile acids are absorbed passively *in vivo* in the duodenum and jejunum, but are absorbed both passively and actively in the ileum.[1] The total transport rate depends effectively on the pK_a of the acid and the pH of the solution. For this reason, taurine-conjugated bile acids ($pK_a \sim 2.0$) are absorbed principally within the ileal segment of the small intestine. For glycine-conjugated bile acids (pK_a 3–4) and unconjugated bile acids (pK_a 5), there is more significant contribution of the passive mechanism to the total transport rate in the ileum. Characteristic of active transport mechanisms, bile acids manifest concentration-dependent and Na-dependent transport rates leading to a maximum rate, which may be ascribed to saturation kinetics similar to the Michaelis-Menten kinetics for enzyme reactions. The rates are inhibited by anaerobiosis or the presence of metabolic inhibitors. Mutual inhibition between bile acids appears to follow kinetic behavior consistent with competition.[2,3] Dihydroxy bile acids are better competitive inhibitors than trihydroxy compounds. From a structural point of view, the Michaelis K_m is apparently related to whether the bile acid is conjugated or unconjugated: unconjugated > glycine conjugate ~taurine conjugate by a factor of two. For practical purposes, the K_m value is about 1 mM. The apparent maximum rates are independent of conjugated or unconjugated bile acids, but depend upon the number of hydroxyl groups: trihydroxyl ≫ dihydroxy > monohydroxy.

Following intestinal absorption, all bile acids are efficiently taken up by the liver, approximately 95% on first pass. Unconjugated bile acids are readily converted to the glycine and taurine conjugates with aid of coenzyme A in the liver so that normal bile consists of only conjugated species. The acids are stored in the gall bladder and ultimately flow into the duodenum via the common bile duct. The dynamics of bile acid absorption by the small intestine and liver and the circulation between them comprise the enterohepatic circulation of bile acids (FIGURE 2). Since the enterohepatic

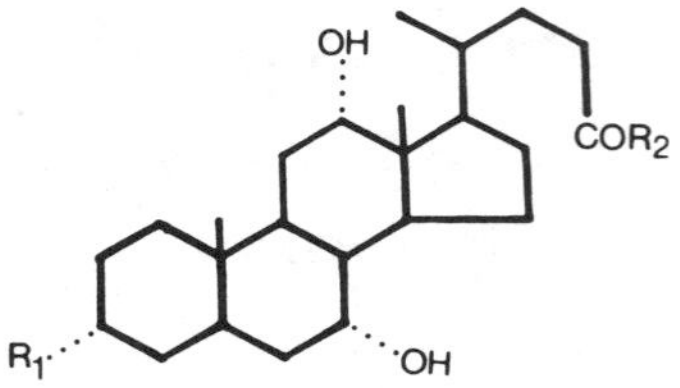

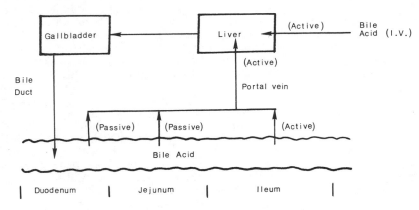

Bile Acid	R_1	R_2
Cholic	OH	OH
Taurocholic	OH	$-NHCH_2CH_2SO_3H$
Glycocholic	OH	$-NHCH_2COOH$

FIGURE 1. Trihydroxy bile acids.

circulation is a relatively closed system, endogenous bile acids are remarkably conserved. Only 10% of the total bile acids is lost in the feces per day. An insignificant amount is found in the peripheral circulatory system in normal humans. The finding of significant bile acid blood levels is indicative of some kind of liver dysfunction. The homeostatic mechanism of the liver mobilizes the bioconversion of cholesterol to bile acids to maintain the total bile acid pool.

On the basis of perfused isolated liver studies in rats, the mechanism of bile acid transport can be summarized as follows.[4–6] The initial step is the transport of bile acid from sinusoidal plasma into the hepatocyte. This is a Na^+-dependent, carrier-mediated mechanism, a saturable process that follows Michaelis-Menten kinetics. It has a capacity far exceeding the demands imposed by the enterohepatic circulation of bile acids. Competition for uptake among conjugated and nonconjugated bile acids is indicative of a common transport system for hepatic uptake. The second step is the movement of bile acid within the hepatocyte toward the bile canaliculi. Here, bile acids are conjugated with glycine and taurine, but conjugation is not essential for biliary excretion. Bile acid binding proteins in the sinusoidal membrane and liver cytosol

FIGURE 2. Schematic diagram of bile acid absorption.

appear to be involved in hepatic uptake and intracellular transport, but this has not been clearly elucidated. The third step is secretion into the bile canaliculi, which appears to be the rate-limiting step in the overall process of hepatic bile acid transport. It is postulated that bile acids are excreted by a carrier-mediated process at the canalicular membrane site.

Structure-Absorptivity Relationships of Bile Acids

Based on *in vitro* absorption studies with everted sacs of rat ileum and *in vitro* isolated liver uptake studies, several generalizations on the structural requirements of bile acids for active transport have been made.[4,7,8]

(1) No single hydroxyl group on the cholanic acid ring structure is essential for transport. (2) The requirement for a single negative charge (sulfonic or carboxylic acid moiety) applies to the region of the C_{17} side chain. Bile acids with two negative charges (dicarboxylic acid) give minimal active transport. However, the addition of an additional negative charge at the C_3 position of the ring structure does not preclude transport. No active transport is observed when the single negative charge on the side chain is replaced with a positive charge (quaternary ammonium group) or amphoteric group (lysine-type). Glycine and taurine conjugates show active transport activity. (3) Substitutions at the C_3 position (for example, 3-chloro-) do not appear to interfere with the active mechanism.

The structural requirements for active transport suggest that three components of interaction are cooperatively involved: (1) an interaction between the steroid part of the bile acid and the carrier; (2) coulombic interaction between the negatively charged side chain and a positively charged element in the membrane or carrier; and (3) a closely positioned function of negative charge on the carrier, which can interact with sodium ions. Although no specific hydroxyl group is required for critical interaction, it influences the interactions of the steroid in the hydrophobic space.[9]

Concept

Based on the rationale that conjugated and nonconjugated bile acids are rapidly and efficiently absorbed in the liver and, consequently, undergo enterohepatic cycling and that the essential molecular requirement of bile acids for active transport is the retention of its acidic side chain function at the 17-position of the ring system, it is postulated that C_3-derivatives and analogs of bile acids (C_3-esters of cholic acid, for example) may also undergo active transport. In other words, we want to exploit the active transport system for bile acids.

Many potential therapeutic applications are foreseen: improvement of the oral absorption of an intrinsically, biologically active, but poorly absorbed hydrophilic drug; liver site-directed delivery of a drug to bring about high therapeutic concentrations in the diseased liver with the minimization of general toxic reactions elsewhere in the body; and gallbladder-site delivery systems of cholecystographic agents and cholesterol gallstone dissolution accelerators.

RESULTS AND DISCUSSION

To establish the concept that bile acids are unique transport carriers of drugs (as C_3-derivatives and analogs of bile acids) across membranes in the intestinal tract and of liver cells, 3-tosylcholic, 3-benzoylcholic, and 3-iodocholic acids were radiosynthe-

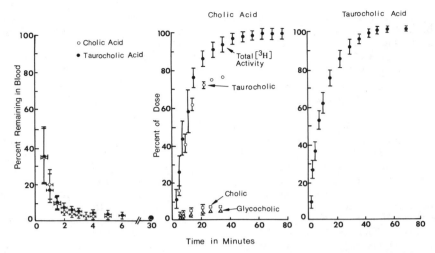

FIGURE 3. Blood disappearance and biliary appearance kinetics following the i.v. administration of bolus dose of tritiated cholic and taurocholic acids. The bars indicate the range from four rats.

sized and employed in *in situ* liver absorption and biliary excretion studies and in rat intestinal perfusion studies of the jejunum and ileum. In general, the model set of compounds includes the drug itself, the bile acid carrier, and the drug-bile acid prodrug represented, for example, by *p*-toluenesulfonic acid, cholic acid, and 3-tosylcholic acid, respectively. Only dilute concentrations of cholic acid, cholic acid derivatives, and analogs ($1–5 \times 10^{-3}$ mM) in isoosmotic, pH 7.5 buffer solutions were used. While the critical micelle concentration of cholate is ~5 mM at these conditions, the expected lower CMC of the more hydrophobic derivatives and analog of cholic acid was not determined.

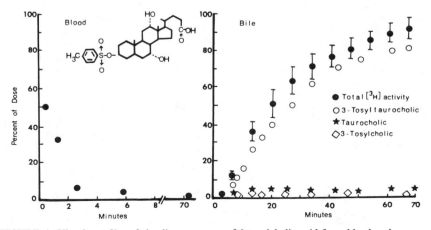

FIGURE 4. Kinetic profiles of the disappearance of 3-tosylcholic acid from blood and appearance of 3-tosylcholic acid and metabolites in bile.

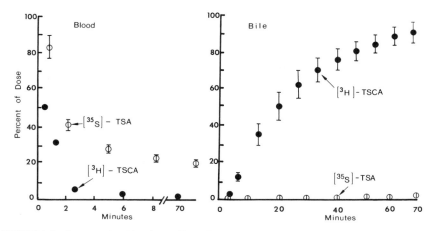

FIGURE 5. Comparative kinetic profiles of the disappearance of p-toluenesulfonic and 3-tosylcholic acids from blood and appearance of their radiolabels in bile.

3-Tosylcholic Acid

Our initial baseline studies emphasized liver absorption and biliary excretion of cholic and taurocholic acids in anesthetized Sprague-Dawley rats wherein the bile duct is cannulated and the jugular vein is intubated to gain access to blood in the right atrium. In turn, the kinetic patterns of these bile acids served as templates by which the kinetics of representative C_3-bile acid derivative and analog compounds are compared.[10,11]

After the intravenous injection of [³H]-taurocholic and [³H]-cholic acids into the rat tail vein in separate experiments, the bile acids are found to be rapidly absorbed by the liver (FIGURE 3). It is noteworthy that within 30 sec of the bolus injection, 50 to 80% of the dose disappeared from the blood. After 5 min, insignificant amounts are detected. FIGURE 3 also shows the cumulative percent of the dose appearing in the bile with time. The blood disappearance and biliary appearance rates are comparable

TABLE 1. Tissue Distribution of Total Radioactivity Following the Intravenous Bolus Dosing of *p*-Toluene-[³⁵S]Sulfonic Acid

Tissue	% Total [³⁵S] Activity	
	6 min	35 min
Blood	18.6	9.6
Brain	—	0.05
Heart	—	0.4
Kidney	4.6	27.2
Liver	7.5	2.8
Lung	—	1.2
Muscle	—	0.34/g
Spleen	—	—
Urine	0.5	33.7
Bladder	—	0.4

among the bile acids. The recovery of the total dose in the bile is remarkably rapid, and is complete within 40–50 min. Following liver absorption, cholic acid (CA) is metabolized to both glycocholic and taurocholic acids with the latter metabolite being the dominant species appearing in the bile.

The results of absorption experiments with 3-tosyl-[³H]-cholic acid (TSCA) provided our first exploration into the liver site-directed, bile-acid carrier concept. The kinetics of disappearance of TSCA from the blood and appearance in bile are shown in

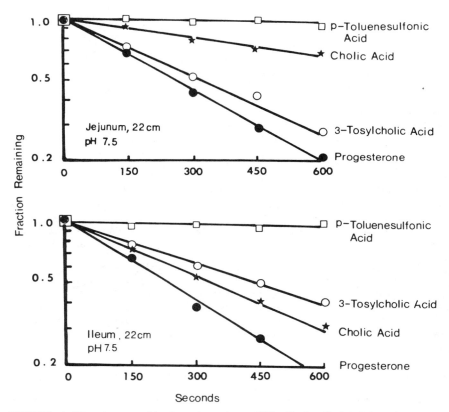

FIGURE 6. Disappearance kinetics of p-toluene-[³⁵S]sulfonic, [³H]cholic, and 3-tosyl-[³H]cholic acids and [³H]-progesterone in the rat jejunum and ileum using the modified Doluisio perfusion technique and phosphate-sodium chloride pH 7.5 buffer.

FIGURE 4. The bile acid derivative is absorbed by the liver just as rapidly and completely as cholic acid (CA) itself. Total biliary recovery of the intravenous dose in terms of total radiolabel activity is attained in about 70–80 min. The presence of four tritium-labeled substances is indicative of liver metabolism of TSCA. Intact TSCA and cholic and taurocholic acid metabolites are present in the bile, but the major metabolite is 3-tosyltaurocholic acid. Metabolic products were identified by thin layer

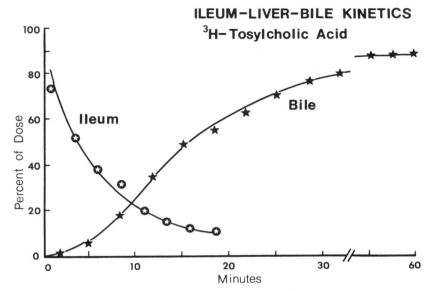

FIGURE 7. Kinetic profiles of the simultaneous absorption of [³H]3-tosylcholic acid in the rat ileum at pH 7.5 and appearance of total ³H label in bile.

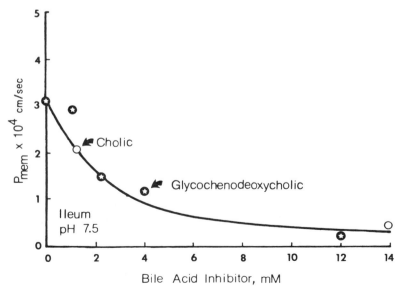

FIGURE 8. Competitive inhibition of active transport of [³H]tosylcholate (5×10^{-3} mM) in the rat ileum by additions of cholate and glycochenodeoxy cholate.

chromatography against authentic samples. It is seen that the ratio of tosyltaurocho-
late to tosylcholate is about 15:1. Expressed in other terms, the yield of intact
3-tosylated bile acid, in the form of tosyltaurocholic and tosylcholic acids, is approximately 85% of the intravenous dose of tosylcholic acid. It does not appear that TSCA is
significantly hydrolyzed in the liver, since the bile concentrations of cholic and
taurocholic acids are very low.

The disappearance of p-toluenesulfonic acid (TSA) from blood and the appearance
of total [^{35}S] activity in bile with time are shown in FIGURE 5. As compared with
3-tosyl-[^{3}H]-cholic acid, the initial disappearance is rapid and slows down considerably
after 8 min. After 2 hr, about 20% of the dose is still found in the blood. In contrast to

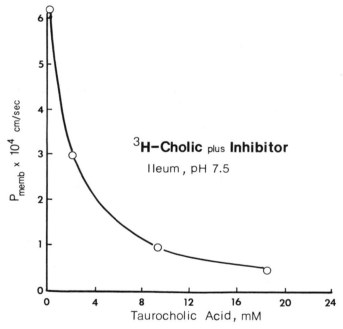

FIGURE 9. Competitive inhibition of active transport of [^{3}H]cholate (1×10^{-4} mM) in the rat
ileum by additions of taurocholate.

the total recovery of [^{3}H] activity in the bile following the i.v. administration of TSCA,
the recovery of [^{35}S] activity in the bile from TSA administration is less than 1%.
TABLE 1 gives the tissue distribution of the [^{35}S] label at various times. The significant
feature is the low amount in the liver. This gives additional supporting evidence to the
concept that cholic acid has carried the TSA as TSCA across the membrane of liver
cells.

We now turn to *in situ* intestinal absorption studies in the isolated jejunal and ileal
segments of the rat. Typical first-order disappearance kinetic plots are shown in
FIGURE 6 for radiolabel tracer concentrations of TSA, CA, and TSCA. Progesterone, a
highly lipophilic solute whose intestinal absorption is already known to be controlled by

TABLE 2. Stability of 3-Benzoyl-[³H]Cholic Acid in Various Media at 37°C

System	Time	Percent Remaining
Liver homogenate	5 min	19.5
	15 min	1.0
Homogenate of ileal tissue	5 min	99.8
in phosphate buffer pH 7.5	15 min	96.0
	20 hr	7.6
Bile	30 min	99.3
	12 hr	99.4
Plasma	30 min	84
	12 hr	0
Isotonic phosphate	30 min	99.5
buffer, pH 7.5	12 hr	99

the aqueous boundary layer,[12,13] is also included to provide the upper limit in transport rates for the hydrodynamic conditions employed.

Differences in the passive absorption rates of CA and TSCA in the jejunum are in accord with their differences in lipophilicity. The absorption of TSCA is more rapid than CA. When compared with progesterone, the absorption rate of TSCA is found to be 75% aqueous boundary layer–controlled. In view of what is known about the transport of taurocholic acid at high pH in the rat jejunum,[12] the transport of other bile acids across the aqueous pore pathway should also be negligible. In contrast to the

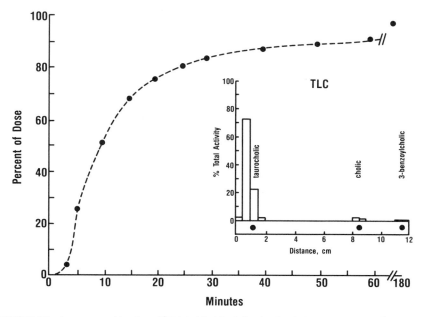

FIGURE 10. Appearance kinetics of ³H label in bile following i.v. bolus of 3-benzoyl-[³H]cholic acid. TLC of 5 min bile sample shows negligible 3-benzoylcholate, 95% taurocholate, and 5% cholate; heavy dots represent authentic samples.

jejunum, the results in the ileum show that the transport kinetics of TSCA are slower (more membrane-controlled) than that for CA. Furthermore, the absorption of TSCA is more efficient in the jejunum than in the ileum, whereas CA is more efficiently absorbed in the ileum than in the jejunum.

It is significant that at pH 7.5 the absorption of p-toluenesulfonic acid is enhanced 25-fold by passive absorption in the jejunum and 35-fold by passive and active absorption in the ileum as the 3-tosylcholic acid. The dramatic differences provide strong support for bile acid having an enhancing effect on the absorption of highly hydrophilic molecules via derivatization at the 3-OH group of the bile acid. Concurrent intestinal absorption from the ileum and liver-to-bile kinetic studies show complete absorption of TSCA (FIGURE 7).

To place the above intestinal absorption studies on a quantitative, physicochemical, and mechanistic level of understanding, we have treated the data using physical models. The first-order absorption rate constant is expressed by:

$$K_u = \frac{A}{V} \cdot P_e, \tag{1}$$

where K_u is the rate constant; A/V is the apparent surface area to bulk solution volume ratio; and P_e is the effective permeability coefficient. For the passive absorption of weak acids in general, the effective permeability coefficient[12] is:

$$P_e = \frac{1}{\dfrac{1}{P_{aq}} + \dfrac{1}{P_o X_s + P_p}}, \tag{2}$$

where P_{aq}, P_o, and P_p are the permeability coefficients of the aqueous boundary layer, lipoidal biophase and aqueous pore pathways of the membrane, respectively; and X_s is the fraction of nondissociated acid species at the membrane surface. For the simultaneous first-order active and passive absorption of bile acids in the ileum,[14]

$$P_e = \frac{1}{\dfrac{1}{P_{aq}} + \dfrac{1}{P_o X_s + P_m^*(1 - X_s)}}, \tag{3}$$

TABLE 3. Permeability Coefficients[a]

			Jejunum at pH 7.5			Ileum at pH 7.5			
Bile Acid	log P.C.[b]	pK$_a$	P_e	$P_o X_s$	P_p	P_e	$P_o X_s$	P_p	$P_m^*(1 - X_s)$
Cholic	0.65	5	0.63	0.83	0	1.82	0.5	0	5.58
3-Tosylcholic	2.30	5	1.92	6.93	0	1.41	0.5	0	2.61
p-Toluenesulfonic	≪1.0	2	0.07	0	0.1	0.07	0	0.1	0
Progesterone[c]	3.99		2.66	>30	0	2.58	>30	0	0

[a]All permeability coefficients have units of 10^{-4} cm/sec.
[b]P.C. is the partition coefficient in n-octanol/pH 7.5 buffer.
[c]The permeability of the aqueous boundary layer, P_{aq}, is 2.66×10^{-4} cm/sec in the jejunum and 2.58×10^{-4} cm/sec in the ileum as determined by progesterone.
[d]P_e is calculated by dividing the first-order rate constant, K_u, by A/V where A/V is equal to 11.2 cm^{-1}.

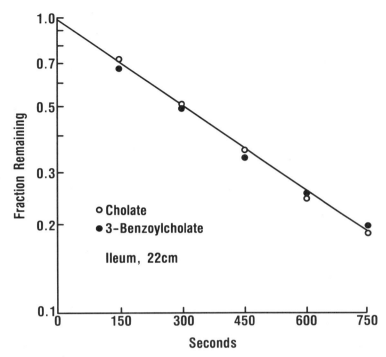

FIGURE 11. Disappearance kinetics of 3-benzoyl-[³H]cholic and [³H]cholic acids in the rat ileum at pH 7.5.

where P_m^* is the membrane permeability coefficient for active transport. It is readily observed in Eqs. 2 and 3 that P_e becomes aqueous boundary layer–controlled when the membrane permeability is much greater than that of the aqueous boundary layer in front of the membrane; that is, $P_e \simeq P_{aq}$. To account for the fact of competitive inhibition of the active transport mechanism among bile acids, the effective membrane permeability coefficient term in Eq. 3 may be written:

$$P_{\mathrm{memb}} = P_o X_s + \frac{P_m^*(1 - X_s)}{1 + [I]/K_i}, \tag{4}$$

where $[I]$ is the bile acid inhibitor concentration and K_i is the Michaelis inhibition constant. Within the limits of high inhibitor concentrations, $P_{\mathrm{memb}} \simeq P_o X_s$, as seen in the competitive inhibition of the active transport of [³H]tosycholate and [³H]cholate by additions of bile salts in FIGURES 8 and 9, respectively.

The delineation of the permeability coefficients of the various solutes into its passive components in the jejunum and its passive and active components in the ileum is shown in TABLE 2. It is observed that tosylation of cholic acid at the 3-OH position has two effects on the effective membrane permeability relative to that for cholic acid itself: (1) increase in $P_o X_s$ for passive absorption in the jejunum by a factor of 20 or more and (2) decrease in the $P_m^*(1 - X_s)$ for active transport in the ileum by a factor of

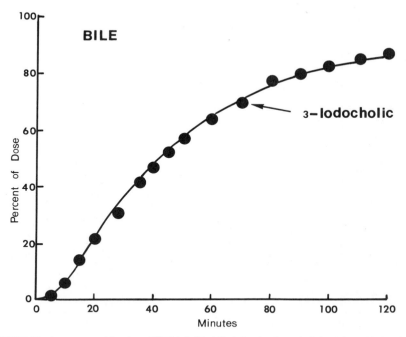

FIGURE 12. Appearance kinetics of [³H] label in bile following i.v. administration of bolus dose of 3-iodo-[³H]cholic acid. TLC analyses of a few samples indicated 5% 3-iodocholate and 95% 3-iodotaurocholate.

2. Also, the passive mechanism in the ileum contributed about 10% to the total membrane transport process.

3-Benzoylcholic Acid

Following intravenous administration of a bolus dose of 3-benzoyl-[³H]-cholic acid, it is seen in FIGURE 10 that the appearance of total ³H activity in the bile is rapid and complete. Upon TLC analysis of the bile collected 5 min after the administration of the intravenous dose, taurocholic acid was found to be the principal metabolite (about 96%). No benzoylcholic acid appeared in the bile. Although benzoylcholic acid is somewhat unstable in plasma (TABLE 3), the hydrolysis rate is relatively slow as compared to the rapid appearance of the total activity in bile. Furthermore, the ester is rapidly cleaved *in vitro* to benzoic and cholic acids in the supernatant liquid of liver homogenates. Taken together, the data suggest that 3-benzoylcholic acid is rapidly absorbed by the liver and, subsequently, rapidly metabolized to cholic acid and, in turn, to taurocholic acid. This is in sharp contrast to the 3-tosylcholic acid, which was relatively nonlabile to liver esterases.

In FIGURE 11 the absorption of 3-benzoylcholic acid in the rat ileum at buffer pH 7.5 is found to be just as rapid as cholic acid. When co-administered with varying concentrations of cholic acid, the active absorption rate of the 3-benzoylcholic acid was depressed.

2-Iodocholic Acid Analog

The appearance kinetics of total radioactivity post i.v. administration of 3-iodo-[³H]-cholic acid indicated complete liver uptake and biliary excretion (FIGURE 12), but was slower than cholic acid (FIGURE 3). Almost 95% appeared as the taurine conjugate and about 5% as the intact 3-iodocholic acid. Since the disappearance kinetics from blood was not followed, it could not be determined whether liver uptake or biliary excretion was the rate-determining step.

The *in situ* absorption of 3-iodocholic acid in the jejunum was efficient (FIGURE 13). From a quantitative mechanistic point of view, the more lipophilic 3-iodocholic acid was passively absorbed faster than cholic acid in the jejunum; however, their active absorption efficiencies are nearly the same in the ileum.

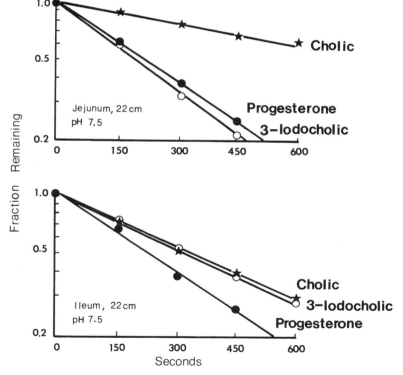

FIGURE 13. Disappearance kinetics of 3-iodocholic acid in rat jejunum and ileum at pH 7.5 as compared to cholic acid and progesterone.

SUMMARY

On the basis of the enterohepatocycling phenomenon of bile acids involving the intestines, liver, and gallbladder, it was conceptualized that bile acids could serve as a molecular carrier of drugs by taking advantage of the bile acid active transport mechanism. It was further proposed that derivatization or analogation of bile acids at the C_3-OH position was the desired route because of the reactive hydroxyl group and, moreover, because of the active transport requirement of retaining the C_{17} side chain with a single terminal acidic function. Using 3-tosylcholic, 3-benzoylcholic, and 3-iodocholic acids, *in situ* liver absorption, biliary excretion, and intestinal absorption studies in the rat were successful in establishing the concept that C_3-derivatives and analogs of bile acids are, potentially, novel molecular delivery systems for intestinal and liver-site directed absorption.

ACKNOWLEDGMENTS

Special recognition is given to Dr. W. Morozowich and S. L. Douglas of The Upjohn Company for the synthesis of the model cholic acid derivatives and analogs and to Dr. R. Chen of The National Taiwan University for the radiosynthesis. The evaluation of the concept was meticulously carried out by Drs. J. Y. Park and M. Mahjour, my former Ph.D. graduate students at The University of Michigan.

REFERENCES

1. DIETSCHY, J. J. 1968. Mechanism for the intestinal transport of bile acids. J. Lipid Res. **9:** 297–309.
2. HOLT, P. R. 1966. Competitive inhibition of intestinal bile salt absorption in the rat. Am. J. Physiol. **210:** 635–639.
3. HEATON, K. W. & L. LACK. 1968. Ileal bile salt transport: mutual inhibition in an in vivo system. Am. J. Physiol. **214:** 585–590.
4. LACK, L. & L. M. WEINER. 1972. Bile acid transport systems. *In* The Bile Acids. P. P. Nair & D. Kritchevsky, Eds. **2:** 33–54. Plenum Press. New York.
5. TAVOLONI, N., J. S. REED & J. L. BOYER. 1978. Hemodynamic effects on determinants of bile acid secretion in isolated liver. Am. J. Physiol. **234:** E584–E592.
6. REICHEN, J. & G. PAUMGARTNER. 1980. Excretory function of the liver. *In* Liver and Biliary Tract Physiology. N. B. Jafitt, Ed. **21:** Ch. 3. University Park Press. Baltimore, MD.
7. TYROR, M. P., J. T. GARBUTT & L. LACK. 1971. Metabolism and transport of bile acids in the intestines. Am. J. Med. **51:** 614–626.
8. ANWER, M. S., E. R. L. O'MAILLE, A. F. HOFMANN, R. A. DIPIETRO & E. MICHELLOTTI. 1985. Influence of side chain change on hepatic transport of bile acids and bile acid analogues. Am. J. Physiol. **249:** G479–G488.
9. LACK, L. 1979. Properties and biological significance of the ileal bile salt transport system. Environ. Health Perspective **33:** 79–90.
10. MAHJOUR, M. 1980. C_3-Derivatives and analogs of bile acids as novel delivery systems for intestinal and liver-site directed absorption. Ph.D. Thesis. The University of Michigan. Ann Arbor, MI.
11. HO, N. F. H., M. MAHJOUR & J. Y. PARK. 1982. Specific liver-site delivery and enhanced intestinal absorption of the drug-bile acid carrier mechanism. *In* Optimization of Drug Delivery. H. Bundgaard, A. B. Hansen & H. Koford, Eds.: 80–92. Munksgaard. Copenhagen.
12. HO, N. F. H., J. Y. PARK, W. MOROZOWICH & W. I. HIGUCHI. 1977. Physical model

approach to the design of drugs with improved intestinal absorption. *In* Design of Biopharmaceutical Properties Through Prodrugs and Analogs. E. B. Roche, Ed.: 136–277. American Pharmaceutical Association. Washington, D.C.

13. HIGUCHI, W. I., N. F. H., HO, J. Y. PARK & I. KOMIYA. 1981. Rate-limiting steps and factors in drug absorption. *In* Drug Absorption. L. F. Prescott & W. S. Nimmo, Eds.: 35–60. Adis Press. New York.

14. HO, N. F. H. & W. I. HIGUCHI. 1974. Theoretical model studies of intestinal drug absorption IV: bile acid transport at premicellar concentrations across the diffusion layer-membrane barrier. J. Pharm. Sci. **63:** 686–690.

Entrapment of 6-Carboxyfluorescein within Cylindrical Phospholipid Microstructures

THOMAS G. BURKE, ALOK SINGH, AND PAUL YAGER

Department of Medical Oncology
City of Hope National Medical Center
Duarte, California 91010

Bio/Molecular Engineering Branch
Naval Research Laboratory
Washington, DC 20375
and
Geo-Centers
Suitland, Maryland 20746

We have employed phase and fluorescence microscopies to demonstrate that micron-size lipid tubules, which form from polymerizable, diacetylene-containing phosphatidylcholines, can entrap the hydrophilic fluorophore 6-carboxyfluorescein (CF). Previous light and electron microscopic observations have shown tubules to be long, thin multilamellar structures (approximately 0.5 microns wide with lengths from 10 to 100 microns), which appear to have large, open-ended central cavities.[1,2] The potential of tubule lumens to retain water-soluble fluorescent probe molecules is examined in this report.

Two different routes to the thermal formation of 1,2-bis(10,12-tricosadiynoyl)-sn-glycero-3-phosphocholine ($DC_{23}PC$) tubules that have been developed in our laboratories are summarized in FIGURE 1. The latter method allows for thorough mixing of the initial vesicle preparation; we used this method here to achieve tubule formation in the presence of CF. Glycerol was included in these studies because interbilayer expansion, known to occur in tubules due to the presence of the solute,[2] could potentially enhance entrapment. Aqueous lipid dispersions were prepared by hydration of lipid films in 50 mM CF at 60°C for 30 min, with or without the presence of 40% glycerol (vol/vol). Small MLVs were formed by vortex mixing near 60°C for 10 min. At rates of 1°C min^{-1}, the lipid dispersions were then cooled to 0°C, reheated to 60°C, and subsequently cooled to ambient temperature. Examination by optical microscopy demonstrated that tubules with lengths of 10 to 50 microns had formed. The tubules were rinsed with 3 × 10 ml distilled water at ambient temperature to remove free dye, the supernatant being decanted from the tubules after low-speed centrifugation. The tubules were then resuspended in distilled water and examined by simultaneous phase contrast and fluorescence microscopies using a Leitz Diavert inverted fluorescence microscope (63× lens) interfaced with a MTI 66 intensified video camera and Panasonic Model NV 8950 video cassette recorder. Photographs were taken directly from a Sony PVM-122 monitor using a 35 mm camera.

Tubules containing intensely fluorescent regions were observed in preparations with or without the presence of glycerol. Phase and fluorescence micrographs of a tubule formed in the presence of glycerol are presented in FIGURE 2. The micrographs demonstrate the presence of several high-intensity fluorescent regions within the tubule lumen. Some of these fluorescent, dye-filled regions exhibited rapid movement,

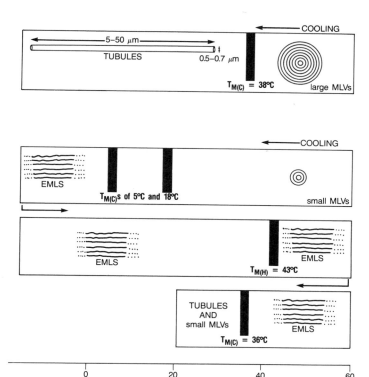

FIGURE 1. A schematic of the thermal phase behavior of $DC_{23}PC$ in aqueous suspension (100 mg ml^{-1}) at scan rates of 1°C min^{-1} is shown (Burke *et al.*, unpublished results). $T_{M(H)}$ and $T_{M(C)}$ refer to the peak temperatures of exothermic or endothermic events observed during differential scanning calorimetric heating or cooling scans, respectively. Calorimetric, freeze-fracture electron microscopic and vibrational spectroscopic investigations have shown that cooling large multilamellar vesicles (MLVs) with outer diameters in excess of 1 µm forms a gel phase with tubule morphology at 38°C, whereas cooling small MLVs (diameters of 0.3 + 0.2 µm) results in the formation of a gel phase with extended multilamellar sheet (EMLS) morphology.[3] Upon reheating the EMLS suspension to 50°C, followed by cooling to ambient temperature, tubules and small MLVs are present in the sample. Accordingly, tubules can be thermally formed by cooling either large MLV or EMLS suspension.

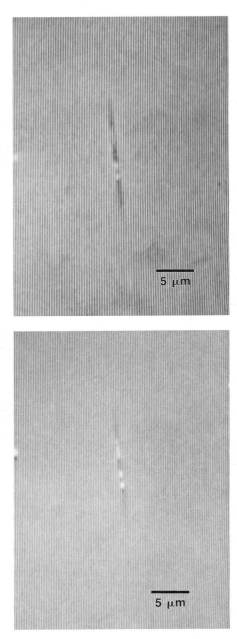

5 μm

5 μm

FIGURE 2. Micrographs demonstrating entrapment of CF in compartments within a tubule. (Left) A 20 μm tubule under simultaneous phase contrast and fluorescence illumination. The light areas of the image represent high-intensity fluorescent regions due to the presence of CF. (Right) A micrograph of the same tubule, but observed with the transmitted light phase illumination source nearly extinguished. A set of fluorescence illumination filters optimized for fluorescein detection were used.

indicative of the presence of intact, diffusing liposomes within the tubule. The departure of liposomes from the ends of tubules was seldom observed during the time course of visual observation (20 min). The majority of tubules in this preparation exhibited fluorescent regions; the number of individual fluorophore-filled compartments and/or liposomes that could be readily observed by eye ranged from one to as many as seven. Our results demonstrate that tubules can accommodate and retain CF-containing liposomes. Tubules can thus serve as carriers of water-soluble molecules, their shape offering a new variable to exploit in applications of lipid microstructures.

REFERENCES

1. YAGER, P. & P. E. SCHOEN. 1984. Mol. Cryst. Liq. Cryst. **106:** 371–381.
2. YAGER, P., P. E. SCHOEN, C. DAVIES, R. PRICE & A. SINGH. 1985. Biophys. J. **48:** 899–906.
3. RUDOLPH, A. S. & T. G. BURKE. 1987. Biochim. Biophys. Acta **902:** 349–359.

Use of a Chemical Redox System for Brain Enhanced Delivery of Estradiol Decreases Prostate Weight

K. S. ESTES, M. E. BREWSTER, AND N. BODOR[a]

Pharmatec, Inc.
Alachua, Florida

Center for Drug Design and Delivery
College of Pharmacy
University of Florida
Gainesville, Florida 32610

A redox-based system of brain-directed drug delivery was recently developed in our laboratories and was shown capable of both enhancing penetration of drugs through the blood-brain barrier (BBB) and maintaining sustained drug concentrations in brain, compared to other tissues.[1,2] The method is designed to biomimic the $NAD^+ \rightleftharpoons NADH$ redox system and utilizes a lipophilic dihydropyridine carrier, which is covalently attached to a relatively hydrophilic drug. The system is designed to function as follows. *In vivo,* the metabolically labile drug-carrier complex is oxidized to the corresponding quaternary salt of the drug-carrier complex. Increased hydrophilicity impedes efflux through the BBB, while facilitating peripheral excretion. The resulting "locked-in"

TABLE 1. Effects of E_2-CDS and Estradiol Valerate on Organ Weights Three Weeks Post-Treatment

Treatment Group	Seminal Vesicles (mg)	Testes (g)	Anterior Pituitary (mg)	Serum E_2 at 24 hr (pg/ml)
Intact control	$1175 \pm 107^{a,d}$ $4/4^b$	3.2 ± 0.0^e	12.7 ± 0.5^c	25 ± 2
Castrate control	182 ± 35^c $0/5$	—	11.5 ± 0.6^c	<20
E_2-CDS, i.v.	305 ± 47^c $3/6$	$2.0 \pm 0.3^{c,d}$	$21.1 \pm 1.9^{d,e}$	1110 ± 48
EV, i.v.	444 ± 69^c $5/6$	$2.1 \pm 0.3^{c,d}$	$18.0 \pm 1.9^{c,d,e}$	3408 ± 677
E_2-CDS, s.c.	799 ± 138^d $5/6$	$3.0 \pm 0.1^{d,e}$	$13.9 \pm 0.8^{c,d}$	243 ± 25
EV, s.c.	339 ± 34^c $2/5$	1.8 ± 0.2^c	23.5 ± 4.0^e	986 ± 94

[a]Mean ± S.E.M.
[b]Fluid or Semen Filled/n.
[c-e]Values with different superscripts are significantly different, $p < 0.05$.

[a]To whom all correspondence should be addressed at Center for Drug Design and Delivery, Box J-487 JHMHC, University of Florida, Gainesville, FL 32610.

334

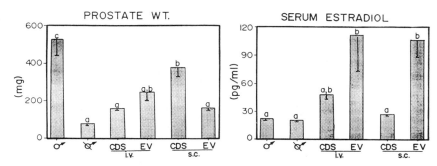

FIGURE 1. Prostate weights (left panel) and serum estradiol values (right panel) 21 days following treatment with estradiol carrier delivery system (E_2-CDS) or equimolar estradiol valerate (EV). Drugs were administered i.v. via tail vein at 5 mg/kg in 0.5 ml/kg volumes or subcutaneously (s.c.) at 1 mg/kg in sesame oil in 1.0 ml/kg volumes. Superscripts that are different designate statistically significant differences at $p < 0.05$.

drug-carrier complex can be hydrolyzed to release free drug and the non-toxic carrier metabolite, trigonelline.

This chemical delivery system (CDS) was recently applied to estradiol (E_2).[3] Although E_2 normally penetrates the BBB, the potential of the CDS to preferentially target E_2 to the brain made this approach attractive. Distribution studies in rats verified that drug-carrier complex half-life was sustained in brain compared to other tissues.[3] Pharmacological investigation demonstrated sustained luteinizing hormone (LH) suppression in castrate rats following treatment with E_2-CDS.[4] Further, the activity could not be attributed to serum E_2 levels.

The results of previous studies suggested that E_2-CDS may be therapeutically advantageous in prostate cancers, which are dependent on LH-stimulated testosterone. We, therefore, examined androgen-dependent tissues three weeks following treatment with E_2-CDS or equimolar estradiol valerate (EV), a long-acting estrogen similarly esterified. Control groups were intact and orchidectomized rats. Treatment groups received 5 mg/kg E_2-CDS via tail vein injection or equimolar EV (0.5 ml/kg). E_2-CDS was formulated in a water-soluble β-hydroxycyclodextrin complex,[5] while EV vehicle was ethanol:water (70:30). Two other treatment groups received 1 mg/kg E_2-CDS or equimolar EV s.c. in oil vehicle. Tissue weights were examined 3 weeks later and sera were evaluated for E_2 (Diagnostic Products Cost-A-Count Kits). Data were evaluated by ANOVA and Student Newman Keuls tests.

Results shown in TABLE 1 and FIGURE 1 are consistent with the CDS concept. Prostate and seminal vesicle weights were not different from castrate control rats in animals treated i.v. with PR-63. However, serum E_2 levels were also not different in these groups. In contrast, rats treated with EV sufficient to decrease testosterone-dependent tissues had elevated E_2 levels. Sustained pharmacological activity following administration of E_2-CDS in water-soluble formulations as well as oil s.c. injections indicates the feasibility of developing the CDC for prostate cancer therapies.

REFERENCES

1. BODOR, N., H. FARAG & M. BREWSTER. 1981. Site-specific, sustained release of drugs to the brain. Science **214:** 1370–1372.

2. BODOR, N. & M. E. BREWSTER. 1983. Problems of delivery of drugs to the brain. Pharm. Ther. **19:** 337–386.
3. BODOR, N., J. MCCORNACK & M. E. BREWSTER. 1987. Improved delivery through biological membranes XXII. Synthesis and distribution of brain-selective estrogen delivery system. Int. J. Pharm. **35:** 47–59.
4. SIMPKINS, J., J. MCCORNACK, K. ESTES, M. BREWSTER, E. SHEK & N. BODOR. 1986. Sustained brain-specific delivery of estradiol causes long-term suppression of LH secretion. J. Med. Chem. **29:** 1810–1812.
5. PITHA, J. & J. PITHA. 1985. Amorphous water soluble derivative of cyclodextrins: Non-toxic dissolution enhancing excipients. J. Pharm. Sci. **74:** 987–990.

Targeting of Neoglycoprotein-Drug Conjugates to Human Tumor Cells via Endogenous Lectins

HANS-JOACHIM GABIUS

Max-Planck-Institut für experimentelle Medizin
Abteilung Chemie
Hermann-Rein-Straße 3
D-3400 Göttingen, Federal Republic of Germany

Endogenous carbohydrate-binding proteins (lectins) of tumors are supposed to partici-pate in recognitive and growth regulatory processes, relevant to tumor growth and spread.[1,2] Because such lectins have been detected in a variety of human tumor cells,[3] they offer a means to address the question of whether tumor lectins may contribute to an improvement of clinical management of tumors by serving in a selective lectin-mediated uptake of therapeutically active glycoproteins. The carrier potential of glycoproteins or synthetic neoglycoproteins in this system of specific carbohydrate-protein interaction can thus be exploited to direct drugs to certain cell types. Whereas carbohydrates on the carrier render it accessible to the lectin-mediated uptake, the cotransported drugs will be released after intracellular proteolysis of the carrier. Experimentally, fluorescent neoglycoproteins are first used to infer the presence of membrane lectins on different types of human tumor cell lines. They comprise for this initial study two different human embryonic carcinoma cell lines, two human colon carcinoma cell lines and a human melanoma cell line. The panel of neoglycoproteins, chemically coupled to etoposide, cis-Pt, FuDr, or methotrexate, reveals that neoglyco-proteins serve as carriers with graduated efficiency, significantly enhancing the carrier capacity of the nonglycosylated carrier. Pronounced uptake that can be drastically diminished by addition of the respective drug-free neoglycoprotein, but not by unrelated neoglycoproteins is seen for those neoglycoproteins that have strongly labeled the cell surfaces. In summary, additional lactose, melibiose, or maltose as entry functions confer an up to 10-fold increase in cytotoxic activity to the conjugate of drug and the carrier serum albumin relative to nonglycosylated albumin or albumin with sugars like cellobiose or mannose-6-phosphate as drug carriers.[4] Melibiose has also been effective in leading to a cytotoxicity of the drug-carrier conjugate by lectin-mediated uptake that resembles the cytotoxicity of the freely diffusible drug at the same concentration for the colon carcinoma lines.[5] In the case of the melanoma line, lactose and mannose prove to be useful entry functions.[6] Because biochemical characterization of the respective tumor lectins demonstrates that they exhibit an at least restricted expression in comparison to other tissues and tumors, the prerequisite for clinical application of differences in the lectin profile appears to be fulfilled. With the preparation of more refined carbohydrate structures on neoglycoproteins, match-ing the specificity of the target lectin, neoglycoproteins can thus become alternatives to monoclonal antibodies as carriers. They have the further advantage over monoclonal antibodies to tolerate high coupling frequencies for drugs without loss of activity. This is especially important for drugs that are poorly taken up by cells and for drug-resistant cells that have a deficiency in drug transport. Furthermore, different neoglycoproteins as carriers, reacting with independently targeted membrane lectins, are useful in

TABLE 1. Inhibition of [³H]Thymidine Incorporation of Human Embryonic Carcinoma Cells by Etoposide, Linked to Lactosylated BSA (lac-BSA), and cis-Pt, Complexed to Maltosylated BSA (mal-BSA) or Mannosylated-BSA (man-BSA) as a Model for Combination Chemotherapy in Drug Targeting

Substance	Concentration (µg/ml)	Inhibition (%)
Etoposide-lac-BSA	7.5	8
	15	19
	30	27
(cis-Pt)-mal-BSA	1.25	1
	2.5	4
	5.0	6.5
(cis-Pt)-man-BSA	1.25	2
	2.5	3
	5.0	5
(cis-Pt)-mal-BSA	1.25 + 7.5	28
+ etoposide-lac-BSA	2.5 + 15	43
(cis-Pt)-man-BSA	1.25 + 7.5	22
+ etoposide-lac-BSA	2.5 + 15	35

combination therapy, as shown by synergistic effects of etoposide and cis-Pt in lectin-mediated endocytosis (TABLE 1). These data underscore that the application of neoglycoproteins as a Trojan horse for drug transport via tumor lectins, although it is at a preliminary stage, appears to warrant further exploration, since "this idea has considerable appeal," as stated in a recent review on drug targeting.[7]

REFERENCES

1. GABIUS, H.-J., K. VEHMEYER, R. ENGELHARDT, G. A. NAGEL & F. CRAMER. 1986. Cell Tissue Res. **246:** 515–521.
2. GABIUS, H.-J. 1987. Cancer Investigation **5:** 39–46.
3. GABIUS, H.-J., R. ENGELHARDT & F. CRAMER. 1986. Anticancer Res. **6:** 573–578.
4. GABIUS, H.-J., C. BOKEMEYER, T. HELLMANN & H.-J. SCHMOLL. 1987. J. Cancer Res. Clin. Oncol. **113:** 126–130.
5. GABIUS, H.-J., R. ENGELHARDT, T. HELLMANN, P. MIDOUX, M. MONSIGNY, G. A. NAGEL & K. VEHMEYER. 1987. Anticancer Res. **7:** 109–112.
6. GABIUS, H.-J. & K. VEHMEYER. 1987. Naturwissenschaften **74:** 37–38.
7. POZNANSKY, M. J. & R. L. JULIANO. 1984. Pharmacol. Rev. **36:** 278–336.

Photoactivation of a Psoralen Derivative Conjugated to Insulin

F. P. GASPARRO, R. M. KNOBLER,[a] D. H. WEINGOLD,
S. S. YEMUL,[b] E. BISACCIA, AND R. L. EDELSON

Departments of Dermatology
Yale University
New Haven, Connecticut 06510

[a]University of Vienna
Vienna, Austria

[b]Columbia University
New York, New York

We have developed a new photochemotherapy for the treatment of the leukemic phase of cutaneous T cell lymphoma. An orally administered photoactivatable drug, 8-methoxypsoralen (8-MOP), is activated in extracorporeally routed blood by irradiation with ultraviolet A light (320–400 nm, UVA), leading to DNA crosslinks that inhibit DNA synthesis and kill lymphocytes. Twenty seven of the first 37 patients treated with this new therapy have shown significant clinical improvement.[1]

Because photoactivated 8-MOP has an active half-life on the order of microseconds the direct effects of this photochemotherapy are limited to target cells, precluding the side effects normally associated with chemotherapy. However, the 8-MOP interacts with all nucleated cells in UVA-irradiated blood. Recently, our efforts have been directed towards the development of more specific phototoxic agents. The presence of

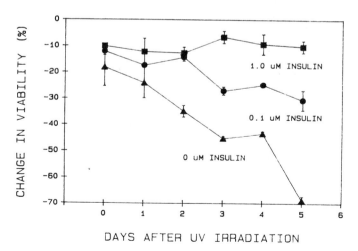

DAYS AFTER UV IRRADIATION

FIGURE 1. Inhibition of AMT-I (10 μM) activity by insulin. Change in viability is measured relative to the viability of cells in PBS treated with 3 J/cm² UVA. ($\blacktriangle$) 10μM AMT-I, ($\blacksquare$) 10 μM AMT-I plus 0.1 μM insulin, ($\bullet$) 10 μM AMT-I, plus 0.1 μM insulin.

insulin receptors on the surface of activated lymphocytes[2] suggested to us that derivatized insulins could be used to deliver photoactivatable moieties to proliferating cells, which could then be activated by UVA irradiation. 4'-Aminomethyl-4,5',8-trimethylpsoralen (AMT) has been chemically conjugated to insulin. The psoralen moiety retains its photochemical reactivity and crosslinks DNA after exposure to ultraviolet light.[3] This chimeric molecule has been used to selectively kill a population of lymphocytes whose expression of insulin receptors has been induced by stimulation with phytohemagglutinin (PHA). The activity of AMT-insulin can be blocked by the presence of native insulin. The hybrid insulin-psoralen molecule is a prototype for a family of phototoxic drugs, which can be selectively delivered to subsets of lymphocytes.[3]

The effect of 10 μM AMT-I and 3 J/cm^2 UVA light on the viability of resting and PHA-stimulated lymphocytes was determined by trypan blue exclusion. The decrease in viability of treated cells is shown in FIGURE 1. While stimulated cells had viability reduced by approximately 70%, resting cells were unaffected by the treatment. FIGURE 1 also shows that the cytotoxic activity of AMT-I can be completely blocked by the presence of 1 μM native insulin, indicating that AMT-I is specifically interacting with the insulin receptor.

Chimeric AMT-I is a photoactivatable drug that affected stimulated lymphocytes. Unstimulated cells were unaffected. The inhibition of AMT-I by native insulin supports a model in which AMT-I binds to the insulin receptor and is then internalized. The compound might then be enzymatically cleaved, which could free the AMT moiety to intercalate with DNA and be activated with UVA light. Alternatively, the entire molecule may interact with DNA.

REFERENCES

1. EDELSON, R. L., et al. 1987. N. Engl. J. Med. **316:** 297–303.
2. MURPHY, R. F., E. BISACCIA, C. R. CANTOR, C. L. BERGER & R. L. EDELSON. 1984. J. Cell Physiol. **121:** 351–356.
3. GASPARRO, F. P., R. M. KNOBLER, S. S. YEMUL, E. BISACCIA & R. L. EDELSON. 1986. Biochem. Biophys. Res. Comm. **141:** 502–509.
4. GASPARRO, F. P., W. A. SAFFRAN, C. R. CANTOR & R. L. EDELSON. 1984. Photochem. Photobiol. **40:** 215–219.

Biosynthesis of Multidrug Resistance-Associated Glycoproteins in J774.2 Multidrug Resistant Cells

LEE M. GREENBERGER, SCOTT S. WILLIAMS, AND
SUSAN BAND HORWITZ

Department of Molecular Pharmacology
Albert Einstein College of Medicine
Bronx, New York 10461

When mammalian cells are selected for resistance to one drug, they can develop cross resistance to structurally and functionally unrelated drugs. There is a reduced level of drug accumulation, which can account for resistance. The cells also overexpress a

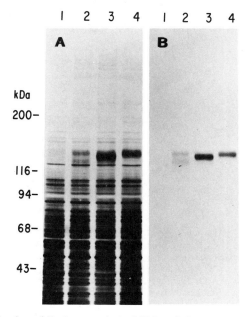

FIGURE 1. Identification of P-glycoprotein in MDR cell lines derived from J774.2 mouse macrophage-like cells. Polypeptides from a plasma membrane-enriched subcellular fraction of wild type and MDR cell lines were resolved by SDS-PAGE (Laemmli 4–10% gradient gel) and silver stained (A) or transferred to nitrocellulose (B). Ten and fifteen micrograms of protein was loaded in each lane of A and B, respectively. Lanes contain material from cells grown in: (1) no drug; (2) 50 μM taxol; (3) 1 μM vinblastine (VBL); or (4) 100 μM colchicine (CLC). Nitrocellulose was probed with a primary rabbit antiserum made against the 135 kD species from VBL-selected cells. Antibody binding species were identified by incubation in rabbit anti-mouse IgG-biotin, followed by avidin-horseradish peroxidase (HRP), and reaction for HRP. Molecular weight markers were myosin, 200 kD; β-galactosidase, 116 kD; phosphorylase b, 94 kD; bovine serum albumin, 68 kD; and ovalbumin, 43 kD. Note that the P-gps were present only in drug-resistant cells and had heterogeneous electrophoretic mobilities.

plasma membrane glycoprotein, referred to as P-glycoprotein (P-gp), and often have amplification of the gene coding for the P-gp. These are the major features of the multidrug resistance (MDR) phenotype.[1] The P-gp is hypothesized to be a drug (efflux) pump that mediates reduced drug accumulation.

Multidrug resistant cells derived from J774.2 (J7) and selected for resistance to colchicine (CLC), vinblastine (VBL), or taxol (TAX) can be distinguished. Each drug-resistant cell line overexpresses antigenically related P-gps with distinct electro-

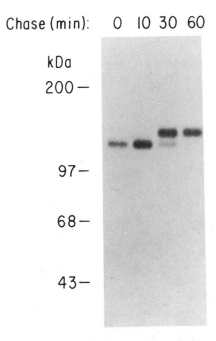

FIGURE 2. Biosynthesis of the P-gp in CLC-resistant cells derived from J7. Multidrug resistant cells maintained in 100 μM CLC were preincubated in methionine-free media, pulsed (5 min) with [^{35}S]methionine, and chased in normal media. Cell lysates were incubated with primary antibody (1:50 dilution) at 4°C for 16 hr followed by Protein A-Sepharose for 15 min at room temperature and 105 min at 4°C. The immunoprecipitated P-gp was then resolved on a gel. All lanes were loaded with equal radioactivity. Prestained molecular weight markers were similar to those in FIG. 1. A precursor of 125 kD was processed rapidly to a mature form of 140 kD.

phoretic mobilities (FIG. 1). They also have unique resistance profiles although resistance is greatest to the agent used for selection.[2]

The basis for P-gp heterogeneity in J7-derived cells has been examined.[3] Comparisons were made with the P-gp expressed in Chinese hamster ovary cells selected for resistance to colchicine. ("CH^{R}C5" cells were a generous gift from Dr. Victor Ling). Cells were pulsed (5 to 60 min) with [^{35}S]methionine, chased for varying periods, and the P-gp immunoprecipitated by a polyclonal antibody specific for the P-gp. Then, the P-gp was resolved by polyacrylamide gel electrophoresis.

J7 cells selected for resistance to CLC or VBL made a 125 kD precursor that was processed to a mature P-gp ($t_{1/2} \sim 20$ min) of 140 and 135 kD, respectively (FIG. 2). TAX-selected cells, when pulsed for 5 min, made a 123–125 kD precursor that was processed by 1 hr to a major species of 140 kD with a smear extending to 125 kD; more than 3 hr were needed before the mature species of 130 and 140 kD appeared. When TAX-selected cells were pulsed for 15–60 min, a second precursor (120 kD) was observed. Tunicamycin-treated cells, which were pulsed for 5 min, made a 120 kD form of the P-gp. Enzymatic removal of N-linked oligosacharides from the precursor form (5-min pulse) or the 2-hr chase material shifted the molecular mass to 120 or 125 kD, respectively. However, a doublet ($\sim$120 and 125 kD) was observed when the mature P-gps of taxol-treated cells were enzymatically deglycosylated. CH^{R}C5 cells made a 120–125 kD precursor that was processed to 155 kD ($t_{1/2}$ greater than 30 min). After removal of N-linked oligosaccharides, the 155 kD form shifted to 125 kD.

We conclude that heterogeneity in the P-gp in J7-derived MDR cell lines is due, at least in part, to N-linked carbohydrate. In taxol-selected cells, the two mature forms of the P-gp may contain distinct polypeptide backbones and/or posttranslational modifications other than N-linked carbohydrate. The major difference between the P-gp expressed in CH^{R}C5 cells and J7 cells is due to N-linked carbohydrate. These data are consistent with the hypothesis that a family of P-gps may play a role in mediating the response of each cell line to different drugs.

REFERENCES

1. GERLACH, J. N., N. KARTNER, D. R. BELL & V. LING. 1986. Multidrug resistance. Cancer Surveys **5:** 25–46.
2. ROY, S. N. & S. B. HORWITZ. 1985. A phosphoglycoprotein associated with taxol resistance in J774.2 cells. Cancer Res. **45:** 3856–3863.
3. GREENBERGER, L. M., S. W. WILLIAMS & S. B. HORWITZ. 1987. Biosynthesis of heterogenous forms of multidrug resistance-associated glycoproteins. J. Biol. Chem. **262:** 13685–13689.

In Vivo Augmentation of Mitogen Response by Liposome-Encapsulated Interleukin-2 in Mice

SULABHA S. KULKARNI, LEELA P. KASI,
SUSAN L. TUCKER, AND ROLAND P. PIZZINI

University of Texas System Cancer Center
M.D. Anderson Hospital
and
Tumor Institute
Houston, Texas 77030

Animal studies have shown that the usefulness of interleukin-2 (IL-2) for *in vivo* augmentation of immune response is limited by the variability of its effect ranging from augmentation, lack of augmentation, or the suppression of immune response.[1-3] Lack of augmentation may be attributed to elimination of IL-2 by IL-2–inhibitory factors[4] or free IL-2 receptor molecules[5] present in the recipient serum. To minimize possible interaction of injected IL-2 with serum factors, we encapsulated IL-2 in liposomes and evaluated its effect *in vivo* on the mitogen response of mice.

Ten units of ^{125}I-labeled IL-2 (NEN Research Products, Boston, MA) were encapsulated in 12 mg of negatively charged multilamellar liposomes (Lipo-IL-2) and injected intravenously into B6D2F1 mice. Saline encapsulated in liposomes (Lipo-Saline), free ^{125}I-labeled IL-2, and sterile saline were used for controls and the response of spleen cells to concanavalin A (Con A), phytohemagglutinin (PHA), and lipopolysaccharide (LPS) was measured at 1, 4, 24, and 48 hr or 24 and 48 hr after injection. Results showed that the proliferative response to Con A of Lipo-IL-2 injected mice was greater than that of Lipo-Saline or saline control mice at 1, 4, 24 and 48 hr after injection but the response was highly significant ($p < 0.01$) only at 4 hr after injection (TABLE 1). Greater, but not significant, response to Con A, PHA and LPS was observed at 48 hr after injection (TABLE 2). Free IL-2–injected mice showed variability in their response to mitogens, ranging from significant augmentation to suppression (TABLES 1 and 2).

These results show that IL-2 can be effectively encapsulated in negatively charged multilamellar liposomes (encapsulating efficiency 65–75%) and IL-2 encapsulated IL-2 can augment mitogen response in mice. The lack of statistically significant response to encapsulated IL-2 at 24 and 48 hours, could be related to the inherent variability of response in mice, and the results might be improved by increasing the number of animals per group. Further studies involving variations in dose, number, and route of injections and composition of the carrier are essential to improve the immune responses obtained in this initial study.

IL-2 mediates its effect on T-cells via hormone-like interactions with IL-2 receptors. The mechanism of action of liposome-encapsulated IL-2 in augmenting the T-cell response is not yet clear but it is possible that the response is due to targeting of encapsulated IL-2 to IL-2 receptor bearing cells via putative surface-associated IL-2 molecules.

TABLE 1. Effect of *in Vivo* Administration of Liposome-Encapsulated Recombinant Human IL-2 (NEN) on Mitogen Response of B6D2F1 Mice. *Experiment 1*: Con A Response at 1, 4, 24, and 48 Hours after IL-2.

[³H]Thymidine Uptake cpm ± SD (SI)[a] at Various Times After IL-2

Treatment[b]	Mouse No.	1-Hour Medium	1-Hour Con A	1-Hour p Value[c]	4-Hours Medium	4-Hours Con A	4-Hours p Value[c]	24-Hours Medium	24-Hours Con A	24-Hours p Value[c]	48-Hours Medium	48-Hours Con A	48-Hours p Value[c]
1. Saline	1	140 ± 39	10,825 ± 266 (77)		166 ± 39	8,518 ± 1,676 (51)		139 ± 13	8,416 ± 1,915 (60)		61 ± 7	2,045 ± 147 (33)	
	2	117 ± 40	6,984 ± 1,757 (60)		145 ± 34	6,606 ± 860 (45)		216 ± 21	120,110 ± 19,291 (556)		71 ± 20	3,075 ± 90 (43)	
	3	117 ± 18	2,524 ± 692 (21)		150 ± 29	1,233 ± 317 (8)		217 ± 16	7,390 ± 1,351 (34)		162 ± 20	5,169 ± 960 (32)	
2. Free-IL-2	1	81 ± 19	2,024 ± 113 (25)		101 ± 18	3,877 ± 76 (38)		197 ± 55	32,176 ± 5,815 (163)		117 ± 23	5,317 ± 935 (45)	
	2	113 ± 18	2,539 ± 90 (22)	0.001[d]	134 ± 18	4,800 ± 536 (36)	0.692[d]	184 ± 34	9,825 ± 3,410 (53)	0.138[d]	223 ± 33	139,610 ± 11,933 (626)	0.028[d]
	3	109 ± 33	1,066 ± 267 (10)		160 ± 28	4,704 ± 722 (29)		140 ± 20	2,523 ± 230 (18)		119 ± 19	3,878 ± 640 (32)	
3. Liposome-Saline	1	106 ± 28	2,216 ± 189 (21)		129 ± 13	1,974 ± 196 (15)		100 ± 6	33,340 ± 9,960 (333)		—	—	
	2	102 ± 7	2,276 ± 520 (22)		129 ± 38	3,558 ± 328 (27)		152 ± 33	39,993 ± 7,449 (263)		—	—	
	3	149 ± 37	3,011 ± 1,029 (22)		165 ± 46	2,542 ± 224 (15)		136 ± 32	3,621 ± 1,214 (24)		—	—	
4. Liposome-IL-2	1	119 ± 10	5,852 ± 496 (49)		169 ± 29	20,404 ± 3,897 (121)		148 ± 10	67,563 ± 31,947 (456)		91 ± 12	15,312 ± 220 (168)	
	2	125 ± 10	5,770 ± 1,245 (46)	0.001, 0.06[e]	119 ± 40	19,468 ± 4,406 (164)	<0.01, <0.01[e]	110 ± 25	25,617 ± 4,074 (233)	0.012, 0.059[e]	224 ± 3	117,865 ± 18,461 (526)	—, <0.01[e]
	3	201 ± 26	75,548 ± 3,143 (376)		171 ± 29	25,578 ± 3,970 (149)		142 ± 16	176,271 ± 69,354 (1,241)		136 ± 17	106,014 ± 1,230 (779)	

[a] Stimulation Index (SI) = cpm of cells + mitogen ÷ cpm of cells + medium.
[b] 10 units of liposome-encapsulated or free IL-2-I[125] (NEN Research Products) was injected in a single intravenous dose.
[c] Significant as evaluated by analysis of variance of logs of observations (cpm) corrected for medium controls.
[d] Compared with saline.
[e] Compared with liposome-saline and saline, respectively.

TABLE 2. Effect of *in Vivo* Administration of Liposome-Encapsulated Recombinant Human IL-2 (NEN) on Mitogen Response of B6D2F1 Mice. *Experiment 2:* Con A, PHA, and LPS Response at 48 Hours.

Treatment[b]	Mouse No.	[³H]Thymidine Uptake cpm ± SD (SI)[a] at 48-Hours After IL-2								
		Medium	Con A	p Value[c]	Medium	PHA	p Value[c]	Medium	LPS	p Value[c]
1. Saline	1	181 ± 63	3,115 ± 596 (17)		109 ± 17	2,205 ± 365 (20)		71 ± 14	1,594 ± 276 (22)	
	2	196 ± 13	706 ± 81 (4)		109 ± 6	629 ± 187 (6)		66 ± 17	441 ± 102 (7)	
	3	154 ± 28	432 ± 101 (3)		117 ± 21	307 ± 142 (3)		120 ± 23	633 ± 234 (5)	
2. Free-IL-2	1	175 ± 64	10,812 ± 1,120 (62)		148 ± 22	83 ± 36 (0.6)		152 ± 51	6,563 ± 939 (43)	
	2	115 ± 35	12,942 ± 371 (11)	<0.05[d]	119 ± 2	35 ± 12 (0.3)	<0.05[d]	103 ± 16	5,153 ± 1,100 (50)	<0.05[d]
	3	111 ± 25	11,750 ± 1,184 (106)		141 ± 20	32 ± 9 (0.22)		188 ± 72	4,931 ± 424 (26)	
3. Liposome-Saline	1	239 ± 107	16,487 ± 1,358 (69)		124 ± 21	2,230 ± 242 (18)		110 ± 15	1,714 ± 173 (16)	
	2	155 ± 21	10,456 ± 1,344 (67)	0.275, <0.05[c]	131 ± 42	3,090 ± 545 (24)	0.275, 0.127[c]	100 ± 24	2,070 ± 497 (21)	0.275, 0.127[c]
	3	180 ± 87	3,062 ± 1,344 (17)		77 ± 17	714 ± 31 (9)		282 ± 54	496 ± 21 (2)	
4. Liposome-IL-2	1	89 ± 17	66,987 ± 15,394 (753)		178 ± 31	7,117 ± 114 (40)		190 ± 11	9,591 ± 1,656 (50)	
	2	42 ± 8	66,246 ± 10,870 (1,577)	0.275, <0.05[c]	204 ± 113	5,789 ± 777 (28)	0.275, 0.127[c]	149 ± 32	10,753 ± 661 (72)	0.275, 0.127[c]
	3	47 ± 25	4,199 ± 1,199 (106)		80 ± 6	2,139 ± 356 (27)		127 ± 33	857 ± 194 (7)	

[a]Stimulation Index (SI) = cpm of cells + mitogen ÷ cpm of cells + medium.
[b]10 units of liposome-encapsulated or free IL-2-I¹²⁵ (NEN Research Products) was injected in a single intravenous dose.
[c]Significant as evaluated by analysis of variance of logs of observations (cpm) corrected for medium controls.
[d]Compared with saline.
[e]Compared with liposome-saline and saline, respectively.

REFERENCES

1. HEFENEIDER, S. H., P. J. CONLON, C. S. HENNEY & S. GILLIS. 1983. J. Immunol. **180:** 222.
2. DONOHUE, J. H., M. T. LOTZE, R. J. ROBB, M. ROSENSTEIN, R. M. BRAZIEL, E. S. JAFFE & S. A. ROSENBERG. 1984. Cancer Res. **44:** 1380.
3. TALMADGE, J. E., *et al.* 1985. J. Immunol. **135:** 2483.
4. HARDT, C., M. ROLLINGHOFF, K. PFIZENMAIER, H. MOSMANN & H. WAGNER. 1981. J. Exp. Med. **154:** 262.
5. RUBIN, L. A., C. C. KURMAN, M. E. FRITZ, W. E. BIDDISON, B. BOUTIN, R. YARCHOAN & D. L. NELSON. 1985. J. Immunol. **135:** 3172.

Poly(L-Lysine) Conjugation: An Efficient Tool for the Introduction of Biologically Active Oligonucleotides in Intact Cells

M. LEMAITRE, C. BISBAL, B. BAYARD, C. WATHY,
J. P. LEONETTI, AND B. LEBLEU

Laboratoire de Biochimie des Protéines
Université de Montpellier II
Place E. Bataillon
34060 Montpellier, France

Gene expression regulation is essentially exerted through specific interactions between nucleic acids sequences or through specific recognition between nucleic acids and proteins. Efficient tools for the introduction in intact cells and tissues of adequately chosen ribo- or deoxyribonucleotidic sequences have thus been searched. They indeed offer the potential of interfering with the expression of normal genes to study their role in cell metabolism or of attenuating the expression of deleterious genes, as for instance viral genes or deregulated oncogenes.

With the exception of plasmids and viruses,[1] little success has been achieved yet in the conception of efficient oligonucleotides delivery systems. We demonstrate here that the chemical conjugation of oligonucleotides to poly(L-lysine) (PLL) allows their efficient internalization in intact cells.

As outlined in FIGURE 1, periodate-oxidized oligoribonucleotides can be conjugated to PLL-amino groups through reductive amination.[2] The introduction of a N-morpholine ring at oligonucleotides 3′ end also stabilizes them against phosphodiesterases.[2] This procedure allows the conjugation of oligonucleotides to exposed amino groups in any natural or synthetic polypeptides, thus allowing (at least in principle) the construction of adducts providing both transmembrane transfer and cell targeting.

As a first example of the validity of this concept, oligoribonucleotides in the $(2'-5')$ $(A)_n$ series were conjugated to PLL. As expected from known intracellular mediators of interferon antiviral action, these $(2'-5')$ $(A)_n$ conjugates significantly protect cultured cells from vesicular stomatitis virus (VSV) infection. (TABLE 1). This antiviral activity is due to the activation of RNase L, the specific target of $(2'-5')$ $(A)_n$, by delivered $(2'-5')$ $(A)_n$ oligonucleotides. Indeed, $(2'-5')$ $(A)_n$-PLL conjugates produce transient inhibition of protein synthesis and rRNAs cleavages, characteristic of RNase L activation.[2]

PLL conjugation also allowed us to internalize efficiently "antisense" oligodeoxyribonucleotides.[3] In these studies, the oligonucleotide sequence was designed to hybridize specifically to the ribosome-binding site of the mRNA coding for the N protein of VSV. This conjugate exerted a reasonably stable and powerful antiviral activity when added to the culture medium prior VSV infection (TABLE 1). The inhibition appeared highly specific since neither the synthesis of cellular proteins nor the multiplication of encephalomyocarditis virus were affected significantly.[4]

Synthetic polypeptides as PLL thus appear as an efficient tool to deliver conjugated oligonucleotides to intact cells at least *in vitro*. Preliminary experiments also indicated that $(2'-5')$ $(A)_n$ asialofetuin conjugates (FIG. 1) provide an antiviral activity in hepatoma cells (HepG2) carrying galactose receptors at their surface.

348

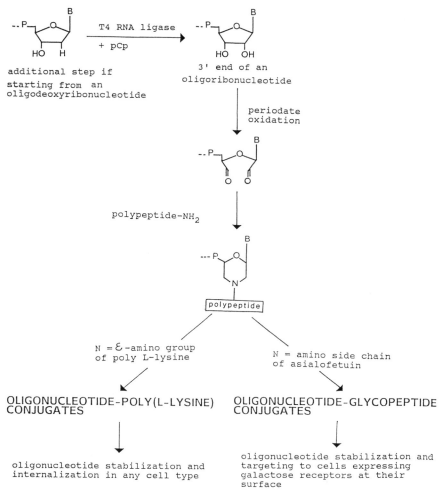

FIGURE 1. Outline of oligonucleotide-polypeptide conjugation. 3'-end oxidation of the oligoribonucleotide with sodium periodate is performed at pH 4.5 in the cold and followed by reductive amination with sodium cyanoborohydride at pH 8.0 in the presence of the appropriate polypeptide. When dealing with oligodeoxyribonucleotides, a ^{32}P-labeled pCp residue is added to their 3'-end with T4 RNA ligase and the terminal phosphate group is removed by bacterial alkaline phosphatase. Such 3'-modified oligodeoxyribonucleotides are then processed essentially as oligoribonucleotides. Details of the procedures are described elsewhere.[2-4] (2'–5') (A)$_n$ oligonucleotides have been synthesized enzymatically and size fractionated as detailed previously.[2] Antisense oligodeoxyribonucleotides have been synthesized with an automated DNA synthesizer using the phosphotriester method and purified by gel electrophoresis.

TABLE 1. Antiviral Activity of Oligonucleotide Poly(L-Lysine) Conjugates[a]

Experiment	Conjugate	Oligonucleotide Concentration (nM)	% of VSV Yield in Control Cells
1	no or PLL alone	0	100
	(2'–5') (A)$_4$ + PLL	1,000	100
	(2'–5') (A)$_4$ – PLL	180	100
	id.	500	5.0
	id.	900	0.6
2	no	—	100
	antisense + PLL	200	100
	antisense – PLL	100	40
	id.	200	2
	id.	400	0.7

[a]L929 (exp. 1) or L1210 (exp. 2) cells were incubated with oligonucleotide-poly(L-lysine) (PLL) conjugates or with a mixture of PLL and 3'-stabilized oligonucleotide at the indicated concentrations. Cells were injected with VSV (multiplicity of infection: 1) 3 hours later and virus yields were determined 18 hr later by titration of the virus output on L929 cells. Control values ranged from 10^7 to 10^8 pfu × ml^{-1}. The "antisense" oligodeoxyribonucleotide has been designed to complement the translation initiation site of the VSV mRNA coding for its N protein as schematized below:

5' ... A A C A G U A A U C A A A A U G U C U G U U ... 3'   N protein mRNA
          T G T C A T T A G T T T T A C   "antisense" sequence

Experiments aimed at studying the mechanisms involved in cell delivery, linking oligonucleotides to various cell targeting moieties, and applying the same approach to the delivery of other sequence- or protein-specific oligonucleotides will obviously be required to evaluate the general relevance of this approach.

REFERENCES

1. GREEN, P. J., O. PINES & M. INOUYE. 1986. The role of antisense RNA in gene regulation. Ann. Rev. Biochem. **55:** 569–597.
2. BAYARD, B., C. BISBAL & B. LEBLEU. 1986. Activation of ribonuclease L by (2'–5') (A)$_4$-poly (L-lysine) conjugates in intact cells. Biochemistry **25:** 3730–3736.
3. LEMAITRE, M., C. BISBAL, B. BAYARD & B. LEBLEU. 1988. Biological activities of a oligonucleotide linked to poly (L-lysine). Nucleosides and Nucleotides **6:** 311–315.
4. LEMAITRE, M., B. BAYARD & B. LEBLEU. 1988. Specific antiviral activity of a poly(L-lysine)-conjugated oligodeoxyribonucleotide sequence complementary to vesicular stomatitis virus N protein mRNA initiation site. Proc. Natl. Acad. Sci. USA **84:** 648–652.

Transcellular Processing of Proteins in Renal Tubular Epithelium

C. HYUNG PARK

Division of Nephrology, Hypertension and Transplantation
College of Medicine
University of Florida
Gainesville, Florida 32610

The kidney plays an important role in the metabolism of proteins that are present in the circulation.[1] Proteins filtered across the glomerulus are endocytosed by the proximal tubule cell across the apical membrane and transported subsequently to the lysosomes for hydrolysis. To study the mechanism of renal tubular handling of proteins, the time course of absorption, accumulation, and hydrolysis of protein and the vectorial nature of these processes were examined in the isolated perfused proximal convoluted tubule of the rabbit kidney.[2] Tubules of 0.7 to 2.1 mm length were perfused at 8 to 15 nl/min with an ultrafiltrate containing tritiated albumin (^3H_3C-Alb) at 36.4 $\mu g/ml$ and bathed in a solution similar to the ultrafiltrate containing 6.5% BSA. The absorption of albumin was determined from the difference between the perfused and collected loads of ^3H_3C-Alb. The hydrolysis of albumin was determined from the ^3H that was released by the tubule into the peritubular bath. The accumulation of albumin in the tubule cell was determined indirectly by calculating the difference between the absorption of albumin and the efflux into the bath of the hydrolysis products or directly by counting the ^3H that accumulated in the tubule. The fate of absorbed albumin was also determined by gel filtration chromatography. The tubule fluid was analyzed for the presence of hydrolysis products by chromatography and the lysosomal enzymes cathepsins B and L using a synthetic substrate, Z-phenylalanyl-arginine-7-amido-4-methylcoumarin by fluorometric ultramicroassay.[3] The absorption of albumin across the apical membrane was constant ($99.9 \pm 4.9 \times 10^{-3}$ ng $\cdot$ min^{-1} $\cdot$ mm^{-1}). In contrast, the accumulation and hydrolysis of albumin in the cells increased nonlinearly with time and reached a plateau. Gel filtration chromatography demonstrated that the bulk of the tritium that accumulated in the cells was associated with intact ^3H_3C-Alb and the remainder was associated with intermediate hydrolysis products. Only the final hydrolysis products that were similar in size to mannitol and soluble in TCA were released from the cells across the basolateral membrane and first appeared in the bath 6 to 7 min after the start of perfusion of the tubule with ^3H_3C-Alb. Neither the intermediate nor the final hydrolysis product was detectable in the tubule lumen suggesting that a release of the lysosomal contents across the apical cell membrane is not significant. Furthermore, the cathepsin activity was not detectable in the tubule fluid collected during 90 min perfusion. The proteolytic activity of the tubule cells was a linear function of the protein load to the cells. This is characteristic of first-order reaction kinetics and a high capacity system. The results suggest that the renal tubular handling of proteins proceeds from the apical to the basolateral aspect of the cell. The transcellular processing of albumin is rapid and complete as early as 6 to 7 min after absorption at the apical membrane. The accumulation of intact protein in the cell and the first-order reaction kinetics of the hydrolysis of the absorbed protein suggest that the rate-limiting step in proximal tubule handling of proteins may be the initial hydrolysis of the protein or resides in steps that precede the hydrolysis.

REFERENCES

1. Maack, T., C. H. Park & M. J. F. Camargo. 1985. Renal filtration, transport, and metabolism of protein. *In* The Kidney: Physiology and Pathophysiology. D. W. Seldin & G. Giebisch, Eds.: 1773–1803. Raven Press. New York.
2. Park, C. H. & T. Maack. 1984. Albumin absorption and catabolism by isolated perfused proximal convoluted tubules of the rabbit. J. Clin. Invest. **73:** 767–777.
3. Olbricht, C. J., J. K. Cannon, L. C. Garg & C. C. Tisher. 1986. Activities of cathepsins B and L in isolated nephron segments from proteinuric and nonproteinuric rats. Am. J. Physiol. **250** (Renal Fluid Electrolyte Physiol. 19): F1055–F1062.

Hydroxymethylketones as Pro-drugs

F. J. PETRACEK, N. SUGISAKA, AND K. F. SWINGLE

Riker Laboratories, Inc.
(A Division of the 3M Company)
St. Paul, Minnesota 55144-1000

The hydroxymethylketone group ($-CO-CH_2OH$) was investigated as an isostere or pro-drug replacement for the carboxyl radical ($-COOH$) in a series of well-known therapeutic acids. Conversion of the HMK group to the acid could occur by an oxidative decarboxylation analogous to some carbohydrate pathways. Advantages of such a pro-drug might accrue from the neutral character of the HMK group concerning oral absorption, transport mechanisms, and overall pharmacokinetics when compared to the parent acid.

The HMKs shown in TABLE 1 were prepared by conventional synthetic routes from the parent acids. The resulting products are stable, crystalline solids that were characterized by the usual spectroscopic and elemental analyses. In some cases the

TABLE 1. Summary of HMK Screening

Parent Acid[a]	HMK[b]	Primary Screening
1. Naproxen	m.p. 92–94°C	See TABLE 2
2. Indomethacin	m.p. 55–60°C	~1/5 activity of parent acid in rat paw carrageenan
3. Ibuprofen	m.p. 28–30°C	Weakly active in rat paw carrageenan
4. Nicotinic acid	m.p. 110–113°C	Acetate ester more active than parent acid in vasodilator screen
5. p-Aminobenzoic acid (PABA)	m.p. 158–166°C (dec.)	Inactive in antibacterial screens
6. α-Methyl-DOPA	m.p. 92–97°C (fumarate)	Inactive as hypotensive
7. Aspirin	Diol m.p. 62–65°C Acetate 62–64°C	Inactive

[a]Other attempted HMKs included clofibrate, 1-DOPA, mefenamic acid, cromoglycic acid, and biotin.
[b]All HMK's were characterized by NMR spectra and elemental analyses.

presence of the chemically reactive HMK group (or precursors) led to rearrangements and/or cyclic intra-molecular reactions, which precluded completion to the desired HMK (TABLE 1). The HMK's of several non-steroidal anti-inflammatory agents (NSAID) possessed sufficient activity in primary screens to warrant extensive pharmacological investigation as potential clinical agents. The HMK of the NSAID naproxen was studied in the well-known acute and chronic animal screens. Toxicological models of gastric irritation were also employed to assess any relative potential clinical advantage of the HMK over the parent acid. These pharmacological studies are summarized in TABLE 2.

The naproxen HMK was, in general, less active in milligram potency than naproxen in the primary acute screens. It appeared to be equipotent, however, in a 25-day adjuvant arthritis test. The lack of activity in the *in vitro* prostaglandin (PG) synthetase screen indicated that the HMK required metabolic conversion to other products for activity.

Efficient conversion of the HMK to naproxen was demonstrated in the rat and guinea pig. Two hours post oral administration, only the acidic naproxen was detected (TLC analysis of plasma extracts). The postulated metabolic intermediate ketoalde-

TABLE 2. Pharmacological Comparison of Naproxen and Naproxen-HMK

Test	Naproxen	Nap-HMK
Carrageenan ED_{50}	1 mg/kg	6 mg/kg
UV-induced erythema ED_{50}	<6	18
Adjuvant arthritis Med	<2	<2
Randall-Selitto ED_{50}	10–15	10–15
PQ Writhing, mouse ED_{50}	8	32
Locomotor activity, inflamed paw, mouse ED_{50}	~30	30
LD_{50}, mouse, i.p.	560	1100

hyde ($-CO-CHO$) and ketoacid ($-CO-COOH$) were not detected. Blood levels of the naproxen HMK were estimated to be one-half those from an equivalent dose of naproxen itself.

A 21-day toxicological comparison of naproxen HMK with naproxen as a control showed the HMK to be less toxic (~half) on a milligram basis. The toxicity profiles were similar with evidence of gastric hyperemia and adhesions at less than lethal doses.

This work has shown that in certain cases the HMK group is an effective pro-drug for therapeutic acids.

Effect of Sofalcone on the Peptic Degradation of Gastric Mucus[a]

J. BILSKI, J. SAROSIEK, A. SLOMIANY,
AND B. L. SLOMIANY[b]

Gastroenterology Research Laboratory
Department of Medicine
New York Medical College
Valhalla, New York 10595

INTRODUCTION

The resilient layer of mucus that tenaciously adheres to the epithelial surfaces of gastric mucosa constitutes the first line of mucosal defense against a variety of exogenous and endogenous insults.[1,2] Under normal physiological conditions, the continuous renewal and viscous nature of this layer efficiently counters peptic erosion of the gel and provides a milieu for neutralization of the diffusing luminal acid by mucosal bicarbonate. The disturbances in this delicate balance lead to the impairment of the protective function of the mucus layer, resulting in gastric disease. Among the promising agents directed towards strengthening the gastric mucosal defense is a recently introduced antiulcer drug, sofalcone.[3,4] Here, we report the effect of this agent on peptic degradation of gastric mucus.

MATERIALS AND METHODS

Gastric mucus, used for peptic activity assays, was isolated from freshly dissected pig stomach by instillation with 2 M NaCl-10 mM sodium phosphate buffer.[1] The recovered instillate was filtered through a Millipore HA (0.45 μm) filter, subjected to intrinsic pepsin inactivation (pH 9.0 at 37°C for 30 min), dialyzed against distilled water, and lyophilized. Results of chemical analysis indicated that such prepared mucus contained 64.2% protein, 15.1% carbohydrate, 17.6% lipids, and 0.3% covalently bound fatty acids.

The peptic activity assays at pH 1.8 consisted of the following components: gastric mucus, 50–500 μg; pepsin, 0.16 μg; and sofalcone (Taisho Pharmaceutical), 0–1.0 $\times$ 10^{-3} M, in a final volume of 0.22 ml. The tubes were incubated at 37°C for 30 min and the reaction was terminated by the addition of 1 ml of 0.2 M borate buffer, pH 9.0. The proteolytic activity of pepsin towards gastric mucus was measured by following the release of α-amino residues by the trinitrophenylation method. All experiments were carried out in duplicate and the results are expressed as means $\pm$ SD.

[a]Supported in part by U.S. Public Health Service Grant AM21684-10 from the National Institute of Diabetes and Digestive and Kidney Diseases, National Institutes of Health.

[b]Address correspondence to B.L. Slomiany, Gastroenterology Research Laboratory, New York Medical College, Munger Pavilion, Valhalla, NY 10595.

355

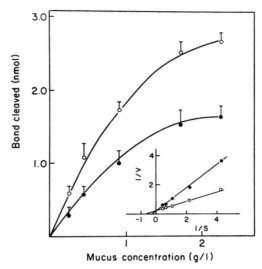

FIGURE 1. Effect of gastric mucus concentration on the proteolytic activity of pepsin in the absence (O) and in the presence (●) of 1.0×10^{-6} M sofalcone. The data show the means ± SD of five separate experiments.

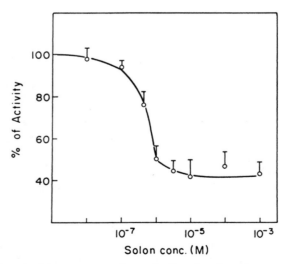

FIGURE 2. Effect of sofalcone concentration on the digestion of gastric mucus with pepsin. The data show the means ± SD of four separate experiments.

RESULTS AND DISCUSSION

The effect of gastric mucus concentration on the proteolytic activity of pepsin is shown in FIGURE 1. Under the assay conditions, the rate of proteolysis was proportional to a mucus concentration up to 300 μg and remained constant with time of incubation for at least 1 hr. The K_m value obtained from the double reciprocal plots for pig gastric mucus was 1.35 g/l. Introduction of sofalcone to the reaction mixture led to reduction of the rate of peptic cleavage (FIGURE 2). The rate of the inhibition of proteolysis was proportional to sofalcone concentration up to 1.0×10^{-5} M at which concentration a 60% decrease in the mucus proteolysis was recorded. The K_I value calculated from Lineweaver-Burk plots for peptic digestion of gastric mucus in the presence of sofalcone was 3.57 g/l. Preincubation of sofalcone with mucus before the addition of pepsin had no deterrent effect of the activity of pepsin towards the mucus. However, when pepsin was preincubated with sofalcone before the addition of mucus a decrease in peptic activity was observed, thus suggesting that the inhibitory effect results from interaction of the drug with pepsin rather than with mucus.

Although the exact sequence of events involved in pathogenesis of peptic ulcer remains elusive, the consensus is that the injury to gastric mucosa occurs when the aggressive forces overcome those responsible for the mucosal defense. Thus, in approach to ulcer therapy, the mucosal healing can be achieved either by reducing aggressive factors or by strengthening the mucosal protective factors. Among the drugs that fall into the latter category is sofalcone. The mechanism of the action of this synthetic analog of sophoradin, an ancient Chinese stomach ache remedy, includes inhibition of the prostaglandin inactivating enzyme, stimulation of the gastric blood flow, and acceleration of the mucosal repair and the biosynthesis of mucin.[4,5] The results of investigation reported herein clearly show that sofalcone also affect the *in vitro* degradation of mucus by pepsin. The data show that the inhibitory effect of sofalcone results directly from its ability to interact with the enzyme protein. By inhibiting the proteolytic activity of pepsin, sofalcone slows down the erosion of the protective mucus layer and thus helps to maintain the integrity of this layer at its best.

REFERENCES

1. SLOMIANY, B. L., A. PIASEK, J. SAROSIEK & A. SLOMIANY. 1985. Scand. J. Gastroenterol. **20**: 1191.
2. SLOMIANY, B. L., W. LASZEWICZ & A. SLOMIANY. 1986. Digestion **33**: 146.
3. SAROSIEK, J., K. MIZUTA, A. SLOMIANY & B. L. SLOMIANY. 1986. Am. J. Gastroenterol. **81**: 858.
4. MURAMATSU, M., M. TANAKA, T. SUWA, A. FUJITA, S. OTOMO & H. AIHARA. 1984. Biochem. Pharmacol. **33**: 2629.
5. SAZIKI, R., I. ARAI, Y. ISOBE, H. HIROSE & H. AIHARA. 1984. J. Pharm. Dyn. **7**: 791.

Interaction of Estramustine with Microtubule Associated Proteins *in Vitro*[a]

MARK E. STEARNS AND KENNETH D. TEW

Department of Pharmacology
Fox Chase Cancer Center
Philadelphia, Pennsylvania 19111

Microtubules and microtubule associated proteins (MAPs) constitute the principle cytoskeletal elements that determine cell shape and regulate intracellular motility events.[1] Studies with drugs that bind tubulin (e.g. colchicine, vinblastine, nocodazole[2]), have established the importance of microtubules *per se*[1] but the involvement of MAPs is incompletely understood.

We have tested the cytoskeletal binding properties of a novel anti-microtubule drug, estramustine (EM). Earlier studies have speculated that EM produced cytotoxicity independently of its constituent nitrogen mustard and steroid moieties.[3] It was found that micromolar levels of EM can produce rapid microtubule disassembly *in vitro*[4,5] and *in vivo*.[6] EM was also found to completely inhibit organelle transport in erythrophores[6,7] and partially inhibit vesicle transport in neurons.[4] We predicted that the primary molecular targets of EM were several high molecular weights MAPs (HMW-MAPs).[6,7] The studies reported here examined the binding affinities of [3H]EM [Estramustine, 2,4,6,7-3H] for MAPs and tubulin.

The [3H]EM binding to proteins was carried out using microtubule proteins isolated from rat brain in the presence in 10 μM taxol according to procedures described by Vallee *et al.*[10] The microtubule associated proteins were extracted from the microtubules with 0.4 M KCl and the taxol-microtubules pelleted by centrifugation to obtain MAPs rich supernatants. Isolated microtubule proteins (MAPs, tubulin) were dialyzed against phosphate buffer containing 1 mM ATP, 2 mM EGTA, 0.1% aprotinin, pH 7.2 for 2 hr, diluted to 1 mg/ml and incubated with 100 μCi [3H]estramustine for 30 min at 23°C. These samples were applied to a phosphocellulose (Whatman PC-11) column (5 × 1.5 cm), eluted with 10 ml phosphate buffer and then eluted with 10 ml phosphate buffer containing 0.4 M KCl at 23°C. Sample fractions were collected in 0.5 ml volumes and the absorbance spectra (A_{280}) measured to determine the protein concentration. Each fraction was split into aliquots (1) to measure protein levels; (2) for SDS-urea gels and, (3) 0.1 ml transferred to a scintillation vial containing 10 ml scintillation solution [2 parts toluene, 1 part Triton X-100, and 5 g/liter Permablend (Packard Ltd.)] and counted in a Beckman liquid scintillation counter. About 95% of the counts (expressed as cpm × 10^3/0.1 ml in FIG. 1) were recovered in peaks 2a, 2b (see below).

The absorbance spectra (A_{280}) from phosphocellulose column fractions show that the proteins were separated in a peak 1, 2a, and 2b fractions, which were eluted with 0.4 M KCl (FIG. 1). About 80% of the [3H]EM binding activity was recovered in peak 2b fractions (FIG. 1) and the remaining counts were recovered in peak 2a fractions. In

[a]Supported by a Helsingborg Research Foundation Grant and National Cancer Institute Grant R01-CA-39373; an institutional grant from the Bristol-Myers Foundation; and an appropriation from the Commonwealth of Pennsylvania.

control studies, 1 mg/ml BSA was incubated with [³H]EM and the preparation eluted on a PC-11 column. [³H]EM eluted in the void volume and did not bind BSA.

The proteins present in peaks 1 and 2b (FIG. 1) are shown on silver-stained SDS-urea gels in FIGURE 2. FIGURE 2 shows that the crude MAPs extract contains tubulin (55 Kd) plus numerous proteins including a prominent 330 Kd band (lane 2). The majority of the [³H]EM binding activity was found in peak 2b and these fractions contained some tubulin, a prominent 330 Kd MAP, and several minor proteins (lane 3). Some [³H]EM binding was observed in peak 2a fractions where the 330 Kd protein represented a minor component in comparison to the many other proteins present (lanes 4 to 6). Virtually no [³H]EM binding was observed in peak 1 fractions where tubulin plus several minor proteins were the principle components. Since tubulin and several minor proteins found in peak 2b fractions (see lane 2, FIG. 2) were also found in

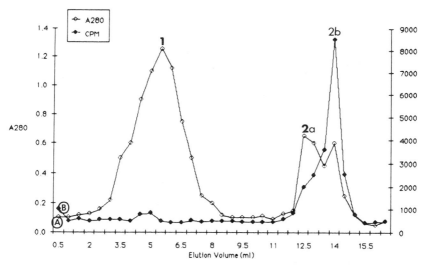

FIGURE 1. Shows the protein absorbance profile (curve A) and the [³H]EM binding activity (curve B) for DU 145 MAPs separated on a phosphocellulose column (PC-11). The proteins were eluted with phosphate buffer in a peak 1 fraction and with 0.4 M KCl in a peak 2 (peaks 2a, 2b) fraction. About 80% of the [³H]EM (cpm × 10⁻³) eluted with the salt fraction in peak 2b and about 15% of the other counts were found in peak 2a fractions.

peak 2a and peak 1 fractions, it was unlikely that the minor proteins were responsible for [³H]EM binding activity. We refractionated the HMW-MAPs (lane 3) to obtain a >95% pure HMW-MAPs preparation (lane 8). [³H]EM co-eluted with the HMW-MAPs (lane 8) and did not bind tubulin (lane 9) or the low molecular weight proteins (lane 10). The specific activity of [³H]EM binding is estimated at 164 pmol/mg for the 330 Kd protein.

From a therapeutic standpoint, a 46 Kd estramustine binding protein appears to promote EM accumulation and to prevent EM diffusion out of prostate cells.[7,8] Consequently, EM is retained intracellularly wherein it can exert long term cytotoxic effects on HMW-MAPs and microtubules in prostatic cells. Certainly, EM is a powerful anti-mitotic agent that prevents prostatic tumor cell division[9] and microtubule-dependent secretory events (unpublished data). By comparison, *in situ* studies have shown that therapeutic dosages of EM produce minimal side effects on neurons and axonal transport[4] presumably because these cells fail to accumulate and retain EM. In conclusion, the selective ability of the prostate to accumulate EM combined

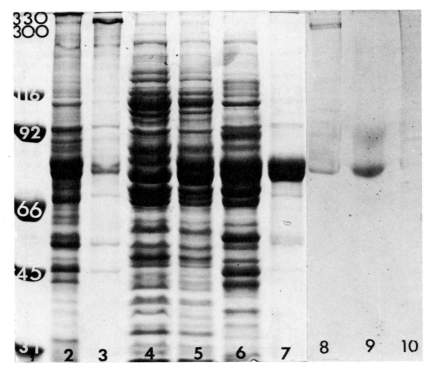

FIGURE 2. Silver-stained SDS-urea gel profiles of protein fractions from peaks 1 and 2a, 2b in FIG. 1. Lane 1, molecular weight standards (Sigma) at 116, 92, 66, 45, 31 Kd; Lane 2, crude MAPs fraction; Lane 3, peak 2b proteins; Lanes 4–6, peak 2a proteins; Lane 7, peak 1 proteins. Peak 2b fractions contain a unique high molecular weight protein (330 Kd), which apparently binds [³H]EM, since low molecular weight proteins in peak 2b (lane 3) were also found in peaks 2a (lanes 4–6), and 1 (lane 7) and these fractions did not appear to bind [³H]EM. Lanes 8–10 show the microtubule associated proteins (from lane 3) after a second re-fractionation on a PC-11 column into three peak fractions. Lane 8, high molecular weight, HMW-MAPs; lane 9, tubulin; and lane 10 low molecular weight MAPs. [³H]EM co-eluted with the HMW-MAPs fraction (lane 8).

with EM's cytotoxic effects on MAPs make it a powerful anti-microtubule tumor drug.

ACKNOWLEDGMENT

We would like to express our sincere gratitude to Donna Platz for typing the manuscript.

REFERENCES

1. HYAMS, J. S. & H. STEBBINGS. 1979. Microtubule associated cytoplasmic transport. *In* Microtubules. K. Roberts & J. S. Hyams, Eds.: 488–510. Academic Press. New York.
2. HOEBEKE, J., G. VAN NIJEN & M. DEBRABANDER. 1976. Interaction of nocodazole (R 17834), a new antitumoral drug, with rat brain tubulin. Biochem. Biophys. Res. Commun. **69:** 319–324.
3. TEW, K. D. 1983. The mechanism of action of estramustine. Sem. Oncol. **10:** 21–26.
4. KANJE, M., J. DEINUM, M. WALLIN, P. EDSTROM, A. EDSTROM & B. HARTLEY-ASP. 1985. Effect of estramustine phosphate on the assembly of isolated bovine brain microtubules and fast axonal transport in the frog sciatic nerve. Cancer Res. **45:** 2234–2239.
5. WALLIN, M., J. DEINUM & B. FRIDEN. 1985. Interaction of estramustine phosphate with microtubule-associated proteins. FEBS Lett. **179:** 238–293.
6. STEARNS, M. E. & K. D. TEW. 1985. Antimicrotubule effects of estramustine, an antiprostatic tumor drug. Cancer Res. **45:** 3891–3897.
7. STEARNS, M. E., D. JENKINS & K. D. TEW. 1985. Dansylated estramustine, a novel probe for studies of estramustine uptake and identification of intracellular targets. Proc. Natl. Acad. Sci. USA **82:** 8483–8487.
8. AUMULLER G., J. SEITZ, W. HEYNS & C. J. FLICKINGER. 1984. Intracellular localization of prostatic binding protein (PBP) in rat prostate by light and electron microscopic immunocytochemistry. Histochemistry **76:** 497–516.
9. HARTLEY-ASP, B. 1984. Estramustine induced mitotic arrest in human prostatic carcinoma cell lines DU 145 and PC3. Prostate **5:** 93–100.
10. VALLEE, R. D., G. S. BLOOM & W. E. THEURKAUFF. 1984. Microtubule-associated proteins: subunits of the cytomatrix. J. Cell Biol. **99:** 38s–46s.

Index of Contributors